The SAGES Manual of Fluorescence-Guided Surgery

Nova Szoka • David Renton
Santiago Horgan
Editors

The SAGES Manual of Fluorescence-Guided Surgery

Springer

Editors
Nova Szoka
Department of Surgery
West Virginia University
Morgantown, WV, USA

David Renton
Division of General Surgery
Ohio State University
Columbus, OH, USA

Santiago Horgan
Department of Surgery
University of California,
San Diego
San Diego, CA, USA

ISBN 978-3-031-40684-3 ISBN 978-3-031-40685-0 (eBook)
https://doi.org/10.1007/978-3-031-40685-0

This Springer imprint is published by the registered company Springer Nature Switzerland AG
The registered company address is: Gewerbestrasse 11, 6330 Cham, Switzerland

Paper in this product is recyclable.

For my family who is my
foundation and my heart.
-Nova Szoka

Introduction

Fluorescence-Guided Surgery (FGS), an innovative technology based on real-time intraoperative image guidance, has been transforming surgical practice in recent years. Currently, the most popular method of FGS uses a near infrared (NIR) fluorescent dye or a NIR emitting light source to identify anatomic structures, target surgical pathology during surgical procedures, or assess perfusion to an area of interest, thus providing surgeons with objective information that can enhance both surgical performance and surgical outcomes.

In this book, we will explore the world of FGS, delving into its history, current applications, and future potential. We will examine the science behind this technique and explore the use of NIR infrared imaging in multiple surgical specialties, as well as examine novel fluorescence agents and modalities. Expert surgeons from a comprehensive list of surgical subspecialties were enlisted to share their experience using FGS, and this manual can be used as a guide for surgeons who are interested in incorporating FGS into their practice.

The first two chapters in this manual introduce the history and science of immunofluorescence and provide a comprehensive review of current fluorescence-guided platforms and devices; the remaining chapters discuss florescence-guided imaging within a specific surgical subspecialty and include background information, indications for use, a technical description of the procedure(s), and a review of potential pitfalls. Each of these chapters also describes the level of evidence for FGS supported by current publications. Chapter content is augmented by color images and videos.

Whether you are a surgeon, a medical professional, or simply someone with an interest in the latest advances in medical technology, this book will provide you with a comprehensive overview of Fluorescence-Guided Surgery, its current applications, and its exciting potential for the future.

The editors would like to thank the authors who contributed to this book, who are pioneers within a blossoming field of surgical imaging, as well as thank SAGES and Springer for supporting this work.

Contents

Contributors

Maxwell Almenoff, MD Department of Cardiovascular and Thoracic Surgery, Vascular Surgery, West Virginia University Heart and Vascular Institute, Morgantown, WV, USA

Ludovica Baldari, MD Department of General and Minimally Invasive Surgery, Fondazione IRCCS Ca' Granda Ospedale Maggiore Policlinico, Milan, Italy

Luigi Boni, MD Department of General and Minimally Invasive Surgery, Fondazione IRCCS Ca' Granda Ospedale Maggiore Policlinico, Milan, Italy

Department of Scienze Cliniche e delle Comunità, University of Milan, Milan, Italy

Sarinya Boonpoapichart, MD Division of Plastic and Reconstructive Surgery, Department of Surgery, Faculty of Medicine, Khon Kaen University, Khon Kaen, Thailand

Michael Bouvet, MD Department of Surgery, UC San Diego, San Diego, CA, USA

VA San Diego Healthcare System, San Diego, CA, USA

Ryan C. Broderick, MD Division of Minimally Invasive Surgery, Department of Surgery, University of California San Diego, La Jolla, CA, USA

Sebastian Brooke, MD Department of Surgery, Division of Plastic, Reconstructive, and Hand Surgery, West Virginia University School of Medicine, Morgantown, WV, USA

Mark A. Burroughs Department of Surgery, Methodist Dallas Medical Center, Dallas, TX, USA

Kevin Carroll, MBBS Department of Surgery, Northwell Health—South Shore University Hospital, Bay Shore, NY, USA

Elisa Cassinotti, MD, PhD Department of General and Minimally Invasive Surgery, Fondazione IRCCS Ca' Granda Ospedale Maggiore Policlinico, Milan, Italy

Department of Scienze Cliniche e delle Comunità, University of Milan, Milan, Italy

Edmund B. Chen, MD Department of Surgery, School of Medicine, Duke University, Durham, NC, USA

Anna Duprée, MD Department of General, Visceral and Thoracic Surgery, University Medical Center Hamburg-Eppendorf, Hamburg, Germany

Amr Elbakry, MD West Virginia University Department of Urology, Morgantown, WV, USA

Michael R. Freund, MD Ellen Leifer Shulman and Steven Shulman Digestive Disease Center, Cleveland Clinic Florida, Weston, FL, USA

Department of General Surgery, Shaare Zedek Medical Center, Faculty of Medicine, Hebrew University of Jerusalem, Jerusalem, Israel

Jack J. Gelman, MD Department of Surgery, Division of Plastic and Reconstructive Surgery, West Virginia University School of Medicine, Morgantown, WV, USA

Barbara Diane Gillis, BS West Virginia University School of Medicine, Morgantown, WV, USA

Courtney Griffiths, DO Division of Gynecology Oncology, Cooper Medical School for Rowan University, Camden, NJ, USA

Santiago Horgan, MD Department of Surgery, University of California, San Diego, San Diego, CA, USA

Donovan Hui, MD Department of Surgery, New York Medical College Metropolitan Hospital Center, New York, NY, USA

Takeaki Ishizawa, MD, PhD, FACS Department of Hepatobiliary-Pancreatic Surgery, Graduate School of Medicine, Osaka Metropolitan University, Abeno-ku, Osaka, Japan

Jillian C. Jacobson, MD Department of Surgery, UT Southwestern Medical Center, Dallas, TX, USA

Brendan Jones, MD Department of General Surgery, West Virginia University School of Medicine, Morgantown, WV, USA

Ranjeet S. Kalsi, MD Division of Pediatric General and Thoracic Surgery, Department of Surgery, University of Pittsburgh Medical Center/Children's Hospital of Pittsburgh, Pittsburgh, PA, USA

Jennifer Knight, MD, FACS Department of Surgery, The Ohio State University, Werner Medical Center, Columbus, OH, USA

Zachary A. Koenig, MD Department of Surgery, Division of Plastic and Reconstructive Surgery, West Virginia University School of Medicine, Morgantown, WV, USA

Sachin Kukreja Department of Surgery, Methodist Dallas Medical Center, Dallas, TX, USA

Dallas-Fort Worth Bariatrics and General Surgery, Dallas, TX, USA

Lioudmila Lipetskaia, MD, MSc Division of Urogynecology, Department of Obstetrics and Gynecology, Cooper Medical School for Rowan University, Camden, NJ, USA

Phachara Longmeewong, MD Division of Plastic and Reconstructive Surgery, Department of Surgery, Faculty of Medicine, Khon Kaen University, Khon Kaen, Thailand

Adam Luchey, MD West Virginia University Department of Urology, Morgantown, WV, USA

Thinzar M. Lwin, MD Department of Surgery, UC San Diego, San Diego, CA, USA

Department of Surgical Oncology, Dana Farber Cancer Center, Boston, MA, USA

Jared Matson, MD Department of Surgery, UC San Diego, San Diego, CA, USA

Derek Muehrcke, MD, FACS Cardiovascular and Thoracic Surgery at Flagler Hospital, Saint Augustine, FL, USA

Samir Pandya, MD Division of Pediatric Surgery, Department of Surgery, UT Southwestern Medical Center, Dallas, TX, USA

David Pechman, MD Department of Surgery, Zucker School of Medicine at Hofstra, Northwell Health—South Shore University Hospital, Bay Shore, NY, USA

Luis Quiroga, MD, MPH Department of Surgery, Division of Plastic, Reconstructive, and Hand Surgery, West Virginia University School of Medicine, Morgantown, WV, USA

David Renton, MD Division of General Surgery, Ohio State University, Columbus, OH, USA

Hannah Rinehardt, MD Department of Surgery, University of Pittsburgh School of Medicine, Pittsburgh, PA, USA

Christina Sanders, DO, MBA, FACS, FASMBS, FACOS Department of Surgery, Jacobs School of Medicine and Biomedical Sciences, State University of New York at Buffalo, Buffalo, NY, USA

Stefan Scholz, MD Division of Pediatric General and Thoracic Surgery, Department of Surgery, University of Pittsburgh School of Medicine, UPMC Children's Hospital of Pittsburgh, Pittsburgh, PA, USA

Keri A. Seymour, DO, MHSc Department of Surgery, School of Medicine, Duke University, Durham, NC, USA

Emanuel Shapera, MD Department of Surgery, SHARP Grossmont Hospital, La Mesa, CA, USA

Iswanto Sucandy, MD, FACS Department of Surgery, Advent Health Tampa, Tampa, FL, USA

Palakorn Surakunprapha, MD Division of Plastic and Reconstructive Surgery, Department of Surgery, Faculty of Medicine, Khon Kaen University, Khon Kaen, Thailand

Nova Szoka, MD, FACS, FASMBS Department of Surgery, West Virginia University, Morgantown, WV, USA

Elwin Tham, MD Department of Surgery, West Virginia University, Morgantown, WV, USA

Andrea Trinh Department of Surgery, Methodist Dallas Medical Center, Dallas, TX, USA

Acara Turner, MD Department of Surgery, Division of Plastic, Reconstructive, and Hand Surgery, West Virginia University School of Medicine, Morgantown, WV, USA

Cristiane M. Ueno, MD Department of Plastic and Reconstructive Surgery, Ohio State University College of Medicine, Columbus, OH, USA

Steven D. Wexner, MD, PhD (Hon) Ellen Leifer Shulman and Steven Shulman Digestive Disease Center, Cleveland Clinic Florida, Weston, FL, USA

Andrew Williams, BS West Virginia University School of Medicine, Morgantown, WV, USA

Apinut Wongkietkachorn, MD, PhD Division of Plastic and Reconstructive Surgery, Department of Surgery, Faculty of Medicine, Mae Fah Luang University, Chiang Rai, Thailand

Supawich Wongkietkachorn, MD Department of Surgery, Police General Hospital, Bangkok, Thailand

Kerri Woodberry, MD, MBA, FACS Department of Surgery, Division of Plastic, Reconstructive, and Hand Surgery, West Virginia University School of Medicine, Morgantown, WV, USA

Department of Surgery, Division of Plastic and Reconstructive Surgery, West Virginia University School of Medicine, Morgantown, WV, USA

Gene Yang, MD Department of Surgery, Jacobs School of Medicine and Biomedical Sciences, University at Buffalo, Buffalo, NY, USA

David Zekan, MD Department of Urology, West Virginia University, Morgantown, WV, USA

History and Science of Immunofluorescence

1

Ludovica Baldari, Luigi Boni, and Elisa Cassinotti

Introduction

The term fluorescence-guided surgery describes a medical technology based on real-time imaging intended to help and guide the surgeon during their operating practice. The first clinical use of fluorescence was in 1947, when it was used for identification of brain tumors during neurosurgery using the dye fluorescein. After the first experience, other applications have been reported in several surgical fields, but fluorescence-guided surgery has exponentially developed and spread only during the last years.

Indeed, recently, many innovations in surgical technique and minimally invasive technologies with laparoscopic, endoscopic, and robotic approaches have greatly improved surgical practice.

L. Baldari (✉)
Department of General and Minimally Invasive Surgery, Fondazione IRCCS Ca' Granda Ospedale Maggiore Policlinico, Milan, Italy
e-mail: ludovica.baldari@policlinico.mi.it

L. Boni · E. Cassinotti
Department of General and Minimally Invasive Surgery, Fondazione IRCCS Ca' Granda Ospedale Maggiore Policlinico, Milan, Italy

Department of Scienze Cliniche e delle Comunità, University of Milan, Milan, Italy
e-mail: luigi.boni@unimi.it; elisa.cassinotti@policlinico.mi.it

N. Szoka et al. (eds.), *The SAGES Manual of Fluorescence-Guided Surgery*, https://doi.org/10.1007/978-3-031-40685-0_1

Nevertheless, despite these constant advances, surgery still relies primarily on the surgeon's vision and on white-light reflectance. The emerging field of fluorescent surgical imaging promises to be a powerful enhancement to improve surgical guidance.

Among all chromophores and fluorophores that could work as probes in medical imaging techniques, near-infrared fluorescence imaging with indocyanine green (ICG) is emerging as the major contribution to intraoperative surgical decisions, and many different applications have already been described in literature. ICG is a dye used in medicine since the mid-1950s for a variety of diagnostic applications in cardiology and ophthalmology and to test the hepatic clearance. However, its fluorescent properties have only recently been applied to new minimally invasive surgical instrumentations. ICG has some peculiar features that promote its widespread use, like low incidence of adverse effects and very high toxic dose for the human body.

Other fluorescent probes already approved for clinical use are methylene blue (MB), fluorescein sodium, and 5-aminolevulinic acid (5-ALA). Moreover, many probes are currently under clinical development.

In addition, fluorescence-guided surgery appears to have a great potential to become a standard in everyday clinical practice due to its multiple different possible applications and its ease of employment.

History of Immunofluorescence

From Semeiotics to Fluorescence-Guided Surgery Through Medical Imaging

In clinical practice, especially in surgery, the development of a new technology needs to meet these critical criteria: to represent a true clinical requirement, the possibility to solve an open issue, and the peculiar ability not to interfere with normal clinical workflow [1].

This is the reason why, before the end of the nineteenth century, the diagnostic and therapeutic process into the surgical field relied on the physician's hands and eyes. In 1895, Wilhelm Röntgen took the first known X-ray picture of his wife's hand, accidentally discovering the X-ray [2]. Since this report, after many decades of improvements in medicine, there are few imaging techniques routinely employed in clinical practice that can be divided into two main segments: optical and radiological imaging [3].

Covering the 36% of the global market, radiological imaging includes X-ray, computed tomography (CT), ultrasound, magnetic resonance imaging (MRI), and positron emission tomography (PET), and only two of these (X-ray fluoroscopy and ultrasound) are used occasionally for image-guided surgery. Indeed, these techniques are mainly used for preoperative imaging that is fundamental to plan the surgery, but it can lead to misinterpretation during the procedure due to distortion of images and the time interval between imaging and surgery (e.g., in cancer patients) [4].

Nevertheless, optical imaging covers 64% of the global market, including endoscopy, microscopy, visual surgery, ophthalmic surgery, medical lasers, and robotics-based surgery. The fundamental of optical imaging is the use of light in the ultraviolet, visible, and near-infrared regions of the electromagnetic spectrum, allowing diagnosis and re-evaluation more frequently as the patient is not exposed to ionizing radiation. Moreover, through varying photon absorption and light scattering from different types of tissue, optical imaging can differentiate suspicious tumoral and healthy tissues, using multiple properties of soft tissue [5]. One of the main areas of optical imaging is fluorescence-guided surgery (FGS) in the field of intraoperative imaging techniques. Intraoperative imaging techniques have been developed to help the surgeon identify areas invisible to the naked eye. The main characteristic of an intraoperative imaging technique is the speed at which visual information is obtained.

The term "fluorescence-guided surgery" describes a medical technology based on real-time imaging intended to help and guide the surgeons during their operating practice. In recent years, technological progress in body imaging and diagnostics has enhanced patient selection for surgical interventions. At the same time, surgery has advanced substantially to decrease patient morbidity and trauma through innovations in endoscopic, laparoscopic, and robotic technologies. Nevertheless, surgical practice is still based on anatomy as seen by the operating surgeon with white-light reflectance. This approach does not allow an accurate differentiation between different tissues: in the body, they appear as various shades of white to pink (bone, nerves, cartilage, fat, connective tissue, and muscle) or red to deep red (blood vessels and more easily visible organs such as the liver, kidney, and spleen), thus leading to potential ambiguity during surgical dissection. Furthermore, open-field surgery depends on the direct visualization of patient tissues, whereas in minimally invasive surgeries (i.e., microscopic, endoscopic, laparoscopic, and robotic surgery), patient's tissues are visualized through an interface (viewed through the ocular eyepiece or using cameras and digital displays). For the minimally invasive surgical procedures, the added hardware that is necessary for fluorescence imaging can be fitted into existing instrumentation. The emerging field of fluorescent surgical imaging promises to be a powerful enhancement to traditional low-contrast white-light visualization, offering real-time highlighted delineation of complex anatomic structures. Improved visualization will lead to more complete removal of disease, decreased inadvertent injuries to vital structures, and improved identification for repair of damaged tissues [6].

In addition, working through an interface with cameras and instruments inserted into body cavities through narrow conduits has also sacrificed tactile feedback of directly working with tissue and dissection along tissue planes. Thus, a medical specialty that is traditionally dependent on touch becomes even more dependent on vision. Thus, enhancing the visual differences between tissues by using fluorescent probes based on structure or disease could be equated to color-coding the surgical field. This is the reason why FGS could represent a major contribution to intraoperative decision-making during surgical procedures [7].

First Reports of Fluorescent Events

The first description of fluorescence dates to 1560 and 1565 by Bernardino de Sahagún and Nicolás Monardes, respectively. They reported an early observation of fluorescence in the lignum nephriticum infusion that was derived from the wood of the following tree species: *Pterocarpus indicus* and *Eysenhardtia polystachya*. The chemical component emitting fluorescence was the matlaline, derived from the oxidation of wood flavonoids.

In 1819 and 1822, mineralogists Edward D. Clarke and René Just Haüy described fluorescence in fluorites, respectively. The phenomenon was described for chlorophyll by Sir David Brewster in 1833 and for quinine by Sir John Herschel in 1845.

In his 1852 article on "Refrangibility," the British physicist and mathematician George Gabriel Stokes, noted for his studies of the behavior of viscous fluids and for Stokes' theorem, described the ability of fluorspar and uranium glass to change invisible light beyond the violet end of the visible spectrum into blue light. This phenomenon was called "fluorescence." The name derives from the mineral fluorite (calcium difluoride) that can contain traces of divalent europium that serves as the fluorescent activator to emit blue light. In a fundamental experiment, a prism was used to isolate ultraviolet radiation from sunlight and he observed blue light emitted by ethanol solution of quinine [8].

Preliminary Use of Fluorescence into Surgical Field

The first clinical use of fluorescence was in 1947, when it was used for identification of brain tumors during neurosurgery using the dye fluorescein [9]. In 1953, Ray and Randall succeeded in detecting cancer cell in vaginal smears through a fluorescent staining. The rationale behind the research was the affinity of the basic fluorochrome dyes (berberine sulfate, acid fuchsin, and acridine) for nucleic acids. As neoplastic cells have an increase in total nucleic and ribonucleic acids, with an increase in protein synthesis, cancer cells were identified. A fluorescent microscope was used to evidence this finding [10].

In 1955, Peck and Mack investigated the affinity of hematoporphyrin for malignant tissue and its capability to evidence the biliary anatomy after biliary excretion through its fluorescent properties. They used different spectra of the hematoporphyrin to visualize malignant tumors and bile ducts. Today, hematoporphyrin is used as an endobronchial tumor indicator to facilitate the bronchoscopic localization of early squamous cell carcinoma of the central tracheobronchial tree [11, 12].

In 1963, Acherman and McFee studied tetracycline fluorescence in benign and malignant tissues. Tetracycline has fluorescent properties in ultraviolet light allowing its detection through yellow color into tissue. The authors demonstrated that few minutes after parenteral administration, the drug is distributed to all body tissues apart from the central nervous system, with the highest concentrations in liver, kidneys, and bones. In 1957 Ral et al., during a study on the effects of fluorescent riboflavin antagonist on breast cancer metastases, observed the presence of fluorescent material in tumor tissue of patients treated with tetracycline some weeks before. Klinger and Katz reported that oral administration of tetracycline for 5 days followed by gastric washing for exfoliative cytology after 36 h and examination of aspirate residue under ultraviolet light could allow the visualization of cancerous cells. Fluorescence was seen in 17 of 18 patients with stomach cancer and was not noted on 42 patients without cancer [13, 14].

In 1965, Whitmore et al. performed ultraviolet light cystoscopy after administration of tetracycline, concluding that this method has higher sensibility to evidence tumor if compared to light cystoscopy. It could identify grade III tumor in patients with positive urinary sediments, but negative visible light cystoscopy. There was no relation between fluorescence occurrence and the grade of histologic malignancy or bladder carcinoma type. Ultraviolet cystoscopy can give a valid guidance for biopsy, facilitating early detection of recurrence in patient with persistent tumor cells in urinary sediments but no tumor at visible light cystoscopy after treatment for bladder cancer [15].

It was only in 1966 that fluorescence was used to evaluate perfusion. Tetracycline was used for evaluation of ischemic changes in renal transplantation. After this evidence, renal spectroscopy was defined as a noninvasive method to determine organ viability in renal ischemia and reperfusion. This conclusion was achieved through a study of fluorescence spectroscopy that used histologic evidence to evaluate ischemic injury and organ viability. Authors stated that there is a strong correlation between fluorescence spectroscopy and histologic changes only in the reperfusion phase after renal ischemia. Thus, the described technique was unable to define the viability of organs before transplantation [16, 17].

After these results, fluorescence was tested in different fields as early detection of brain and rynolaringologic tumors. Nessel tested tetracycline fluorescence in rhinolaryngologic malignant tumors' surgery, and Golghahn in brain tumors [18, 19].

After studies on renal ischemic changes in transplant surgery, fluorescence was evaluated in cardiac surgery. There were published studies on the use of fluorescence for defining the degree of revascularization of the heart in surgical treatment of experimental cardiac ischemia and tetracycline fluorescence in experimental necrotizing cardiopathies and in the macroscopic delimitation of experimental acute myocardial ischemia before and after revascularization [20, 21].

This field of research has been in constant development since the 1950s, leading to three Nobel Prizes in Chemistry for the organic chemist and marine biologist Osamu Shimomura, the scientist Martin Chalfie, and the biochemist Roger Yonchien Tsien for the discovery and development of green fluorescent protein in 2008 [8].

The main field of current research and clinical applications of fluorescence in surgery will be extensively described in the following chapters of this book.

Basic Principles of Fluorescence

Fluorescence is the emission of electromagnetic radiation at one wavelength, especially of visible light, stimulated in a substance after absorption of incident radiation, at a different wavelength, which ceases once the incident radiation stops. From a chemical point of view, the light absorbed by an atom or a molecule causes the transition of an electron from the ground state to a certain excited state. After a brief period (nanosecond scale), the electron relaxes to its ground state, emitting part of this energy at a different wavelength. This energy is emitted in the form of photons and

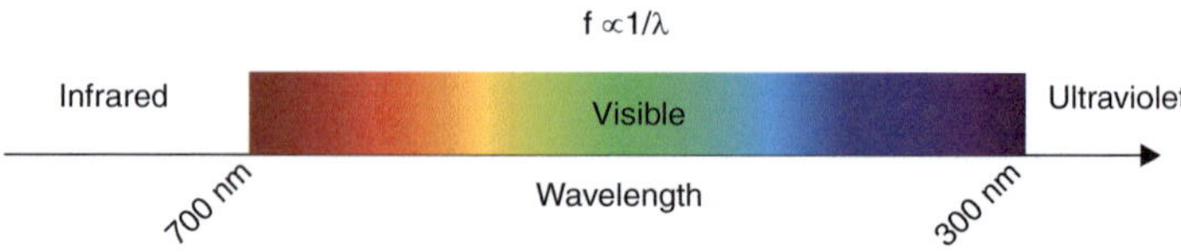

Fig. 1.1 Electromagnetic spectrum and its relation to visible, ultraviolet and infrared light: wavelength (*λ*), frequency (*f*) (nm nanometer)

it is lower, thus corresponding to longer wavelength, than the absorbed photons (and energy).

The wavelengths associated with fluorescence and energy absorption are in the range of 200–1000 nm and can be divided as follows:

- Ultraviolet range: 200–400 nm.
- Visible range: 400–600.
- Near-infrared (NIR) range: 600–1000 nm (Fig. 1.1).

Fluorophores

Molecules that emit fluorescence are called "fluorophores." Their chemical structure is usually made of merged or conjugated aromatic groups. There are several fluorophores available: organic molecules, minerals, nanoparticle, and transition complex metals.

To be used in vivo, fluorophores should demonstrate fluorescence when stimulated by different wavelength light sources and should also have good solubility and photophysical characteristics (brightness, peak excitation, and photostability). Owing to their hydrophobicity, fluorophores often demonstrate poor solubility and aggregation in solution, which can lead to changes in their excitation and emission ranges, as well as quenching of fluorescence [22–24].

When using a fluorophore, four parameters have to be known in order to obtain information of fluorescent signal into the microenvironment:

- Fluorescence intensity that changes according to excitation energy.
- Emission wavelength: emission energy is lower than the excitation one, with emission wavelength that is higher than the excitation one.
- Fluorescence lifetime: the mean time the fluorophore spends into the excited state before photon emission.
- Fluorescence polarization: describes the polarization of the emission compared to the absorption. It gives information about viscosity of the medium and molecular size.

Fluorescence has been exploited in several areas, and, as aforementioned, during the last decades, it reached the medical and surgical field, giving birth, with the development of new technologies, to fluorescence-guided surgery. If this specific molecule allows to study and gives information about the structure and/or a system, it is named "fluorescent probe" [8, 25, 26]. As aforementioned, fluorescence-guided surgery needs fluorescent probes to be performed.

Chromophores in Surgical Practice

A chromophore can basically be defined as an "optically active" substance. Chromophore-containing molecules are widely used in conventional surgical practice because of their capability to enhance human vision; their application is demonstrated across several medical specialties, ranging from skin marking ink and sentinel lymph node biopsy (SLNB) to methylene blue for urinary tract lesions [27].

Surgeons increasingly demand for real-time sensory input to achieve a more accurate identification of tissues during their practice. Enhanced visual differentiation of anatomical structures becomes even more important, especially when considering new minimally invasive surgical technology where there is a loss of tactile feedback and everything the surgeon sees is "filtered" from the screen.

In a conventional operating setting, even if the use of some kind of chromophore in medical practice is already established, surgeons have always relied on which is visible to the naked eye (390–700 nm) [28]. While this principle contributes to the mainstay of conventional surgery, it suffers from several drawbacks including multiple light shadowing, dependence on the operating surgeon, and experience [29]. Furthermore, the unmet clinical need in surgery stems from the fact that visible light cannot penetrate blood and tissue more than a few hundred microns, due to high photon attenuation from absorbance and scatter. Thus, when a surgeon looks at the surgical field, he only sees surface features. The implications of this are significant since there are over 40 million surgical procedures performed in the United States (US) each year, and even small improvements in outcome, or reductions in morbidity, will affect large patient populations [1]. FGS can obtain a fundamental role in preservation of normal tissues such as lymphatics, ureters, bile ducts, and blood vessels that are visualizable using untargeted tracers such as ICG [7].

The need to find new applications for chromophores in diagnostics and operative settings led to the development of specific dyes and probes that could be seen in target tissues beyond the visual spectrum, through the use of special light sources ranging from ultraviolet (UV) to near-infrared (NIR) wavelengths.

Fluorescent Probes

Fluorescent probes are contrast agents able to enhance a specific structure of tissue from surrounding ones. Based on their fluorescence emission spectra, clinically evaluated dyes can be separated into three groups. The first group includes probes emitting fluorescence in the visible part of the light spectrum (400–650 nm) with fluorescein sodium being one of the most widely used visible dye in clinical care today. The second group consists of dyes emitting in the far-red region of the light spectrum (650–750 nm). Here, an interesting development has been the clinical introduction of the relatively bright cyanine dye named Cy5. The last group consists of near-infrared emitting cyanine dyes (750–1000 nm) such as indocyanine green (ICG) [8, 30].

There are two main types of fluorescent probes: intrinsic and extrinsic.

Intrinsic Probes

Intrinsic probes have the intrinsic property to become fluorescent in their native form. They can be found in nature components and into the human body. The main advantages are that they do not need any external probe to fluoresce, and they need less regulation in order to be used in clinical practice. The main disadvantage is that the resulting fluorescence intensity is low, ending with low contrast between target structures and surrounding tissues. Indeed, the penetration depth is low and many other endogenous fluorophores can fluoresce under the same condition. Thus, to date, endogenous fluorophores are not currently used in fluorescence-guided surgery, but only as research topic [31]. However, they seem to have high potential, so they will be used probably in clinical practice in the future. The most used endogenous fluorophores are described below (Table 1.1):

Table 1.1 Characteristics of the main endogenous fluorophores

Fluorophore	Absorption peak (nm)	Emission peak (nm)	Average lifetime (ns)
Collagen	325	400	5.3
Elastin	290, 325	340, 400	2.3
NADH/NADPH	340	450	0.4
FAD	450	535	2.3–4.7
Lipofuscin	340–395	430–460	1.34

- Collagen, a structural protein of connective tissue, and elastin, a protein of the extracellular matrix. These proteins fluoresce at low wavelength, so they can be used in superficial sites. For example, they can be used to identify necrosis of bones, allowing a precise removal from healthy tissue [4].
- Nicotinamide adenine dinucleotide (NADH), a key factor in cellular energy metabolism, nicotinamide adenine dinucleotide phosphate (NADPH), and flavin adenine dinucleotide (FAD). These two species, i.e., NADH and NADPH, are spectrally identically fluorescing at the same wavelength, with peak emission at ~450 nm, so they cannot be distinguished in living cells. FAD is involved in cellular energy metabolism too and fluoresce with peak emission at ~535 nm. This different peak emission allows a simultaneous use of fluorescent properties of NADH/NADPH and FAD. For example, they can be used for intraoperative tumor margin analysis [4].
- Lipofuscin, which accumulates in granules in retinal pigment epithelium with age, especially in patients with visual disease, has a peak emission at ~578 nm and can be used to study eye surface [32].

Extrinsic Probes

Extrinsic probes are molecules designed to fluoresce under specific conditions in order to obtain a fluorescent signal that it would not exist otherwise. Compared to intrinsic probes, the main advantages of the extrinsic ones are better fluorescent properties, like intensity, and major control in choosing the structure where the probe has to concentrate or be labeled to gain the specific signal. They can be distinguished based on the wavelength they require to be excited and seen and can be classified as "targeted" and "untargeted" [7]. In current clinical practice, non-targeted fluorophores are the most common.

Usually, the choice of a fluorophore must take into consideration the following specifics [1, 6, 7]:

- Dose (quantity needed to achieve the desired effect).
- Time between administration and visualization.
- Pharmacodynamics.
- Way of administration (e.g., systemic vs. local).

Severe regulatory requirements are necessary to have a fluorescent dye approved for clinical use. Thus, some probes are already available on the market, while some others are still being tested and developed.

Currently Approved Extrinsic Probes

Due to multiple possible applications, many groups around the world are developing novel fluorophores and targeted fluorophores. Nevertheless, the reality is that first-in-human testing of a new chemical entity has a minimum lag of about 2 years, and commercial availability of a new chemical entity has a minimum lag of 2–5 years. For the foreseeable future, there are only four molecules approved for by the FDA (Food and Drug Administration) and thus clinically available for study: fluorescein sodium, methylene blue (MB), indocyanine green (ICG), and 5-aminolevulinic acid (5-ALA). Interestingly, methylene blue (MB) and indocyanine have been used for the last decades as visible dyes, and for this reason, there is a large amount of clinical data regarding their safety when used at millimolar concentrations [1] (Table 1.2). All these approved fluorescent probes are untargeted.

Table 1.2 Characteristics of the main extrinsic probes approved by FDA

Fluorophore	Absorption peak (nm)	Emission peak (nm)	Average lifetime (ns)
Fluorescein sodium	490	510	4.0
Methylene blue	665	685	0.6
Indocyanine green	780	830	0.16
5-ALA	410	630	15

- **Fluorescein sodium.** It is a manufactured organic compound that is FDA approved with peak excitation at ~ 490 nm and peak relaxation at ~ 510 nm [4]. The first clinical application of fluorescein sodium was for the identification of brain tumor in 1948. It is still used for the same purpose in neurosurgery and also widely used as a fluorescent tracer for many other applications, like in ophthalmology and optometry (retinal angiography and angioscopy), detection of oral dysplasia and cancer, and detection of tumors of peripheral nerve sheath. Fluorescein sodium is the designated fluorophore to obtain images through confocal microscopy and its related applications, such as flow cytometry [33]. The relative low cost and the possibility to visualize fluorescein sodium with the naked eye are advantages if compared to other probes. The main disadvantage is that it fluoresces within the visible spectrum, overlapping with endogenous fluorophores. [4].
- **Methylene blue.** Compared to visible spectrum, the near-infrared (NIR) range is more favorable in surgery, as light is less absorbed by tissue and allows greater penetration depth. One clinically approved dye with beneficial properties in the visible and NIR spectrum is methylene blue. It is a hydrophilic phenothiazine derivative with peak excitation at ~665 nm and emission at ~685 [34]. Its fluorescent performance is inferior to the ICG one (below described), due to a lower quantic energy (ratio between the number of electrons emitted and the number of incident photons), and exhibits an extinction coefficient and QY far below those of the indocyanines [1] (Figs. 1.2 and 1.3).

  It is partially excreted through urine and, for this reason, could be useful for ureteral visualization in surgery [35]. Due to the unique biodistribution and fluorescent properties of MB, its application in identifying vital structures, such as assessment of cardiac perfusion and detection of several types of tumors, including neuroendocrine tumors, fibrous pancreatic tumors, paragangliomas, and parathyroid adenomas, sentinel lymph node mapping, has been demonstrated by several inves-

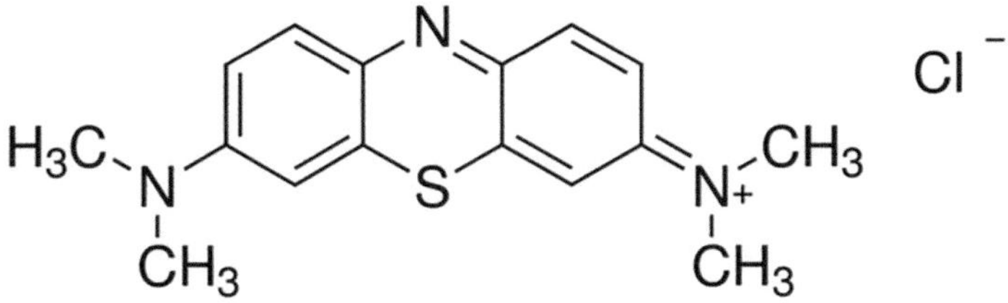

Fig. 1.2 Chemical composition of methylene blue

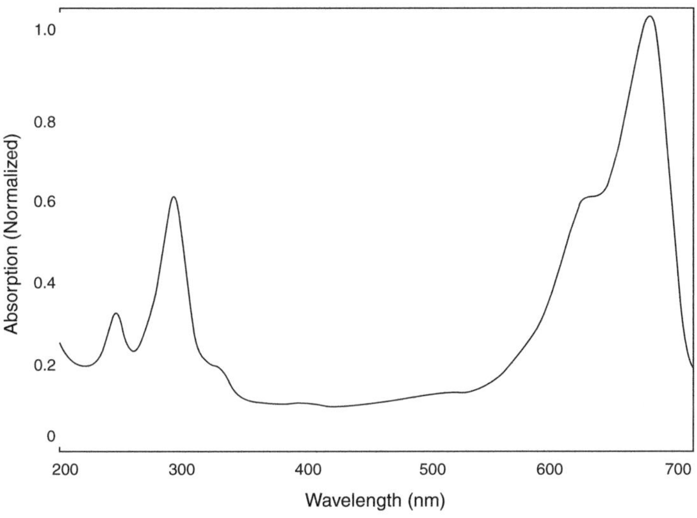

Fig. 1.3 Absorbance spectrum of methylene blue

tigators. However, the tumor-targeting properties of methylene blue remain poorly understood and based on small studies and reports. Moreover, methylene blue has a low fluorescence yield and no functional group for adding ligands [4].

- **Indocyanine green.** It is a water-soluble tricarbocynanine dye that has been used clinically for over 50 years for hepatic clearance, cardiovascular function testing, and retinal angiography on the basis of its dark green color. ICG dye was developed for near-infrared photography by the Kodak Research Laboratories in 1955 and was approved for clinical use already in 1956. However, it took over 10 years before ICG was used for angiography. It has been used for retinal angiography since the early 1970s [36].

Indocyanine green is a negatively charged ion that belongs to the large family of cyanine dyes, having a molecular weight of 751.4 Da. Dry ICG is stable at room temperature. In aqueous solutions, ICG molecules tend to aggregate, which influences their optical properties. The aggregation depends on concentration and time. The spectral stabilization is fastest when ICG is dissolved in distilled water, and thus some authors do not recommend adding isotonic saline and/or albumin to the injectate, when fast spectral stability is essential, for example, when using ICG for quantitative purposes. IGC is hydrophobic and, thus, it frequently bounds to proteins in plasma (especially albumin), which confines ICG to the intravascular space and makes it especially suited for angiographic applications [26, 27]. ICGbased angiography and lymphography have been used in a variety of clinical indications, such as perfusionbased imaging of the liver and blood vessels of the eye and assessment of lymphatic vessel drainage. The important property of fast binding to plasma proteins, especially lipoproteins, makes repeated intraoperative applications of ICG possible. The binding to plasma proteins does not seem to alter protein structures, which is one sign of nontoxicity. Binding to blood proteins also shifts slowly, taking several minutes, the absorption peak at 780 nm toward longer wavelengths, to 805 nm. The absorption peak maximum was observed at 810 nm in the epidermal cell cultures and at 805–810 nm in the human skin in vivo (Figs. 1.4 and 1.5).

ICG does not have any known metabolites, and it is quickly extracted by the liver into bile juice. The transport is done by a protein called glutathione *S*-transferase without modification. The protein spectra of different liver diseases also affect ICG protein binding in blood. It has a quick clearance rate of 18–24% per minute by the liver, which is the result of both the

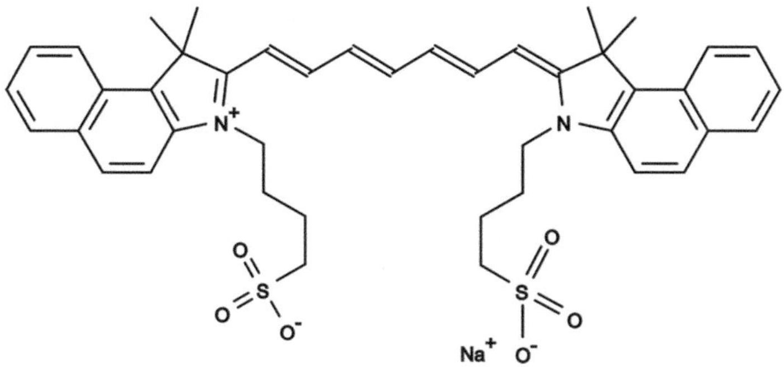

Fig. 1.4 Chemical composition of indocyanine green

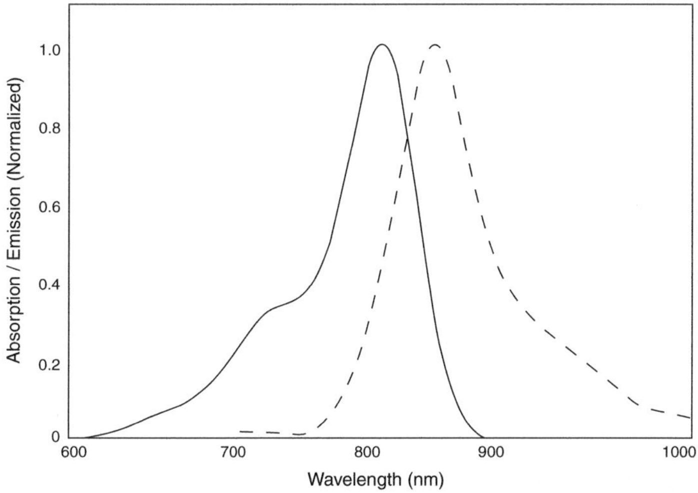

Fig. 1.5 Absorbance and fluorescence-emission spectra of indocyanine green. Continuous and dotted lines show absorbance and emission spectra respectively

compound's confinement to the intravascular space and that the decomposition products of ICG are not metabolites. The dye is cleared from the system exponentially in the first 10–20 min after application, with a half-life of generally

3–4 min depending on the vascularization of the organ of interest [26, 27, 36].

The typical dye concentrations used for in vivo retinal angiography are in the range of 20–25 mg/mL of ICG applied by injection into a peripheral arm vein. For studies of hepatic function, an intravenous injection dose is calculated on the basis of 0.5 mg/kg of body weight. In cardiac output and blood volume monitoring, the total dose of dye injected should be kept below 2 mg/kg. Peculiar feature is the low toxicity (LD50 after single IV dose of 50–80 mg/kg for animals). No significant toxic effects have been observed in humans with the high dose of 5 mg/kg of body weight. ICG for injection contains sodium iodide and should be used with caution in patients who have a history of allergy to iodides because of the risk of anaphylaxis. ICG was not found to be mutagenic in the tests performed. No studies for reproduction, teratogenicity, or carcinogenic properties in animals are available, but decades of experience in humans have not revealed any incidence of these properties.

To date, ICG is the first and only clinically approved fluorophore that displays NIR fluorescence. Because ICG has no functional groups for conjugation to targeting moieties for molecular imaging application, it is a nonspecific contrast agent. The commercially available instrumentation used for ICG detection is adjusted for the characteristics that ICG displays in plasma (peak excitation wavelength of 807 nm and peak emission wavelength of 822 nm) [36, 37].

- **5-aminolevulinic acid**. 5-ALA is an amino acid that acts as a fluorophore processed by high metabolic active cells. Indeed, it is a precursor of protoporphyrin IX that is involved in the pathway of heme synthesis. After 5-ALA administration, protoporphyrin IX accumulates in malignant glioma tissue, which became fluorescent, due to an abnormality in porphyrin metabolism.

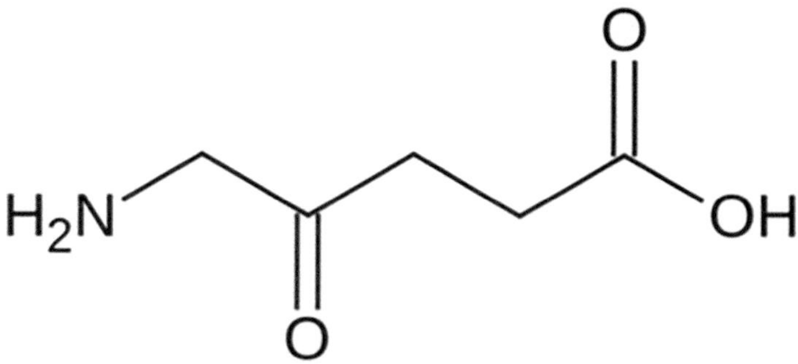

Fig. 1.6 Chemical composition of 5-aminolevulinic acid

It exhibits a fluorescence absorption peak of 405 nm, and an emission peak in the red visible light range (635 nm), permitting fluorescence imaging on the surface of tissues and in a depth range of millimeters. This fluorescence spectrum outside the NIR window is a disadvantage for surgical application, but it has minimum toxicity and 5-ALA is naturally present in the body (Figs. 1.6 and 1.7).

Approved in 2017 by FDA, it is used mainly for FGS for guided ablation of malignant glioblastoma-based. In addition, 5ALA has also been used in clinical settings for the photodynamic detection and photodynamic therapy of many superficial skin lesions, and its use is being investigated in several cancer types [4, 38].

The main limit of extrinsic probes is the limited approved number for clinical use. The approval process is long, because a good fluorescent probe should have good fluorescent properties, low toxicity, great quantum yield, and short half-life. Indeed, depending on the fluorophore uptake from the target tissue, the greater the quantum yield is, the smaller the dose to achieve effectiveness. Moreover, short half-life implicates rapid clearance so the possibility to repeat fluorophore administration for further intraoperative evaluation.

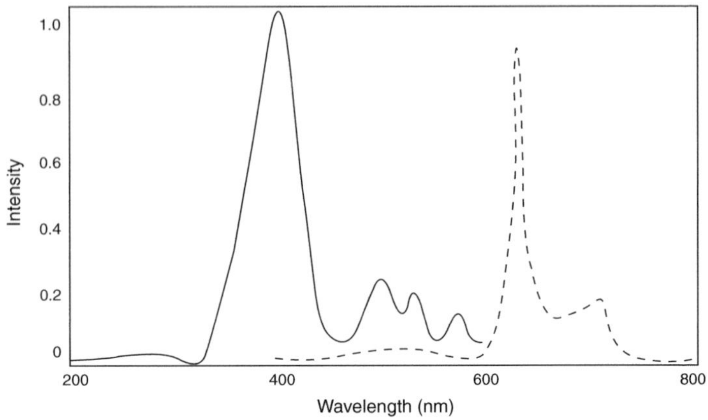

Fig. 1.7 Absorbance and fluorescence-emission spectra of Protoporphyrin IX. Continuous and dotted lines show absorbance and emission spectra respectively

Extrinsic Probes Under Clinical Development

Even if the approval process is long and difficult, there is high interest in fluorophore development for clinical use. A recent review reported that a total of 85 trial have been registered to test 39 new contrast agents for fluorescence-guided surgery. Some of these probes under development utilize target like antibodies or peptides to obtain highly specific fluorescent signal. For example, optically active probes can specifically label intra- and extracellular biomarkers of cancer. Targeted fluorophores actually under development aim mainly to identify cancer cells in order to diagnose tumor early and to verify that tumor dissection is complete. Other untargeted probes generate fluorescent signal through enzymatic process. Others have fluorescent properties themselves [4, 39].

Some of these probes for fluorescence-guided surgery have reached phase III clinical trials:

- **SGM-101**. It is a target antibody for carcinoembryonic antigen (CEA) linked with a NIR fluorophores. It has been tested in colorectal tumors, showing high specificity in primary tumor tissue and in metastases [40].

- **BLZ-100.** It is a chlorotoxin peptide linked to ICG, with affinity for metalloprotease 2. It has been studied for pediatric central nervous system tumor, showing specificity for tumor tissue and correlation with fluorophore dose and cancer grade [41].
- **OTL38.** It is composed of folic acid and NIR fluorophore S0456. It has demonstrated high sensitivity for ovarian cancer tissue [42].

Several other probes under development are in phase II or phase I clinical trials. Some of these contrast agents are BBN-IRDye800CW for brain cancer, fluorescein-conjugated *Wisteria floribunda* for colon cancer, and EC17 for renal carcinoma.

Clinically approved fluorescence imaging systems are compatible with FDA-approved contrast agents. Thus, most of the systems are set for ICG, with excitation and emission wavelength around 800 nm. Few imaging systems have capability for fluorescein and 5-ALA fluorescence, and only two systems have the possibility to perform fluorescence surgery with methylene blue in the spectrum of 700 nm. As a result, because fluorescence is centered around 800 nm, the most used fluorophore for contrast agents under development is the IRDye800CW. Thus, there is a gap between fluorescent properties of new contrast agents and imaging possibility with approved imaging systems [4].

Clinical Imaging Systems

Fluorophores with excitation and emission spectra in the near-infrared wavelength range (700–900 nm) have attracted the most attention owing to their improved depth penetration range compared with fluorophores that emit electromagnetic radiation of shorter wavelengths. Within this NIR window, the absorption of most biomolecules (i.e., deoxyhemoglobin, oxyhemoglobin, water, and lipid) reaches minimal levels, and scattering and autofluorescence are relatively low. Since NIR fluorescent light is essentially invisible to the human eye, special imaging systems are required to excite the NIR fluorophores within the surgical field and to collect emitted photons. Well-designed NIR fluorophores are needed to highlight the specific structures desired by the surgeon. The commercial development of these agents for clinical application has synergized with concurrent improvements in detection instrumentation and software [1].

ICG becomes fluorescent once excited with NIR light or with a dedicated laser beam. The fluorescence can be detected using specific scopes and cameras and then transmitted to a standard monitor allowing identification of anatomical structures where the dye is present (i.e., biliary ducts, vessels, lymph nodes, etc.) [43] (Fig. 1.8).

ICG is the only NIR fluorophore employed to date for human use. As described previously, it had widespread uses in hepatic, cardiac, and ophthalmologic studies, and its use is recently reported in analyzing tissue perfusion and identifying lymph nodes in cancer patients. It has several clinically excellent properties, which has been thoroughly verified during its long clinical use [36]:

- Patient safety (nontoxic, nonionizing).
- Ideal for angiography because it binds efficiently to blood lipoproteins and does not leak from circulation; ideal for bile duct study because it is excreted selectively through the bile.
- Short lifetime in blood circulation allowing repeated applications.
- Good signal-to-background ratio (SBR): there is not much NIR autofluorescence in tissue where the exogenous dye is not present.
- Deep imaging with possibility to see beyond the surface, at a depth of several millimeters.
- Simple and relatively cheap imaging devices.

Components of Fluorescence-Based Surgical System

Fluorescence technology used in surgical system is based on methodology already defined in fluorescence microscopy and spectroscopy [44]. The system is made of an excitation source, a

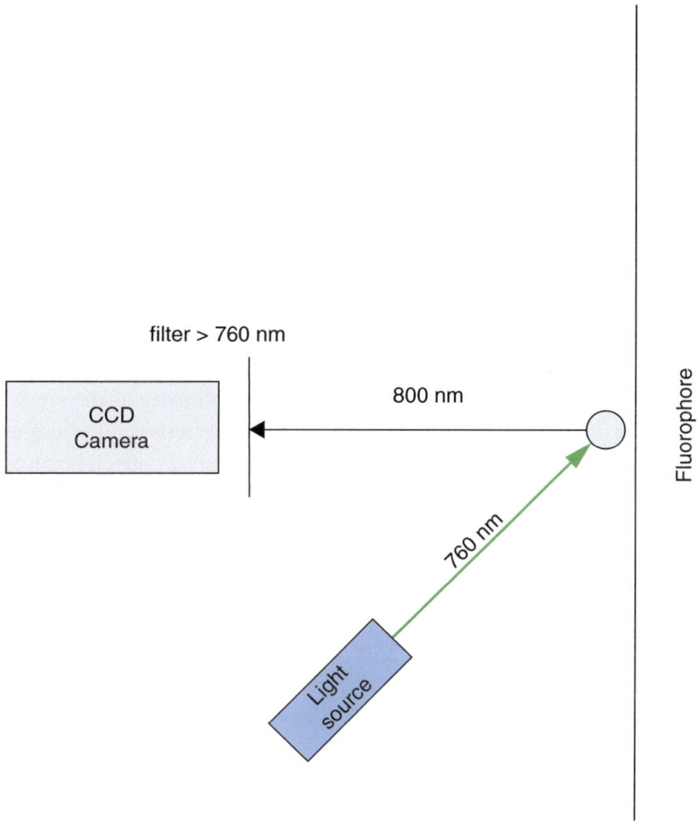

Fig. 1.8 Operating principle of Fluorescence Guided Surgery (FGS)

fluorescent probe (described above), filters, and fluorescent detector.

Excitation Source

The excitation source to obtain a fluorescent signal is a light that can be generated by xenon lamps, light emitting diodes (LEDs), and laser diodes. Even if lamps are flexible, allowing a wide range of wavelength, they are not the ideal source as they produce heat, requiring a warm-up period, and deteriorate with use with a consequent decrease of brightness. LEDs are more diffused. If compared to xenon lamps, LEDs have longer lifetimes, do not need warm up period, have lower consumption, and have a narrow bandwidth. Laser diodes have a narrower wavelength and higher intensity compared with the other two sources. Laser source is more expensive than LED ones, so they are less diffused [4].

Fluorescence System Filters

Excitation and emission filters are necessary to select wavelengths and unwanted signal. For example, emission filters can be used to narrow the fluorescent signal collected to the spectrum of interest. Emission filters' features should be clearly defined and balanced, as a large band allows higher intensity of the signal but less specificity resulting in lower contrast between the target and the background. Moreover, the filter has to be chosen according to the Stokes shift of the fluorophore, that is the difference (in wavelength or frequency units) between positions of the band maxima of the absorption and emission spectra of the same electronic transition [4].

Fluorescence System Detectors

The aim of the detector is to quantify the fluorescence of the single photons according to quantum efficiency, that is the ability to convert the incident light to excited electron, and internal gain, that is the ability to amplify the signal in a large electrical signal.

To date, several systems are currently used to detect photons in surgical field:

- Photomultiplier tubes absorb the incident photons and produce electrons to obtain the signal.
- Microchannel plate photomultipliers absorb the incident photons and produce electron with an amplification of the signal and improved time resolution of the detection system.
- Charge-coupled devices are made of pixel array that produce a signal proportional to exposure time of incident light, resulting in high sensitivity.
- Single photon avalanche photodiode generates current quickly

after photon absorption, thanks to a multiplexed pixel array. The main advantage is the higher quantum efficiency.

Each of these detectors has advantages and disadvantages, and even if single photon avalanche photodiode has high potential for fluorescence lifetime use, photomultiplier tubes and charge-coupled devices are still currently used [4].

Currently Available Devices for Fluorescence-Guided Surgery

Nowadays, a growing number of companies are developing new systems for FGS. These systems that are suitable for both near-infrared (NIR) fluorescence and white-light (WL) imaging, integrating the aforementioned technology, available for both open and minimally invasive surgery.

Each system differs from others on some key features:

- The "exciting" light source type (neon light, LED, or laser beam).
- The system of signal detection.
- The wavelength emitted and captured.
- The optimal distance to visualize fluorescence signal.
- The strength of SBR.
- The possibility of directly overlaying the NIR images to the WL ones.

The different features that characterize each device (field of vision, zoom capability, type of light source, NIR wavelength emitted and captured, etc.) will have an impact on system performance during surgery. During surgical procedures, the alternate exposure from WL to NIR light (ICG mode) is used to identify anatomical structures, blood perfusion, and other details. The fluorescence imaging systems allow to obtain fluorescent images in real-time setting. They are quite unexpensive, if compared to some other technological equipment widely adopted in surgery [45].

Table 1.3 reports some of the most widely adopted devices both for conventional and minimally invasive/robotic surgery (Table 1.3).

Table 1.3 Some of the most widely adopted NIR imaging systems both for conventional and minimally invasive/robotic fluorescence-guided surgery

Imaging system		Image resolution	Use	Visualization mode
Stryker	1688 advanced imaging modalities	4k	Laparoscopic	– Green overlay mode
				– SPY-ENV mode
				– SPY-contrast
				– IRIS
	Pinpoint with SPY-PHI	Full HD	Open	– Green overlay mode
				– Color-segmented fluorescence mode
				– SPY-fluorescence mode
Karl Storz 1 S™	Image 1S™	HD xenon light source	Laparoscopic	– Optical illumination and contrast-enhanced modality
				– No overlay mode
	Image 1S™ Rubina™	4k and 3D	Laparoscopic	– Overlay mode
		Laser-free LED light source		– Intensity map
				– Monochromatic
Arthrex	Synergy *ID* System	4k	Laparoscopic	– Overlay mode
				– Monochromatic
Da Vinci Surgical System (Intuitive)	Firefly camera system integrated into Da Vinci Si and Xi	3D	Robotic	– Normal imaging and fluorescent modes
		LED light		– No overlay mode

Conclusion

In conclusion, since its first clinical application in surgery, fluorescence underwent huge development and spread among specialties. Among all the fluorophores, indocyanine green is the most diffused, thanks to its peculiar features that promote its widespread. Many probes are currently under clinical development and will be on the market soon.

A growing number of companies are developing systems for fluorescence-guided surgery. This imaging system is in constant evolution with many features like overlay visualization and the second near-infrared window (1000–1700 nm), enhancing the power and increasing applications of this technology.

References

1. Gioux S, Choi HS, Frangioni JV. Image-guided surgery using invisible near-infrared light: fundamentals of clinical translation. Mol Imaging. 2010;9(5):237–55.
2. Howell JD. Early clinical use of the x-ray. Trans Am Clin Climatol Assoc. 2016;127:341–9.
3. Pogue BW. Optics of medical imaging: optics plays dominant role in medical imaging market. In: SPIE professional, 2018. p. 6–8.
4. Stewart HL, Birch DJS. Fluorescence guided surgery. Methods Appl Fluoresc. 2021;9:4.
5. National Research Council. Medical optical imaging mathematics and physics of emerging biomedical imaging. Washington DC: National Academy Press; 1996. https://doi.org/10.17226/5066.
6. Orosco RK, Tsien RY, Nguyen QT. Fluorescence imaging in surgery. IEEE Rev Biomed Eng. 2013;6:178–87.
7. Nguyen QT, Tsien RY. Fluorescence-guided surgery with live molecular navigation--a new cutting edge. Nat Rev Cancer 2013;13(9): 653–662.
8. Dip FD, Ishizawa T, Kodudo N, Rosenthal RJ. Fluorescence imaging for surgeons concepts and applications. Basel: Springer; 2015. p. 3–23. ISBN: 978-3-319-35213-8.
9. Moore GE. Fluorescein as an agent in the differentiation of normal and malignant tissues. Science. 1947;106:130–1.
10. Lay CL, Randall LM. Fluorescent staining for detection of cancer cells in vaginal smears. Surg Forum. 1953:321–7.

11. Raymond J, Lanzafame MD, David W, Rogers BS, John O, Nairn MS, et al. Hematoporphyrin derivative fluorescence: photographic techniques for the localization of malignant tissue. Lasers Surg Med. 1986;6(3):328–35.
12. Ahlquist RE Jr, Figge FH. Fluorescence of the extrahepatic biliary system following parenteral hematoporphyrin administration. Surg Forum. 1956;6:356–8.
13. Ackermann NB, Mc Fee AS. Tetracycline fluorescence in benign and malignant tissues. Surgery. 1963;53:247–52.
14. Sandlow LJ, Allen HA. The use of tetracycline fluorescence in the detection of gastric malignancy. Ann Intern Med. 1963;58(3):409–13.
15. Whitmore WF Jr, Bush IM. Ultraviolet cystoscopy in patients with bladder cancer. Trans Am Assoc Genitourin Surg. 1965;57:149–55.
16. Málek P, Kolc J, Pultr V, Zástava V. Tetracycline fluorescence test in evaluation of ischemic changes in kidney transplantations. Rozhl Chir. 1966;45(4):252–6.
17. Cassini MF, da Costa MM. Fluorescence spectroscopy in renal ischemia and reperfusion: noninvasive evaluation of organ viability. Transplant Proc. 2013;45(5):1715–9.
18. Nessel E, Wiggermann W. The tetracycline fluorescence test in surgery of malignant tumors; rhinolaryngologic experiences. HNO. 1965;13(12):346–9.
19. Goldhahn WE. Fluorescence studies of brain tumors. Beitr Neurochir. 1966;13:126–9.
20. Khutsishili TS, Milaeva MA. The use of the fluorescent method for determining the degree of revascularization of the heart in the surgical treatment of experimental cardiac ischemia. Grudn Khir. 1965;7(6):11–2. Russian.
21. Loisance D, Sadony V. Value of fluorescence in the macroscopic delimitation of experimental acute myocardial ischemia before and after revascularization. Arch Mal Coeur Vaiss 1973;66(6):701–707.
22. Zhang RR, Schroeder AB, Grudzinski JJ, Rosenthal EL, Warram JM, Pinchuk AN, et al. Beyond the margins: real-time detection of cancer using targeted fluorophores. Nat Rev Clin Oncol. 2017;14(6):347–64.
23. Mordon S, Devoisselle JM, Soulie-Begu S, Desmettre T. Indocyanine green: physicochemical factors affecting its fluorescence in vivo. Microvasc Res. 1998;55:146–52.
24. Desmettre T, Devoisselle JM, Mordon S. Fluorescence properties and metabolic features of indocyanine green (ICG) as related to angiography. Surv Ophthalmol. 2000;45:15–27.
25. Valeur B, Berberan-Santos MN. Molecular fluorescence: principles and applications. Weinheim: Wiley-VCH; 2012. ISBN: 978-3-527-32837-6.
26. Lakowicz JR. Principles of fluorescence spectroscopy. New York, NY: Springer; 2010. ISBN: 978-1-4615-7658-7.

27. Azzopardi EA, Owens SE, Murison M, Rees D, Anne Sawhney M, Francis LW, et al. Chromophores in operative surgery: current practice and rationalized development. J Control Release. 2017;249:123–30.
28. Rashid A, Warnakulasuriya S. The use of light-based (optical) detection systems as adjuncts in the detection of oral cancer and oral potentially malignant disorders: a systematic review. J Oral Pathol Med. 2015;44(5):307–28.
29. de Boer E, Harlaar NJ, Taruttis A, Nagengast WB, Rosenthal EL, Ntziachristos V, van Dam GM. Optical innovations in surgery. Br J Surg. 2015;102(2):e56–72.
30. Fernandez-Suarez M, Ting AY. Fluorescent probes for super-resolution imaging in living cells. Nat Rev Mol Cell Biol. 2008;9(12):929–43.
31. Mondal SB, et al. Real-time fluorescence image-guided oncologic surgery. Adv Cancer Res. 2014;124:171–211.
32. Marmorstein AD, Marmorstein LY, Sakaguchi H, Hollyfield JG. Spectral profiling of autofluorescence associated with lipofuscin, Bruch's membrane, and sub-RPE deposits in normal and AMD eyes. Invest Ophthalmol Vis Sci. 2002;43(7):2435–41.
33. Shin D, Vigneswaran N, Gillenwater A, Richards-Kortum R. Advances in fluorescence imaging techniques to detect oral cancer and its precursors. Future Oncol. 2010;6:1143–54.
34. Selvam S, Sarkar I. Bile salt induced solubilization of methylene blue: study on methylene blue fluorescence properties and molecular mechanics calculation. J Pharm Anal. 2017;7:71–5.
35. Matsui A, Tanaka E, Choi HS, Kianzad V, Gioux S, Lomnes SJ, Frangioni JV. Real-time, near-infrared, fluorescence-guided identification of the ureters using methylene blue. Surgery. 2010;148:78–86.
36. Alander JT, Kaartinen I, Laakso A, Pätilä T, Spillmann T, Tuchin VV, et al. A review of indocyanine green fluorescent imaging in surgery. Int J Biomed Imaging. 2012;2012:940585.
37. Schaafsma BE, Mieog JS, Hutteman M, vad der Vorst JR, Kuppen PJ, Lowik CW, et al. The clinical use of indocyanine green as a near-infrared fluorescent contrast agent for image-guided oncologic surgery. J Surg Oncol. 2011;104:323–32.
38. Stummer W, Pichlmeier U, Meinel T, Wiestler OD, Zanella F, Reulen HJ. Fluorescence-guided surgery with 5-aminolevulinic acid for resection of malignant glioma: a randomised controlled multicentre phase III trial. Lancet Oncol. 2006;7(5):392–401.
39. Staderini M, Megia-Fernandez A, Dhaliwal K, Bradley M. Peptides for optical medical imaging and steps towards therapy. Bioorg Med Chem. 2018;26:2816–26.
40. Hoogstins CES, Boogerd LSF, Sibinga Mulder BG, Mieog JSD, Swijnenburg RJ, van de Velde CJH, et al. Image-guided surgery in patients with pancreatic cancer: first results of a clinical trial using SGM-

101, a novel carcinoembryonic antigen-targeting, near-infrared fluorescent agent. Ann Surg Oncol. 2018;25:3350–7.
41. Patil CG, Walker DG, Miller DM, Butte P, Morrison B, Kittle DS, et al. Phase 1 safety, pharmacokinetics, and fluorescence imaging study of Tozuleristide (BLZ-100) in adults with newly diagnosed or recurrent gliomas. Neurosurgery. 2019;85:E641–9.
42. Randall LM, Wenham RM, Low PS, Dowdy SC, Tanyi JL. A phase II, multicenter, open-label trial of OTL38 injection for the intra-operative imaging of folate receptor-alpha positive ovarian cancer. Gynecol Oncol. 2019;155:63–8.
43. Luo S, Zhang E, Su Y, Cheng T, Shi C. A review of NIR dyes in cancer targeting and imaging. Biomaterials. 2011;32:7127–38.
44. Engelborghs Y, Visser AJWG. Fluorescence spectroscopy and microscopy: methods and protocols. Methods Mol Biol. 2014. https://doi.org/10.1007/978-1-62703-649-8.
45. Sevick-Muraca EM, Houston JP, Gurfinkel M. Fluorescence-enhanced, nearinfrared diagnostic imaging with contrast agents. Curr Opin Chem Biol. 2002;6:642–50.

Current Fluorescence-Guided Platforms and Devices

2

Donovan Hui, Kevin Carroll,
Christina Sanders, and David Pechman

Introduction

Fluorescence-guided surgery (FGS) enables clinicians to visualize fluorescence-enhanced images in real time to assist in surgical procedures. Its use has transformed the way surgeons visualize structures that may not be apparent under visible light alone [1]. The wavelength of visible light is between 380 and 780 nm. Near-infrared (NIR) extends from a wavelength of 780–2500 nm with penetration of tissues ranging from 5 to

D. Hui
Department of Surgery, New York Medical College Metropolitan Hospital Center, New York, NY, USA

K. Carroll
Department of Surgery, Northwell Health—South Shore University Hospital, Bay Shore, NY, USA

C. Sanders
Department of Surgery, Jacobs School of Medicine and Biomedical Sciences, State University of New York at Buffalo, Buffalo, NY, USA
e-mail: cs328@buffalo.edu

D. Pechman (✉)
Department of Surgery, Zucker School of Medicine at Hofstra, Northwell Health—South Shore University Hospital, Bay Shore, NY, USA

N. Szoka et al. (eds.), *The SAGES Manual of Fluorescence-Guided Surgery*, https://doi.org/10.1007/978-3-031-40685-0_2

8 mm [2, 3]. The depth of penetration and the working distance of each device determine which structures can be identified with fluorescence imaging.

FGS utilizes a specialized camera with an NIR detector to relay images in real time. An excitation light source is used to activate fluorophores within target tissue [4, 5]. Excitation and emission wavelengths are specific for each device. These wavelengths are generally within a similar range and are limited by clinically available fluorophores [2, 3, 6, 7].

Fluorescence imaging requires a fluorophore or an NIR-emitting LED to create near-infrared images. Fluorophores are compounds that release light with excitation and are the primary means for visualizing key structures in FGS. In 2021, available fluorophores include fluorescein, methylene blue (MB), 5-aminolevulinic acid (5-ALA), and indocyanine green (ICG) [8]. ICG is the most frequently used fluorophore due to its ease of use and low side effect profile. It is easy to mix and administer intravenously in the pre-op or intraoperative setting. Its emission wavelength does not overlap with visible light; this minimizes scattering effect and background noise that may obscure visualization [8–10].

Fluorescein has an excitation wavelength of 495 nm and an emission wavelength of 519 nm. MB has an excitation wavelength of 668 nm and an emission wavelength of 688 nm. 5-ALA has an excitation wavelength of 380–440 and an emission wavelength of 620–634 nm, depending on the acidity of its solution. Fluorescein, MB, and 5-ALA have emission wavelengths within the visible light wavelength and are therefore not ideal fluorophores for FGS. The excitation and emission wavelengths of ICG are 740–900 and 800–860 nm ranges, respectively, and are ideal for use with NIR cameras [11–13].

Fluoroscopic devices have become increasingly prevalent in the opening room since the Food and Drug Administration (FDA) approved the Novadaq SPY imaging system in 2005 [6, 12]. FGS has shown utility in a wide range of procedures, including intraoperative angiography, perfusion assessment, tissue plane identification, biliary structure identification, and lymphangiography [5, 14]. As the technology to fluorescently label specific tissues continues to advance, FGS devices will become increasingly more commonplace in the operative suite [8, 9].

Indocyanine Green (ICG) Dye

Indocyanine green (ICG) was developed in 1955 by Kodak Research Laboratory for NIR photography. It was approved for clinical use in 1959 for assessment of cardiac output. It was later found to be excreted exclusively by the liver with uptake by hepatocytes and excretion via bile which prompted its use in the assessment of hepatic function [15]. ICG was found to be useful in the assessment of choroidal blood flow and has since been utilized in an increasing number of angiographic and lymphangiographic modalities [11]. Use of ICG is heavily favored for fluorescence-guided surgery as it is a water-soluble dye with emission wavelength of approximately 800 nm. The autofluorescence at this wavelength in normal tissue is low which increases the signal-to-noise ratio and improves sensitivity of visualized target anatomy following excitation. ICG has a relatively low toxicity profile with a half-life at approximately 3 min. It readily binds lipoproteins in the blood without systemic effects and is very well tolerated by patients [16, 17]. It is non-nephrotoxic and has a low side effect profile. It can be used multiple times during the same surgery. ICG requires fresh preparation with 6 h of viable use.

Contraindication for use of ICG is anaphylaxis. Recommended dosing, mode of administration, timing for administration, and timing for visualization are per manufacturer recommendations [17]. General recommendations are as follows:

- Angiographic perfusion: 2.5 mg given intravenously during surgery with visualization in less than 1 min.
- Biliary assessment: 5 mg given intravenously up to 1–7 h before surgery with direct visualization.
- Lymph node mapping: 2.5 mg given directly around target tissue during surgery with visualization in 15–30 min.

Fluorescence-Guided Systems and Devices

The first FDA-approved system for FGS is the Novadaq SPY system developed in 2005. Many of the first FGS systems were used in open surgery via a cart-based platform that contained an excitation laser and imager to capture NIR light. These cart-based systems have largely been replaced by handheld devices and have been adapted to laparoscopic, robotic, and microscopic systems. As FGS continues to advance, devices may integrate with augmented reality systems and wearable technology.

Open Surgical Systems

The two categories of open FGS systems are cart-based and handheld devices. Cart-based systems offer visualization of key structures while freeing the surgeon's hands to manipulate tissue and operate while assessing in real time. The working distance for such devices is fixed, but offers a wide area of visualization in assessing overall perfusion in reconstructive procedures. Handheld devices also offer visualization of key structures in real time with some systems having the option for mounting the imager on an adjustable securing arm. The size and convenience of handheld devices offer a greater degree of freedom and maneuverability with a flexible working distance [1, 3, 6].

Cart-Based Platform

SPY Elite System [Spy Elite Intraoperative Perfusion Assessment System (LC3000, SP 3000)]—Stryker, Kalamazoo, Michigan, USA

The SPY Elite System (Fig. 2.1a) is the updated version of the first clinically available FGS platform, the SPY System. The SPY Elite System consists of a mounted imaging head that can be positioned above the surgical field in order to obtain NIR images.

SPY Elite System Components

The system includes the following: imaging console (radiation source and mage detector), dual display (1080p resolution),

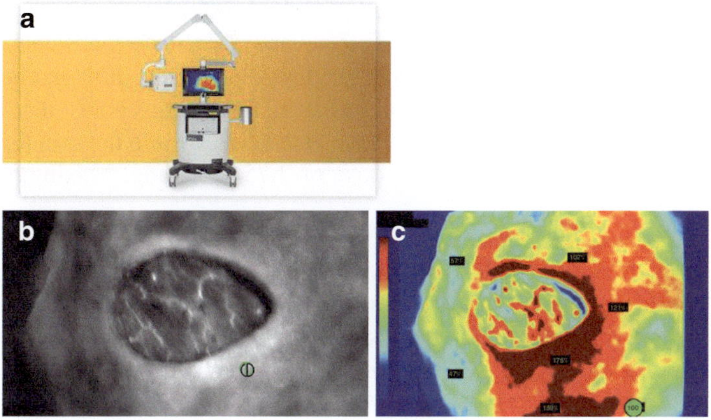

Fig. 2.1 (**a**) SPY Elite cart-based fluorescence system—Photo courtesy of Stryker. (**b**) SPY Elite fluorescence image—Photo courtesy of Stryker. (**c**) SPY-Q image captured for qualitative assessment of tissue perfusion—Photo courtesy of Stryker

CINEVAQ Software, sterile drape, and SPY AGENT GREEN (ICG)—25 mg vials.

For use, the SPY Elite System should be positioned in the operating room to provide optimal visualization of the monitor located on the cart. The imaging console is sterilely draped, using the included clear drapes, and positioned over the surgical field. The imaging console is attached to a flexible arm mount connected directly to the cart system, which can be easily positioned and removed from the operative field while maintaining sterility. The working distance of the imaging console is 30 cm and is the ideal distance from the target anatomy to obtain accurate fluorescence images. SPY mode fluorescence is activated from the cart or the "laser on" button on the left side of the imaging console. The radiation source is a class 3R laser that activates a fluorophore to produce emission wavelengths between 825 and 850 nm. NIR images are captured through a charge-coupled device camera and relay real-time images on the display attached to the system cart. The preferred fluorophore with SPY Elite System is SPY AGENT GREEN (ICG), and its timing for use depends on the indication for use [18, 19].

Dosing, Timing, and Route of Administration

For angiography and assessment of tissue perfusion, ICG can be given immediately intraoperatively as an intravenous bolus injection of 1.25 to 5 mg. ICG can be injected directly into the skin for reconstructive surgeries in a dose of 3.75 to 10 mg. Maximum dose is 2 mg/kg.

For visualization of extrahepatic biliary duct for use in patients ages 12 and older, ICG should be administered at least 45 min prior to surgery as an intravenous bolus injection of 2.5 mg.

For lymphangiography, visualization of lymph nodes, and lymphatic mapping, ICG can be injected directly into target tissue as a direct injection of 5 mg or divided into four 1.25 mg injections around target tissue.

As the first clinically available FGS system, the SPY System established the clinical utility of FGS but has largely been replaced by handheld devices and other newer systems. The FDA has determined the SPY Elite System was substantially equivalent to the predicate SPY System device as a fluorescence imaging system for use in imaging blood flow in plastic surgery (microscopic and reconstructive), gastrointestinal surgery, transplant surgery, cardiovascular surgery, and vascular surgery [20].

The SPY Elite System is able to provide real-time monochromatic images of fluorescent tagged structures (Fig. 2.1b) for the assessment of perfusion. SPY Elite contains updated processing and image acquisition software (CINEVAQ) that is able to overlay a color intensity gradient to the grayscale NIR image. This color intensity image can be recorded and reviewed to assess perfusion via SPY mode (Fig. 2.1c). SPY mode analyzes differences in near-infrared color intensities to offer objective values on estimated perfusion in the form of absolute perfusion units (APUs) to assess how well-perfused structures are during surgery [18–20].

The cart-based SPY Systems have been used across many surgical specialties since its clinical debut in 2005. Within the field of plastic surgery, it is used to assess tissue perfusion in reconstruction. SPY Elite laser angiography can help predict tissue necrosis following microvascular and reconstructive procedures such as facial reconstruction and nipple-sparing mastectomies [21–23]. Using the SPY proprietary software, absolute perfusion units (APUs) offer objective data on tissue perfusion with studies showing APUs of less than 24 associated with increased risk of tissue necrosis [24, 25]. A randomized double-blinded controlled study on complex abdominal wall reconstruction using the SPY Elite System displayed that real-time perfusion assessment could predict intraoperatively which patients were at increased risk for wound complications [26].

The SPY Elite System has been used for laser angiography of gastrointestinal anastomosis. SPY Elite angiography has displayed utility in assessing bowel perfusion when creating gastrointestinal anastomoses, but there have been no randomized controlled studies to assess whether its use decreases anastomotic failure [27–31]. The system has been used as an adjunct to assess graft patency following bypass in open heart surgery [32]. Recently, lymphangiography during sentinel lymph node biopsies has shown a non-inferior capability to identify lymph nodes compared to traditional approaches (radiofrequency labeling and application of dyes) [33, 34].

Pearls and Pitfalls

- SPY mode relies heavily on the quality of near-infrared images. Tissue should be in plane with the imager at an ideal distance of 30 cm.
- SPY perfusion assessment can be used in real time or saved for later review.

Handheld Devices

SPY Portable Handheld Imaging (PHI): HH9000—Stryker, Kalamazoo, Michigan, USA

SPY PHI (Fig. 2.2a) was initially developed by Novadaq Technologies as a handheld system approved for fluorescence-guided surgery in open surgical procedures. SPY PHI is the handheld version of the first clinically available fluorescence-guided

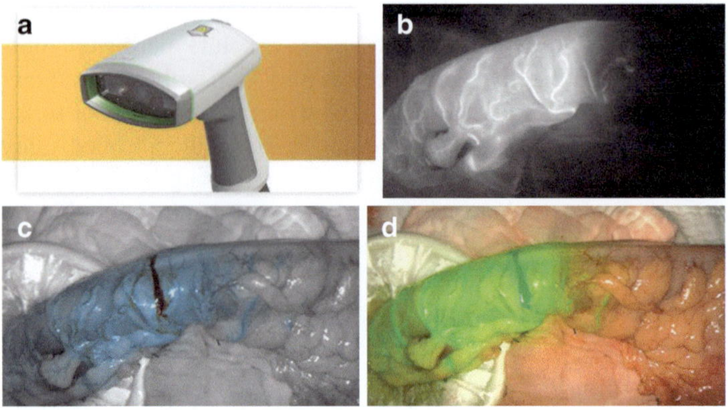

Fig. 2.2 (**a**) SPY PHI handheld device—Photo courtesy of Stryker. (**b**) SPY PHI in SPY mode—Photo courtesy of Stryker. (**c**) SPY PHI in color-segmented mode—Photo courtesy of Stryker. (**d**) SPY PHI in overlay mode—Photo courtesy of Stryker

surgical system, the SPY System. The system consists of a handheld imager that is directly manipulated by the surgeon at target anatomy in order to obtain NIR images.

SPY PHI System Components

The system includes the following: SPY PHI imager with integrated light cable, video processor/illuminator (VPI), display (1080p resolution), SPY PHI Fluorescence Assessment Software (SPY-QP), sterile drape, and SPY AGENT GREEN (ICG)—25 mg vials.

During use, SPY PHI platform is positioned for optimal visualization of the monitor. The handheld imager is connected to the video processor/illuminator with a light cable and camera cable. The imager is then sterilely draped, using the included clear drapes, and is now free to position sterilely in the operative field. The working distance of the imager is 10–40 cm. The green illumination button on the handheld device activates the light source and NIR laser for fluorescence excitation. The camera is able to detect full-color visible light and NIR images with the default image in overlay mode. The preferred fluorophore with SPY PHI System is SPY AGENT GREEN (ICG) with identical dosing and timing as with the SPY Elite System [35, 36].

Novadaq (now part of Stryker) developed its handheld fluorescence imaging system in 2017 with model HH9000. The currently available system is the SPY PHI model HH9000 now with SPY-QP Fluorescence Assessment Software. The FDA has determined the current system was substantially equivalent to the predicate SPY Elite System for use in imaging blood flow in plastic surgery (microscopic and reconstructive), gastrointestinal surgery, transplant surgery, cardiovascular surgery, and vascular surgery. SPY PHI provides real-time visible and NIR imaging with multiple modes. SPY mode (Fig. 2.2b), color-segmented fluorescence (CSF) mode (Fig. 2.2c), and overlay mode (Fig. 2.2d) can be toggled using button "A" on the handheld device. SPY mode is a pure fluorescence image, displayed in monochromatic format to detect only NIR images. Color-segmented fluorescence (CSF) mode displays visible light in grayscale with fluorescence overlay in different color intensities to display fluorescence ranges (blue being the lowest to yellow and then red as the highest). Overlay mode allows for real-time visualization in the visible and NIR spectrum simultaneously, with fluorescence overlaid in green. SPY-QP software can be accessed from the handheld device via button "B" or through the VPI console. SPY-QP provides fluorescence assessment via relative percentage values (Fig. 2.2e) compared to a user set reference point and by color mapping similar to CSF mode [35–37].

Much like the SPY Elite System, the SPY PHI System has shown utility in a variety of clinical situations, including flap reconstruction, bowel anastomosis creation, and sentinel lymph node tracing [38, 39]. Because it is a handheld device, it has a more compact design that is user friendly in the operating room.

Pearls and Pitfalls

- Plug in device to the VPI prior to turning the system on to prevent "camera cable not detected" error.
- Easy-to-use handheld controls to toggle fluorescence on and off (green button) and adjust focus of captured image (up and down blue buttons).

- The VPI menu accessed from button “B” allows users to access SPY-QP and make adjustments such as flipping the image and capturing stills or video. Additionally, the reference point for SPY-QP assessment can be changed via this menu.
- The device has a wide range working distance (10–40 cm). It is recommended that the user starts further away for better clarity in perfusion assessment.
- SPY-QP should be activated prior to administration of ICG with recommendation to not change fluorescence mode during the timed perfusion assessment window (indicated by a red arrow and timer on the bottom right of the monitor).

Photodynamic Eye (PDE)-neo II infrared fluorescence imager: C10935-400—Hamamatsu Photonics K.K, Higashi-ku, Hamamatsu City, Japan

PDE-neo II (Fig. 2.3a) was developed by Hamamatsu Photonics as a handheld system approved for fluorescence-guided surgery in open surgical procedures. PDE-neo II is a handheld system designed to visualize ICG in the blood or lymph systems in real time. The system utilizes a handheld imager that can be directly held or mounted to a flexible arm to manipulate over the desired anatomy.

PDE-Neo II System Components

The system includes the following: camera unit with attachable camera cable, controller box, remote controller, TEAC recording box, monitor, sterile drape, ICG dye, and PDE FlexArm.

During use, the PDE-neo II platform is positioned for optimal visualization of the monitor located on the cart. The controller box is turned on and the camera unit is plugged directly into the input access on the far right. The TEAC recording box can be turned on to allow for video and image capturing but is not essential for use of the device. The camera unit is then sterilely draped and locked into the foam lens cover attached to the drape. An optional rail or clamp attachment for the flexible arm mount can

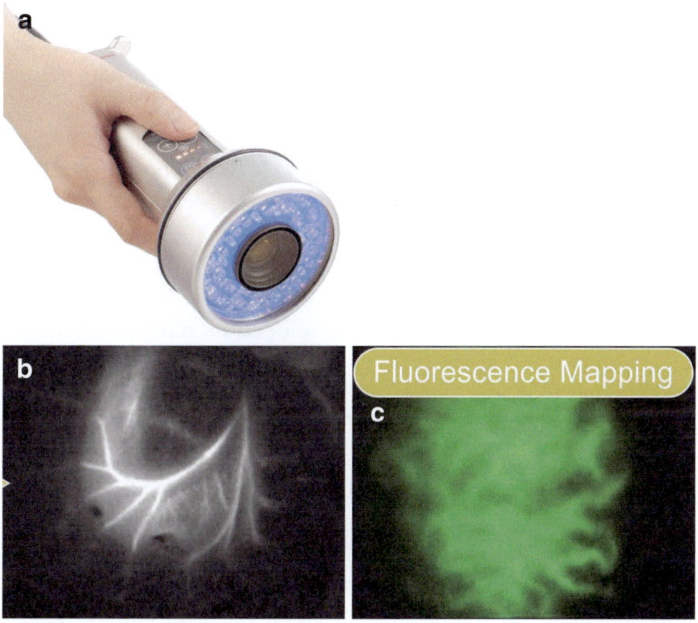

Fig. 2.3 (**a**) PDE-neo-II handheld device—Photo courtesy of Hamamatsu. (**b**) PDE-neo-II in fluorescence mode—Photo courtesy of Hamamatsu. (**c**) PDE-neo-II in fluorescence mapping mode—Photo courtesy of Hamamatsu

be secured to allow for hands-free operation of the camera unit. The working distance of the camera unit is 5–30 cm and image clarity can be obtained using the adjustable focus ring. A non-sterile assistant can then turn on the white light and fluorescence mode using the remote controller. The handheld camera unit can then toggle between color and fluorescence at the discretion of the surgeon. Fluorescence excitation is achieved using a class 1M LED that produces infrared emissions at a wavelength of 820 nm. These infrared images can be captured via the camera unit with ambient room lights on but may scatter and produce poorer images if direct sunlight is present in the room. The timing and dose administration of a 2.5 mg/mL concentration of ICG varies depending on indications for use [29–37].

Dosing, Timing, and Route of Administration

For angiography and assessment of tissue perfusion, ICG can be given immediately intraoperatively as an intravenous bolus injection of 3.3 mL to 10 mL. For lymphangiography, visualization of lymph nodes, and lymphatic mapping, ICG can be injected into target tissue as a direct subcutaneous or intradermal injection of 0.5 mL around target tissue.

PDE-neo II was originally developed by Hamamatsu Photonics with distribution within the United States via Mitaka USA Inc. Hamamatsu initially developed its handheld fluorescence imaging system in 2014 with the Hamamatsu PDE and subsequent PDE-neo. The currently available system distributed by Mitaka since 2016 is the PDE-neo II. The FDA determined that the system was substantially equivalent to the predicate PDE-neo device for use in viewing fluorescence images of blood flow. PDE-neo II has two video channel outputs that can toggle between color mode and fluorescence mode (Fig. 2.3b). The fluorescence mapping mode (Fig. 2.3c) digitally enhances NIR images with green color which can define structures containing fluorescence compared to surrounding structures. The resulting image quality can be adjusted by using the brightness, contrast, and infrared intensity dials located on the remote controller [40–42].

PDE-neo II was designed as a fluorescent angiographic system for use in assessing tissue perfusion. It is commonly used in reconstructive surgery for flap assessment and has been found to assist clinical judgment when determining whether to resect additional tissue [43–45]. PDE-neo II can also assist in identifying resection margins in pulmonary and hepatic wedge resections [46]. PDE-neo II was able to successfully identify tumor margins during lung segmentectomy to maximize tissue preservation. PDE-neo II provides enhanced visualization of the thoracic duct during mediastinal lymphadenectomy to prevent chyle leak in thoracic surgery [47]. The device can also be utilized to evaluate patients with lymphedema for lymphaticovenous anastomosis and postoperatively to evaluate for anastomosis patency [48].

Pearls and Pitfalls

- Simple, lightweight handheld device with adjustable focus ring with surgeon control over infrared intensity and image toggling.
- Remote controller separate from handheld device can adjust contrast and brightness to enhance visualization.
- With initial use, recommend that the contrast, brightness, and infrared intensity dials are placed in their default locations marked on the remote controller..
- Visualization of halos during fluorescence mode may indicate infrared intensity is too high.

Fluobeam LX—Fluoptics, Grenoble, France

The Fluobeam LX (Fig. 2.4a) was developed by Fluoptics as a handheld system approved for FGS in open surgical procedures. Fluobeam LX is Fluoptics' newest handheld system designed to visualize ICG fluorescence in blood vessels and tissue perfusion as well as autofluorescence from parathyroid tissue.

Fluobeam LX System Components

The system includes the following: optical head with light cord, control box, touchscreen display, Fluosoft software, and sterile drape.

For use, the Fluobeam LX is positioned with the touchscreen monitor in view of the surgeon. The controller box is turned on and the optical head with light cord is plugged directly into the input access on the far left. The optical head is sterilely draped with the optical window of the sterile drape attaching directly to the lens of the optical head. The fluorescence imaging system is now free to use with control of fluorescence imaging via the power button on the touchscreen display or accessed from the handheld joystick control. The system offers a high depth of field >5 cm with variable working distances with autofocus and up to 10× zoom. Fluorescence is achieved via class 1M laser which excites fluorophores with emissions in the range of 800–900 nm.

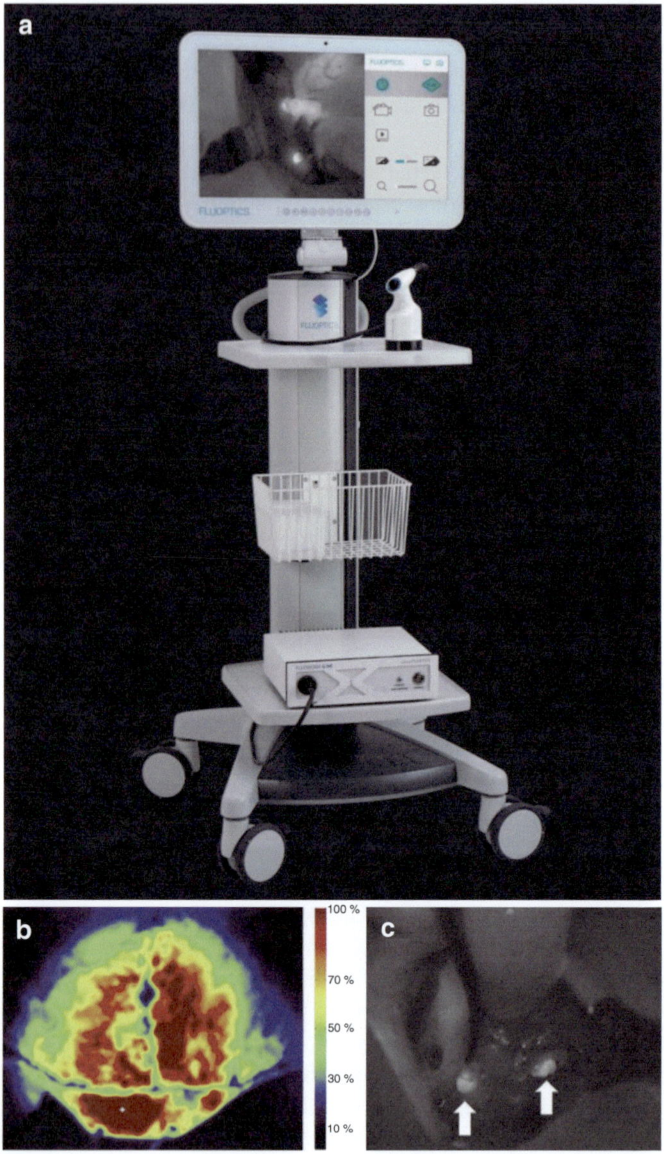

Fig. 2.4 (**a**) Fluobeam LX system—Photo Courtesy of Fluoptics. (**b**) Fluosoft quantification analysis—Photo Courtesy of Fluoptics. (**c**) Fluobeam LX image of parathyroid autofluorescence—Photo Courtesy of Dr. Marco DeMarchi

Infrared images can be captured via the camera unit with ambient room lights on. There are no device-specific recommendations for ICG dosing or timing with use of this device. Autofluorescence from parathyroid tissue does not require ICG [49, 50].

Fluoptics developed its handheld fluorescence imaging system in 2014 with the Fluobeam 800 Clinic Imaging Device. Although the Fluobeam 800 remains clinically available, the Fluobeam LX is the most recent system created by Fluoptics with emphasis on parathyroid surgery. The FDA has determined the current system is substantially equivalent to the predicate Fluobeam device as a fluorescence imaging system for use as an adjunctive method to evaluate tissue and organ perfusion used in plastic surgery (microscopic and reconstructive) and transplant surgery [51–53]. Additionally, it has been FDA approved to observe autofluorescence of parathyroid glands without the injection of ICG. Fluobeam provides real-time NIR imaging with fluorescence mode with Fluosoft optimization of images. Fluosoft available on Fluobeam 800 provides quantification analysis that overlays color representation of relative tissue perfusion (Fig. 2.4b). The relative tissue perfusion shows maximal reference perfusion in red and lower relative perfusion in black/blue. Perfusion assessment has been shown to be effective even with angulation of the optical head from 60 to 90° to the tissue (#). Image quality is automatically optimized by Fluosoft software and contrast of images can be adjusted by the surgeon via joystick controls [50].

Fluobeam LX was designed as a fluorescence system for use as an adjunctive visual assessment in parathyroid surgery. Fluobeam is commonly used in endocrine surgery during parathyroid and thyroid surgery with its ability to detect parathyroid autofluorescence without the use of ICG [50, 54]. Fluobeam LX has been successful in the fluorescence visualization of parathyroid adenomas (Fig. 2.4c) for resection and parathyroid tissue for preservation during thyroidectomy [55, 56]. With ICG, Fluobeam LX is able to intraoperatively identify lymphatics and sentinel lymph nodes for biopsies and is equivalent in accuracy to radioactive tracing [53]. Perfusion assessment using Fluobeam with associated Fluosoft quantification analysis during reconstructive surgery has shown that relative perfusion of less than 30% to likely be nonviable tissue [52].

Pearls and Pitfalls

- If autofocus produces distorted images, adjust the zoom to decrease magnification for clearer images.
- Touchscreen display has many options to adjust image for fine-tuned assessment of captured image which can all be toggled using the handheld joystick on optical head.
- Images and video can be easily accessed using playback mode.
- ICG is not needed with autofluorescence of parathyroid tissue, but may still be used to additionally visualize blood vessels to aid in tissue dissection.

Endoscopic Surgical Devices

Fluorescence in minimally invasive procedures has been used in clinical settings since 2009. FGS has become more prevalent in minimally invasive surgery. The first endoscopic system was the PINPOINT System developed by Novadaq. Its use as the first endoscopic FGS device has been well-documented. The PILLAR (perfusion assessment in left-sided/low anterior resection) trial displayed that the PINPOINT System allowed for successful visualization of perfusion using ICG; however, it did not display a significant difference in anastomotic leak rate with use of ICG angiography [57]. Indications for all minimally invasive FGS devices include the identification of vessels, extrahepatic bile ducts, and lymphatics and assessment of tissue perfusion [57, 58].

PINPOINT Endoscopic Fluorescence Imaging System: PC9000—Stryker, Kalamazoo, Michigan, USA

PINPOINT System (Fig. 2.5a) was initially developed by Novadaq Technologies as an endoscopic fluorescence system for use in minimally invasive surgical procedures. PINPOINT was the first clinically available endoscopic fluorescence-guided surgical system. The system consists of a handheld camera head that attaches to a laparoscope for capturing visible light and near-infrared light images obtained in minimally invasive surgical procedures.

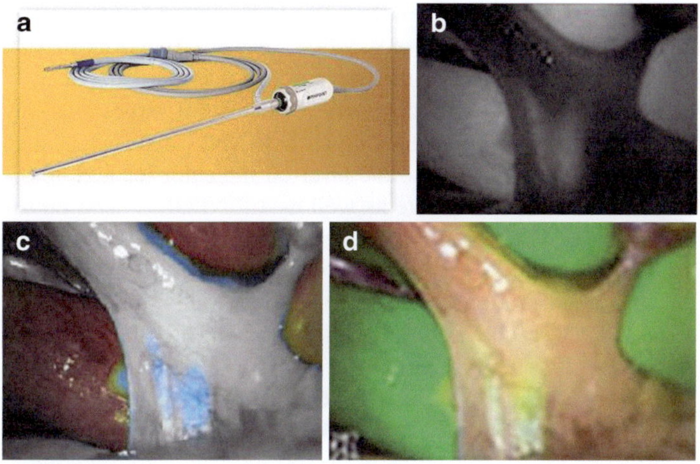

Fig. 2.5 (**a**) PINPOINT: laparoscope—Photo courtesy of Stryker. (**b**) PINPOINT SPY mode—Photo courtesy of Stryker. (**c**) PINPOINT color-segmented mode—Photo courtesy of Stryker. (**d**) PINPOINT overlay mode—Photo courtesy of Stryker

PINPOINT System Components

The system includes the following: video process/illuminator (VPI), PC9001; camera head with light guide cable, PC9002/PC9004; camera (resolution 1080p); fluorescence imaging laparoscopes, SC9000 series (5 mm, 10 mm), 0 and 30° scopes; PINPOINT Cart with 1080p HD monitor and optional recorder and printer; and SPY AGENT GREEN (ICG)—25 mg vials.

To use, PINPOINT is set up similar to any other laparoscopic surgical system with placement of monitors depending on surgical indications. The camera head with light guide cable and laparoscopes are autoclavable and will be handed to the surgeon sterilely. The laparoscope eyepiece is attached to the camera head and the light cable attached to the laparoscope via threaded connector. The light cable and camera cable are then handed off to a non-sterile assistant to plug into the VPI with light cable inserted into the far left, orange-colored input, and the camera cable inserted into the far right, green-colored input. After the cable inputs have been plugged in, the VPI can be turned on for use as a laparoscopic camera with only white light on. The working distance is not specified for this device, but it is recommended to image in PINPOINT mode further away from target anatomy prior to advancing the laparoscope. PINPOINT mode is activated by pressing button "1," and the laser-on indicator located on the camera head will illuminate as well as a PINPOINT icon on the main display. PINPOINT contains a dedicated light source with a light-emitting diode (LED) array for visible light and an NIR laser diode for near-infrared. Fluorescence excitation is achieved using a class 3R laser which produces excitation wavelength at 805 nm and near-infrared emissions from 700 to 770 nm. The preferred fluorophore with PINPOINT System is SPY AGENT GREEN (ICG), and its use in angiography should be given intraoperatively as a weight-dependent bolus delivered intravenously. Maximum dose is 2 mg/kg body weight. Fluorescence will appear within blood vessels in the field of view within 5–15 seconds after the injection [21, 59, 60].

Dosing, Timing, and Route of Administration

For patients less than or equal to 90 kg, use 0.5 ml of a 2.5 mg/ml concentration. For patients greater than 90 kg, use 1–1.5 ml of a 2.5 mg/ml concentration.

Novadaq (now a part of Stryker) developed its endoscopic fluorescence-guided systems in 2009 with the SPY Scope: SC8000. The currently available system is the PINPOINT System: PCS:9000. The FDA has determined the current system is substantially equivalent to the predicate PINPOINT System and SPY Scope as an endoscopic fluorescence imaging system for use in endoscopic assessment of vessels, blood flow, and tissue perfusion as well as fluorescence imaging of biliary ducts. PINPOINT provides real-time visible and NIR imaging with an operating principle of SPY mode (Fig. 2.5b), color-segmented fluorescence (CSF) mode (Fig. 2.5c), and overlay mode (Fig. 2.5d), which can be toggled using button "2" on the camera head. SPY mode is a pure fluorescence image, displayed in monochromatic format to detect only NIR images. Color-segmented fluorescence (CSF) mode displays visible light in grayscale with fluorescence overlay in different color intensities to display fluorescence ranges (blue being the lowest to yellow and then red as the highest). Overlay mode allows for real-time visualization in the visible and NIR spectrum at the same time with fluorescence overlaid in green. Parallel display will show all operating principles on one display [59, 60].

PINPOINT System is widely known as the progenitor fluorescence-guided surgical system that allows for fluorescence visualization as a laparoscope. It was intended for use in minimally invasive surgical cases and was designed as an adjunctive visual assessment in tissue perfusion and biliary ducts with fluorescence labeling. It is not intended as a standalone visualization of the biliary ducts in lieu of cholangiography. Most recently, it has been approved for use in lymphatic visualization with ability to fluorescence image lymph nodes and lymphatic vessels such as during lymphatic mapping of the uterus and cervix [61].

Pearls and Pitfalls

- Parallel display can show singular overlay images or multiple images that display both white light and NIR light images together without overlay.
- Damage to the laparoscope tip or light cable tip can affect apertures for NIR emission causing a scattering effect.
- If the entire image shows strong fluorescence signal throughout, the laparoscope may be an HD laparoscope instead of a fluorescence laparoscope.
- Image quality settings (sharpness, brightness, color saturation) can be adjusted via the display monitors, but adjustment of the focus is via the up and down arrows located on the camera head.

Synergy ID Near-Infrared Fluorescence 4K Imaging Platform—Arthrex, Munich, Germany

SynergyID (Fig. 2.6a) was developed by Arthrex to complement its endoscopic system with the capabilities of fluorescence-guided surgery in minimally invasive procedures. The basis for Arthrex

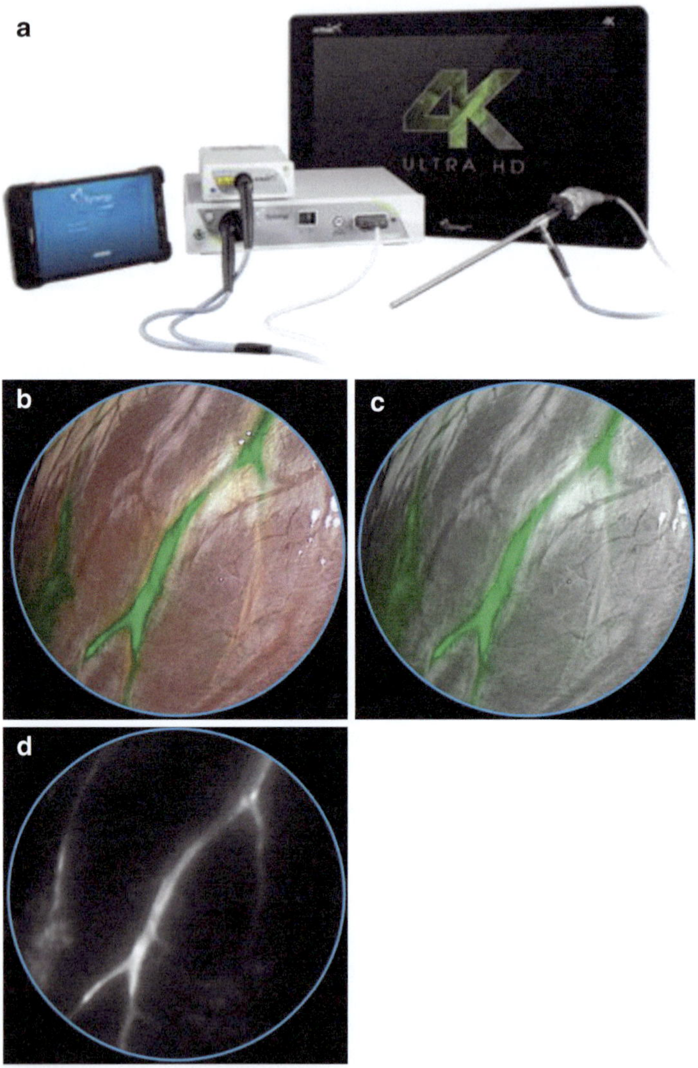

Fig. 2.6 (**a**) SynergyID System—Photo courtesy of Arthrex. (**b**) SynergyID System—Photo courtesy of Arthrex. (**c**) SynergyID System—Photo courtesy of Arthrex. (**d**) SynergyID System—Photo courtesy of Arthrex. (**e**) SynergyID System—Photo courtesy of Arthrex

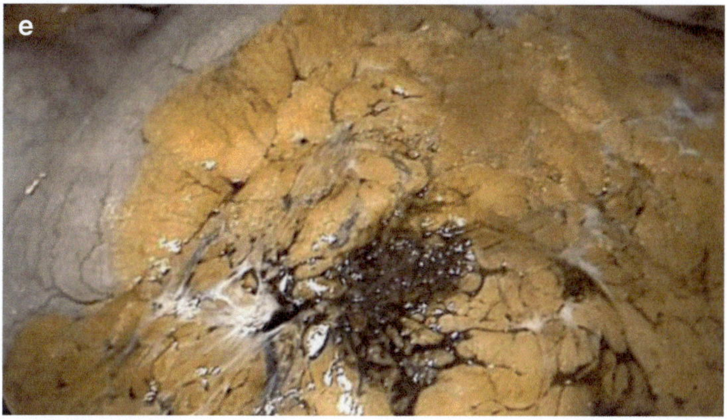

Fig. 2.6 (continued)

fluorescence-guided surgical device is the high-quality imaging using UHD4 camera system. The current SynergyID System consists of a camera head with 4 chip image processing to provide high-definition standard light and near-infrared light images.

SynergyID Endoscopic Imaging System Platform Components

The system includes the following: imaging console/camera control unit, AR-3200-0025; camera head option for fluorescence, 4K SynergyID; synergy laser light source and light cable, AR-3200-1018; laparoscope, AR-3351 (5 mm high magnification, 10 mm) with 0, 30, and 45° scopes; and tablet controller (Digital Doc Tablet).

The tower for the Synergy ID contains the imaging console/camera control unit and the synergy laser light source. The unit is initially turned on via the green switch in the back of the power unit. The tablet controller can then connect to the console and users can select cases and patient lists for optimizing image settings. The tablet controller offers a unique way for surgeons to set up preferences and review cases for planned surgical interventions. Once the patient is prepped and ready for a procedure, the autoclavable camera head, light cables, and laparoscopes can be connected to one another and input cables connected to the tower. The camera cable is plugged into the input on the far right, while the light cable, which has a split output (one for the imaging console for standard light and one for the laser light source), can be connected accordingly. Fluorescence mode for the SynergyID can be activated from either the tablet or the programmable buttons located on the camera head. The SynergyID laser light source contains a class 3R laser with 8 mm of penetration and generates infrared emission wavelength at 785 nm. There are no device-specific recommendations for timing or dosing of ICG.

Arthrex developed the SynergyID device in 2020. The FDA determined that the system was substantially equivalent to the predicate Arthrex UHD4 System and Novadaq's PINPOINT for use as a camera system in all endoscopic procedures and a fluorescence-guided surgical system for the visual assessment of vessels, blood flow, extrahepatic bile ducts, and tissue perfusion. The SynergyID System offers 4K standard light images and NIR images. The default operating principle while in fluorescence mode is overlay mode (Fig. 2.6b). The different fluorescence images can be cycled by pressing the programmed buttons on the camera head with grayscale visible and NIR overlay (Fig. 2.6c) or NIR-only (Fig. 2.6d) imaging [62–64]. The color of fluorescence can be changed from green to other colors, such as red, cyan, and magenta. The SynergyID System can further enhance the high-definition images via its augmented reality features [65]. This allows users to filter red colors that can enhance visualization (Fig. 2.6e) as an additional customizable view for the surgeon [65, 66].

The Arthrex SynergyID system is intended to be used as an endoscopic video camera for a variety of surgical procedures. These can range from orthopedic, laparoscopic, urologic, sinuscopic, and plastic surgical procedures including microscopic surgery. The laser light source allows SynergyID to visualize NIR images for use in general FGS procedures such as in the visualization of blood vessels, extrahepatic bile ducts, and lymphatics with 4K high-resolution imaging [62, 66].

Pearls and Pitfalls

- UHD4 camera system with 4K high-resolution images offers greater depth perception and color clarity.
- The rotatable turret for the light guide has a number of light inputs compatible with different cables. Ensure the correct port is aligned with the LED prior to inserting light cable.
- Camera has programmable buttons to allow surgeon to easily toggle desired display settings.
- Digital Doc Table can be used to store and configure case preferences remotely.

Visera Elite II Infrared Imaging System—Olympus, Fukushima, Japan

The Visera Elite II Infrared Imaging System (Fig. 2.7) was developed by Olympus as an endoscopic system for fluorescence-guided minimally invasive surgery. The Visera Elite II Infrared Imaging System attaches to a xenon arc lamp excitation source. This light source allows for infrared (IR) illumination that is visualized via specialized IR endoscopes.

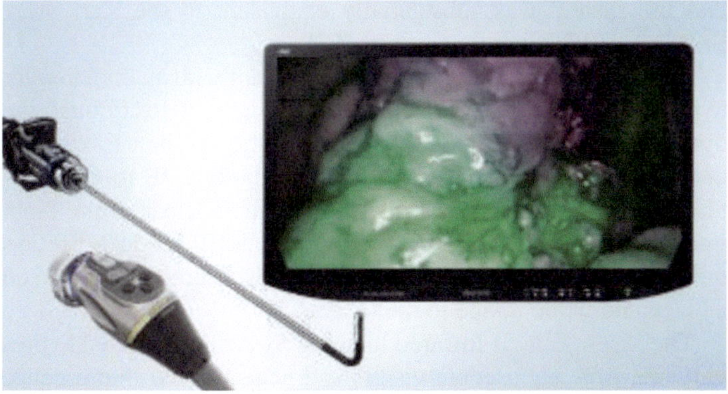

Fig. 2.7 Visera Elite II Infrared System—Photo courtesy of Olympus

Visera Elite II Components

The system includes the following: Visera Elite II Video System Center; infrared imaging system; xenon light source; autoclavable camera head, CH-S200-XZ-EB; and the telescope IR/ultra (specialized IR endoscope).

The device consists of the source circuit, control circuit, illumination lamp, and optical filter. The control circuit is connected to the diaphragm to control light intensity with the source circuit supplying power to the illumination lamp. After the control unit is activated, the IR endoscope is connected. The IR endoscopes are rigid and consist of an image relay system of rod lenses that transmit either a 2D or 3D image for standard laparoscopy. The IR endoscopes are reusable and fully autoclavable. There are no device-specific recommendations for dosing or timing of ICG injection [67, 68].

Olympus developed the Visera Elite II Xenon Light Source Olympus (CLV-S200-IR) in 2020. Olympus initially developed an FGS device after the acquisition of Quest Photonic Devices. Quest innovations, based in the Netherlands, was established in 1998 and specialized in fluorescence and multispectral technologies to offer enhanced visualization of tumor margins during oncological surgery. This was the foundation for the eventual production of the Visera Elite II product line. The FDA determined that the system was substantially equivalent to the Karl Storz Endoscopic ICG imaging system [67].

The Visera Elite II utilizes a control circuit with an optical filter to provide a clear image. The fluorescent light passes through the optical filter in the endoscope, allowing the surgeon to work in one of two IR modes: IR mode 1 and IR mode 2. IR mode 1 displays fluorescent illumination overlaid on a clear white light image the visualization of detailed structures. IR mode 2 displays the pure fluorescence image with the highest degree of contrast on a black and white image [67, 68].

The Visera Elite II Infrared Imaging System is intended to provide real-time endoscopic visible and near-infrared fluorescence imaging. These endoscopes are intended to be used for endoscopy and endoscopic surgery within the thoracic and peritoneal cavities including the female reproductive organs. The device is also indicated for visualization of transanal and transvaginal natural orifice surgery. The system is approved for use in the assessment of vessels, tissue perfusion, and biliary anatomy [67].

Pearls and Pitfalls

- The system includes a compact video system center in one modular device that is compatible with 3D laparoscopes.
- A 3D image rotation function maintains the horizon as 30° scopes are rotated.
- The lightweight camera head can control and toggle between desired infrared imaging modes.

Open/Endoscopic Devices

A number of recently updated systems have been able to integrate open and endoscopic systems with fluorescence capabilities into one platform. These systems are able to integrate interchangeable cameras or scopes to enable use for both open and minimally invasive surgical procedures.

1688 Advanced Imaging Modalities (AIM) 4K Platform—Stryker, Kalamazoo, Michigan, USA

1688 AIM 4K Platform (Fig. 2.8a) was initially developed by Stryker as a platform capable of endoscopic fluorescence imaging for use in minimally invasive surgical procedures as well as handheld fluorescence imaging in open surgical procedures using SPY PHI. 1688 AIM is the endoscopic portion of the platform. The endoscopic system consists of a handheld camera head that attaches to a laparoscope for capturing visible light and NIR light images obtained in minimally invasive surgical procedures.

1688 4K Platform Components

The system includes the following: 1688 4K camera control unit with advanced imaging modalities 1688 4K resolution camera head options, camera head with AIM; microscope head, pendulum head, or inline head; L11 LED light source and safelight cable; AIM HD laparoscope; display (4K resolution); connected OR hub (optional for recording and customizing visualization settings); SPY PHI System for handheld/open procedures; and SPY AGENT GREEN (ICG)—25 mg vials.

a

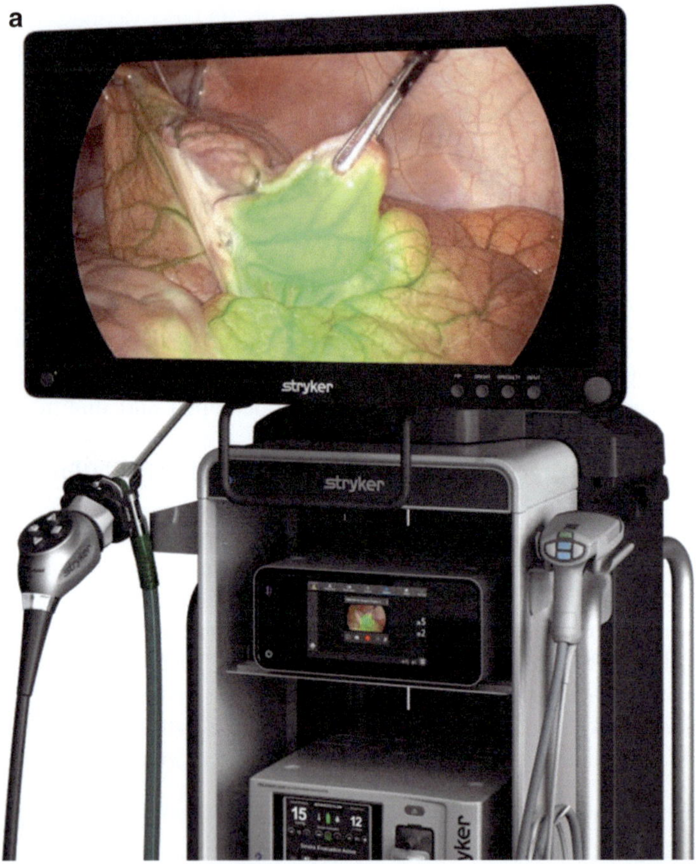

Fig. 2.8 (**a**) AIM 1688 with SPY PHI System—Photo courtesy of Stryker. (**b**) AIM 1688 overlay mode—Photo courtesy of Stryker. (**c**) AIM 1688 contrast mode—Photo courtesy of Stryker. (**d**) AIM 1688 ENV mode—Photo courtesy of Stryker

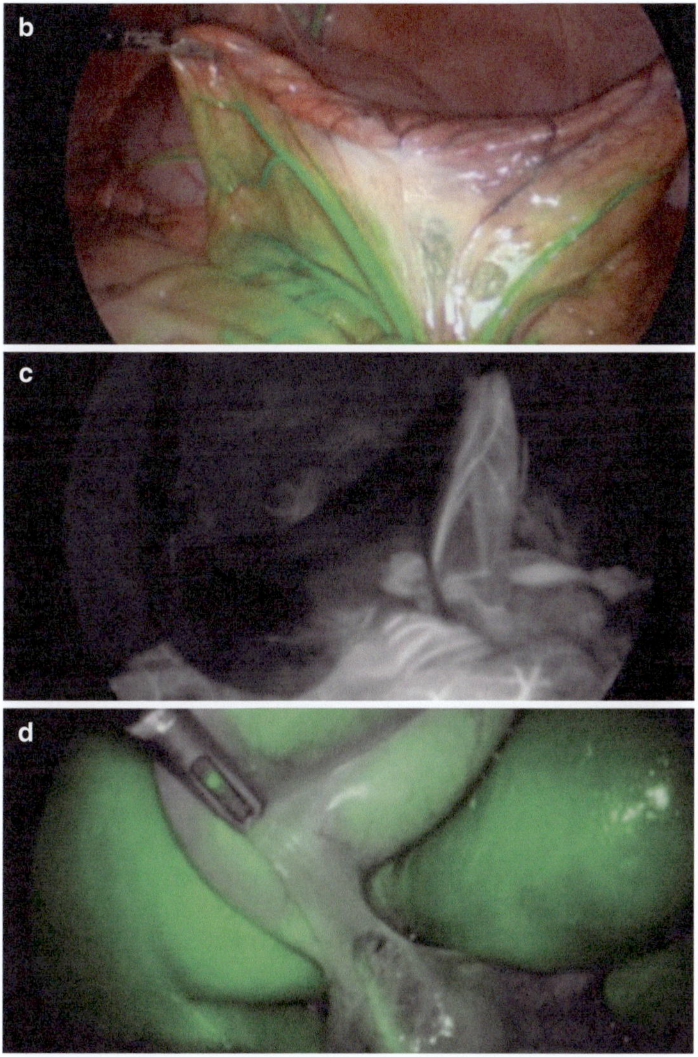

Fig. 2.8 (continued)

For use, 1688 AIM's connected operating room cart is set up similar to any other laparoscopic surgical system with placement of monitors depending on surgical indications. The camera head with light guide cable and laparoscopes are autoclavable and will be handed to the surgeon sterilely. Depending on the type of camera head, a coupler may need to be installed to connect the camera head to the laparoscope eyepiece. The laparoscope eyepiece is attached to the coupler on the camera head and the light cable attached to the laparoscope via the threaded connector. The light cable and camera cable are then handed off to a non-sterile assistant. The camera cable connector is protected by a soaking cap which is removed, and the connector is plugged into the input on the camera control unit. The safelight cable is plugged into the L11 LED light source. From the camera control unit, the type of surgery can be selected from an option of nine different surgical specialties which individually optimize the camera settings based on the desired surgical procedure. The specialty selected on the camera control unit should be "laparoscopy" or "standard"; otherwise, fluorescence mode will not activate. After the cable inputs have been plugged in, the camera can be white balanced and "auto" light setting can be turned on if desired. Auto light will automatically adjust the brightness as needed throughout the case. SPY mode is the fluorescence mode of the 1688 AIM and is controlled by pressing "AIM" on the camera control unit. Additionally, SPY mode can be activated by the surgeon by pressing the menu button on the right of the camera head. The L11 LED light source for the 1688 AIM System utilizes both RGB (red, green, blue) LEDs and a class 1M laser for excitation with wavelength of 806 nm for NIR fluorescence. The preferred fluorophore with AIM 1688 is SPY AGENT GREEN (ICG) with similar timing and dosing as with SPY Elite [69, 70].

Dosing, Timing, and Route of Administration

For angiography for visualization of blood vessels and tissue perfusion, ICG can be given immediately intraoperatively. For patients less than or equal to 90 kg, use 0.5 ml of a 2.5 mg/ml concentration. For patients greater than 90 kg, use 1–1.5 ml of a 2.5 mg/ml concentration. Maximum dose is 2 mg/kg.

For visualization of extrahepatic biliary duct for use in patients ages 12 and older, ICG should be given at least 45 min prior to surgery as an intravenous bolus injection of 1 ml of a 2.5 mg/ml concentration. For lymphangiography, visualization of lymph nodes, and lymphatic mapping, ICG can be injected directly into target tissue as multiple direct injections of 0.5 ml of a 2.5 mg/ml concentration as needed.

1688 AIM 4K Platform was developed by Stryker and is the endoscopic portion of the system that includes the SPY PHI handheld device. Stryker developed an endoscopic fluorescence device in 2014 with the Stryker Infrared Fluorescence (IRF) Imaging System. The currently available system is the 1688 AIM 4K camera system with L11 LED light source. The FDA determined that the system was substantially equivalent to the predicate devices 1588 AIM and Stryker IRF for use as a camera system in all endoscopic procedures and as an FGS system approved for the visual assessment of vessels, blood flow and tissue perfusion, biliary ducts, and lymphatic vessels and nodes. The L11 LED light source is also intended to attach to Stryker's IRIS Ureteral Kit to transilluminate the ureters producing NIR emissions at 830 nm for open and laparoscopic cases. 1688 AIM provides real-time visible and NIR imaging with fluorescence activated in SPY mode. The operating principle for SPY mode is overlay mode (Fig. 2.8b), contrast mode (Fig. 2.8c), and ENV mode (Fig. 2.8d). The different SPY modes can be changed by pressing the up button on the camera head. Overlay mode allows for real-time visualization in the visible and NIR spectrum simultaneously with fluorescence overlaid in green. Contrast mode is a pure fluorescence image, displayed in monochromatic format to detect only NIR images as white color. ENV mode displays visible light in grayscale with fluorescence overlay in green [68–70].

The 1688 AIM camera system can be used with and without fluorescence. There are nine surgical specialties that can be supported by this system and are selectable from the camera control unit for specific image optimization. The nine specialties for use with the camera system are general laparoscopy, ENT/skull endoscopy, arthroscopy, cystoscopy, flexi-scope, hysteroscopy, laser, microscope, and standard use. The fluorescence functionality is only available for laparoscopy and standard and intended for use in minimally invasive surgical cases as an adjunctive visual assessment in tissue perfusion, biliary ducts, and lymphatic mapping. Open surgical cases can use the SPY PHI attached to the platform. The L11 LED light source can connect to IRIS ureteral stents for transillumination of the ureters in open and laparoscopic cases. This has proven beneficial in difficult pelvic dissections to visualize the ureters and prevent injury [71].

Pearls and Pitfalls

- The platform has an independent handheld fluorescence-guided system, SPY PHI, which can be used in conjunction with 1688 AIM.
- The system displays images in 4K resolution.
- The display can show singular overlay images or multiple images in parallel that display both white light and NIR light images together without overlay.
- Specialty select on the camera control unit should be set to "laparoscopy" or "standard" in order for fluorescence SPY mode to activate.
- L11 LED light source needs to be connected to the camera control unit for auto light to work.
- If image quality remains poor, the coupler may not be attached correctly to the camera head and laparoscope eyepiece.

Image 1S Rubina—Karl Storz, Tuttlingen, Germany

The Image 1S Rubina (Fig. 2.9) was developed by Karl Storz as a fluorescence capable, modular system for use in minimally invasive and open surgical procedures. Rubina builds on the Image 1S Camera System and can incorporate 4K, 3D, NIR/ICG, and LED components as needed. The fluorescence-guided surgical system consists of a Rubina camera head that attaches to a laparoscope or exoscope for capturing visible and NIR images in minimally invasive and open surgical procedures, respectively.

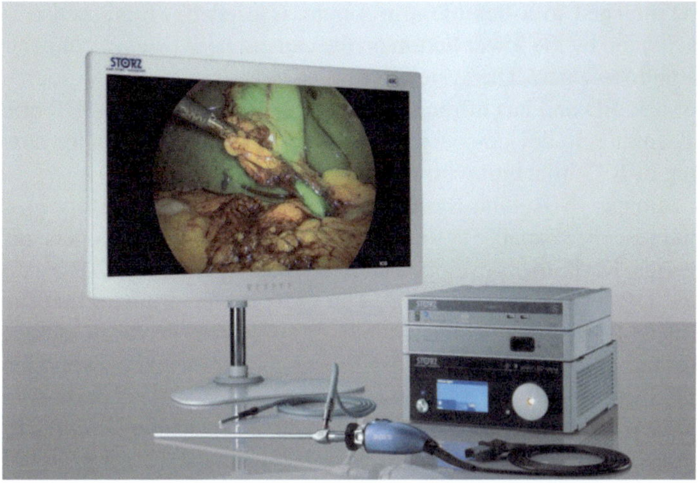

Fig. 2.9 Image 1s Rubina System—Photo courtesy of Karl Storz

Rubina: ICG Imaging System Components

The system includes the following: Rubina LED light source; camera control unit, TC201US; TC 304US; light cable; camera head options, OPAL 1 (NIR/ICG); IMAGE 1S Rubina (4K, NIR/ICG); TIPCAM 1 Rubina (4K/3D, NIR/ICG); laparoscope, Hopkins ICG/NIR (5 mm, 10 mm); exoscope, VITOM II ICG; footswitch; monitors with 4K or 4K/3D resolution; and 3D clip on glasses.

For use, the Image 1S Rubina's operating room cart is set up similarly to any other laparoscopic surgical system, with monitors placed for optimal visualization. 4K and 4K/3D displays can be used. The camera head with light cable and scopes are autoclavable and will be handed to the surgeon sterilely. There are multiple camera head options that provide NIR/ICG images. The camera head, scope, and light cables are attached to one another, and the camera and light cables are then handed off to a non-sterile assistant. The camera cable inserts into the camera control unit and the light cable inserts into the Rubina LED light source. For open surgical procedures, the exoscope and camera head can be attached to a flexible arm mount as needed. Fluorescence is activated by the lower button on the camera head or via a connectable footswitch. The system utilizes a laser-free excitation source of an LED and has infrared emission wavelength at 720–810 nm. There are no device-specific recommendations for timing or dosing of ICG injection with this system.

Image 1S Rubina System was developed by Karl Storz as a fluorescence capable system for minimally invasive and open surgeries. Karl Storz developed an ICG imaging system in 2016 with the OPAL ICG/NIR systems. The FDA has determined that the Image 1S Rubina is substantially equivalent to predicate device for use as a camera system in all endoscopic procedures and as an FGS system approved for assessment of vessels, tissue perfusion, biliary ducts, and lymphatic vessels and nodes. Rubina is compatible with a variety of camera head options to allow for standard imaging, NIR imaging, and imaging in 4K or 4K/3D. The camera system can be fitted for both endoscopes in laparoscopic cases and an exoscope with flexible arm mount for open cases. For NIR images, the system can accommodate an overlay of white light and NIR images on a single display with either green or blue NIR-enhanced images. Intensity map displays the intensity of signals in an overlay image while removing white light images to maximize visualization of fluorescently labeled structures. Monochromatic NIR imaging can overlay NIR images and black and white visible light images for visual contrast [72–74].

The compatibility of the system with multiple camera heads and scopes allows for high-definition and 3D-compatible imaging which can be used for laparoscopic and arthroscopic procedures. The Image 1S Rubina can be used with and without fluorescence imaging. Indications for use with fluorescence include assessment of blood vessels, tissue perfusion, visualization of the biliary system, and lymphatic tracing [75, 76].

Pearls for Use

- Image 1S camera compatible with both laparoscope and exoscope for minimally invasive and open surgery.
- System includes a foot pedal for toggling fluoroscopic imaging.

- System is compatible with 4K and 4K/3D imaging.
- System can display NIR images in two colors (blue and green).
- User can modulate intensity of NIR images to optimize visualization.

EleVision IR Platform—Medtronic, Dublin, Ireland

EleVision (Fig. 2.10) was developed by Medtronic as a fluorescence capable surgical system for use in minimally invasive and open surgical procedures. The system is able to be used in both minimally invasive and open surgery by having a camera capable of attaching to either a laparoscope or a microscope.

EleVision IR Platform Components

The system includes the following: fluorescence camera, Visionsense 3 Iridium (VS3-IR); Iridium Module Scope, Visionsense 3 Miniature Microscope (VS3-MMS); camera control unit; laser light source (LLS); xenon light source; touchscreen monitor; VS3 Iridium Endoscopes (5 mm, 10 mm); VS3 Light Cable and Iridium Light Beam Combiner; sterile drapes for VS3-MMS; VS3-IR Fluorescence ICG Kit; and Iridium software.

The EleVision IR Platform tower's main components for fluorescence imaging are the camera control unit and laser light source. For minimally invasive surgery, the camera head, scopes, and light cable are autoclavable and are handed to the surgeon sterilely. The camera is assembled and the camera cable and light cable are handed to a non-sterile assistant. The camera cable has a protective cap which is removed prior to insertion into the camera control unit with its input located on the left side of the unit. The light cables are attached to the laser light source and the xenon light source (which is the standard light for use in general laparoscopy). For open surgery, the VS3-IR camera is attached to a non-autoclavable iridium module scope: VS3-MMS which can be handheld or attached to a cart-mounted arm for positioning over a surgical field with a working distance of 17–50 cm. It must be sterilely draped prior to use during operative procedures with fixation of the drape window to the scope. Fluorescence can be activated and controlled from the handheld camera head. The

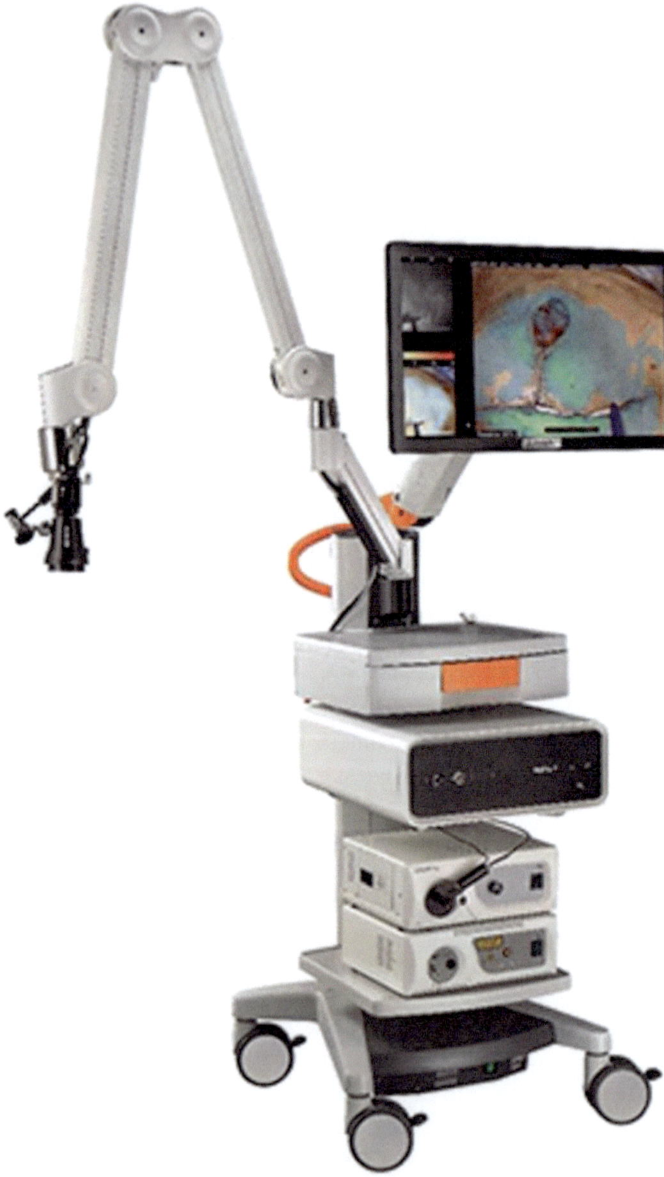

Fig. 2.10 EleVision IR System—Photo courtesy of Medtronic

device utilizes a laser excitation light source and has infrared emission wavelengths at 785–805 nm with penetration 3–5 mm of tissue. There are no specific timing or dose recommendations for injection of the ICG [77, 78].

EleVision IR Platform was developed by Medtronic as a fluorescence capable system for minimally invasive and open/microscopic surgeries. Visionsense, now a part of Medtronic, had developed its endoscopic and handheld fluorescence device in 2014 with the VS3-IR and VS3-MMS, respectively. This system has since been integrated into Medtronic's EleVision IR Platform as of 2018, and the FDA determined that the system was substantially equivalent to predicate devices for use as a camera system in FGS, approved for the visual assessment of vessels, tissue perfusion, biliary ducts, and lymphatic vessels and nodes. Both cameras utilize a dual-channel camera system for imaging of both standard visible light and NIR light images at high resolution up to 4K. Fluorescence images are displayed in monochromatic NIR imaging, in false color NIR imaging, and in overlay mode. False color NIR assigns different colors based on NIR intensity (blue being the lowest to yellow and then red as the highest). Infrared intensity can also be assessed by the Iridium software which offers quantitative and qualitative measurements of infrared signal intensity based on absolute and relative pixelations of images. This software can offer real-time relative quantitative values regarding tissue perfusion with heat mapping [77–79].

The compatibility of the VS3-IR camera with a laparoscope or miniature microscope allows the system to be used in laparoscopic and open cases. EleVision IR Platform can be used with and without fluorescence imaging. Indications for use of fluorescence using the EleVision IR are for the assessment of vessels, tissue perfusion, visualization of the biliary system, and lymphatic tracing.

Pearls for Use

- Available as either open, minimally invasive, or combined system.
- Capable of 4K high-resolution images.

- Iridium software can analyze images in real time to provide both quantitative and qualitative information on perfusion.
- Display can show singular overlay images or multiple images that display both white light and NIR light images together without overlay.
- Two separate channels for the camera each require focus adjustment as needed.

Quest Spectrum—Olympus Surgical Technologies, Hamburg, Germany

Quest Spectrum (Fig. 2.11) was developed by Quest Photonic as a fluorescence capable surgical system for use in minimally invasive and open surgical procedures. The system consists of a camera head, which can attach to one of two different scope

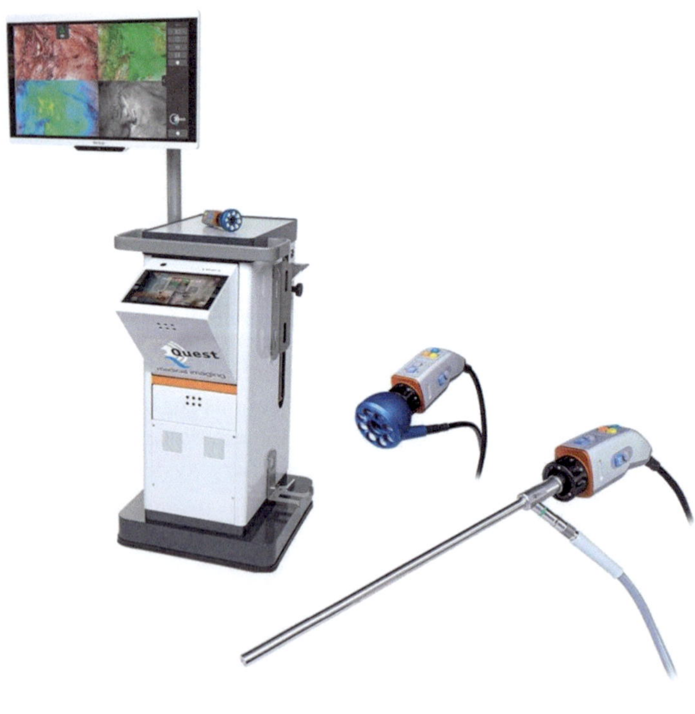

Fig. 2.11 Quest Spectrum System—Photo courtesy of Quest and Olympus

components. These components are easily interchangeable and can be exchanged during a procedure.

Quest Spectrum Components

The system includes the following: Quest Spectrum camera with video cable, ring light with light cable, laparoscope with light cable, display monitor and control tower, light engine, and sterile drapes.

Quest Spectrum utilizes a common camera head for minimally invasive and open surgical procedures. For minimally invasive surgery, the camera head and laparoscope base are sterilely draped to allow for attachment of the laparoscope and light cable. The camera cable will have already been connected to the system and the light cable can be inserted into the light engine on the far right. For open surgery, the ring light and light cable are attached to the camera and are sterilely draped with fixation of the connecting lens to the ring light. The device can then be used as a handheld device or attached to a flexible arm mount over a surgical field with a working distance of 5–30 cm. Fluorescence can be activated from the camera control or cart console. The camera contains two NIR channels and thus ultimately captures three different images: white light image and two different NIR images. The light engine produces the LED light for visible light images, while the modular laser light source produces laser for excitation with capturable infrared emission wavelengths at 700–830 mm and 830–1100 nm. There are no device-specific recommendations for timing or dosing of ICG injection [80, 81].

Quest Spectrum was originally developed by Quest Photonic Devices (now part of Olympus Corporation) as an open and endoscopic system in 2015. At that time, it was initially known as the Artemis Handheld System and was compatible with a ring light for open surgery and laparoscopes for minimally invasive surgery. The FDA determined that the Quest Spectrum system is substantially equivalent to the predicate Artemis system for use as a camera system in FGS, approved for assessment of vessels, tissue perfusion, biliary ducts, and lymphatic vessels and nodes. The system monitor can display visible light, monochromic fluorescence, and overlay of colored fluorescence on visible light images. Since the system has two NIR channels, the overlay mode can display two different NIR emission wavelengths in two different colors to identify multiple fluorescent tagged structures [79].

The Quest Spectrum can be used in both laparoscopic and open cases and can be used with and without fluorescence imaging. Indications for use of fluorescence are for the assessment of vessels, tissue perfusion, visualization of the biliary system, and lymphatic tracing [81, 82].

Pearls and Pitfalls

- System includes a single camera with interchangeable attachments for use in either open or minimally invasive surgery.
- Both open and laparoscopic uses of the system will require sterile drapes to cover the camera head.
- The system includes two channels for two NIR images with ability to toggle between wavelengths in green and blue image enhancement.
- The display can show singular overlay images or multiple images that display both white light and near-infrared light images together without overlay.

Robotic Surgical Systems

Firefly—Intuitive Surgical, California, USA

Firefly (Fig. 2.12a) was developed by Intuitive Surgical to add fluorescence-guided capabilities to its minimally invasive robotic surgical platform. Firefly is a standard integrated feature with Da Vinci Robotic Systems and does not require additional modules or attachments to utilize.

Firefly Components

The system includes the following: 8 mm 0° and 30° endoscopes (PNs 470,026 and 470,027), endoscope controller (PN 372601),

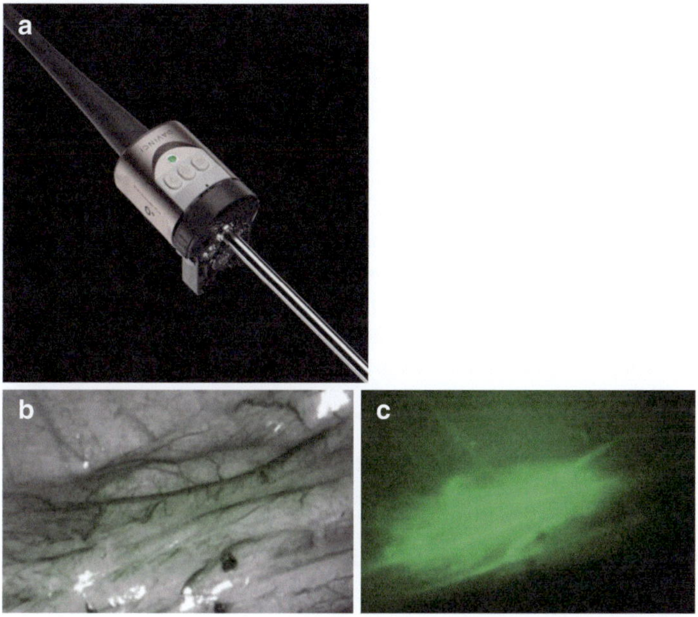

Fig. 2.12 (**a**) Da Vinci Xi Endoscope Plus with fluorescence capability—Image courtesy of Intuitive. (**b**) Firefly mode—Image courtesy of Intuitive. (**c**) Firefly sensitive mode—Image courtesy of Intuitive

fluorescence imaging kit (K101077) (PN 950156), and Da Vinci Xi Robotic Components.

Instructions for Use

The Da Vinci Xi Robotic System is set up in its usual sterile fashion. Once the robot is docked, the surgeon has full access to the Firefly system. The console allows easy switching between normal illumination and fluorescence imaging modes. The camera head optics are optimized to visualize a fluorescence signal. The surgeon will then have full control over near fluorescence imaging. The camera unit is a 3D stereoscopic scope and cable that contains an LED light source, excitation light, and camera. The

Firefly system utilizes an excitation source of a class 3R laser and has infrared emission wavelength at 805 nm. The working distance is 2–14 cm. The visualization of near-infrared frequency can easily be toggled from the operative console and offers LED illuminated black and white visualization with green color-enhanced fluorescence (Fig. 2.12b). Additionally, sensitive mode (Fig. 2.12c) will toggle off the visible light LED to better enhance visualization of deeper near-infrared structures up to 8–10 mm in depth. In sensitive mode, the system automatically adjusts signal intensity and brightness to allow for a consistent image regardless of the distance between the endoscope and tissue. The imaging LED illuminator emits a laser to excite ICG.

Dosing, Timing, and Route of Administration

The recommended dosing for ICG is 0.5–1.5 ml at 2.5 mg/ml concentration with the maximum daily dose not to exceed 2 mg/kg body weight. ICG has a half-life of 2–5 min. It should be used within 6 h of reconstitution.

ICG stays within blood vessels for seconds and one should see fluorescence dye within 5–50 seconds. ICG stays within the kidney for 20 min with visibility within 1 min, the liver for 1–2 h with visibility within less than 2 min, and bile for 1–2 h with visibility within tens of min [83–86]. This timing of onset of visibility and the time it lasts can be used by the operating surgeon as to when to administer the ICG based on the operative case and target tissue to be visualized.

Intuitive developed a robotic fluorescence device in 2011 with the Da Vinci Si platform. Intuitive collaborated with Novadaq to incorporate fluorescence imaging into its robotic surgery platform. The current system available is Firefly and is a component of the Intuitive Da Vinci Xi platform. This system includes a 1080i 3D stereoscopic fluorescence camera with LED illuminator and laser generator.

The indications for Firefly include the assessment of vessels and tissue perfusion and the evaluation of the extrahepatic biliary system [87, 88].

Pearls and Pitfalls

- Firefly is easy to control from the surgical console.
- Firefly can be activated using the finger clutch at the robotic console, so visualization can be maintained as fluorescence is turned on and off.
- A surgeon can activate sensitive mode for greater visualization of NIR images and for visualization of deeper structures.
- Overlay mode not currently available.

ActivSight™—Activ Surgical, Boston, MA, USA

ActivSight™ is an FDA-approved modular imaging device that integrates with the standard laparoscopic vision system to provide multimodal visual intelligence beyond the human visual spectrum. ActivSight™ has three components: the imaging module (IM), the light engine (LE), and the bifurcated light guide (LG). The IM is placed between the laparoscope and standard white light camera. The IM contains a sensor that captures light within the infrared spectrum while passing light in the visual spectrum to the white light camera. The LE illuminates the surgical field with white light and wavelengths of light in near-infrared (NIR) spectrum. The images obtained from the white light and infrared cameras are combined to create overlay images that display real-time tissue perfusion.

ActivSight™ provides two modes for assessing tissue perfusion, a dye-less ActivPerfusion™ mode and a dye-mediated ActivICG™ mode. ActivPerfusion™ mode represents a dye-free imaging method using coherent monochromatic light, known as laser speckle contrast imaging (LSCI), to detect blood flow and tissue perfusion. When a red blood cell is illuminated with coherent laser light, a speckle pattern or random interference pattern is created [89]. Because red blood cells are in motion, the speckle pattern fluctuates in time. In areas where there are more red blood cells in motion, the camera will display more blurring of the speckles. The wavelength of light used for LSCI is significantly less important than with imaging methods that rely on contrast absorption because LSCI is solely based on scattering. A limitation of LSCI is motion artifact. The respiratory and cardiac cycles can produce physiologic motion artifacts. However, image processing methods can compensate and minimize the effect of these artifacts [89–91].

In ActivPerfusion™ mode, tissue perfusion is displayed as a heatmap using a red-green-blue color (RGB) model. Warmer colors in the red spectrum indicate areas of high perfusion, while cooler colors within the blue spectrum indicate areas of relatively less perfusion. There are two imaging displays available within the ActivPerfusion™ mode, overlay and contrast. In the perfusion overlay mode, LSCI perfusion signals from light in the NIR spectrum are viewed over the white light display of the anatomy. The perfusion contrast mode displays only the LSCI perfusion signals to allow finer assessment of tissue perfusion without the interference of colors from the white light spectrum.

The ActivICG™ mode uses NIR technology to detect ICG and superimposes the image on tissue in real time. The advantage of the ActivPerfusion™ mode over contrast-based imaging is that the data provided is instantaneous and reproducible. With ActivPerfusion™, the perfusion signal is lost immediately after vessel occlusion. In contrast, if the vessel is transected or occluded after ICG is given, the image will not change due to the presence of residual dye resulting in false-positive data. This represents a pharmacokinetic limitation of ICG and additional perfusion assessments cannot be made until the 3–4-min half-life of ICG has passed [92]. Repeat dosing of ICG is also necessary and the accuracy may be reduced due to the presence of residual ICG.

Transillumination Systems

Green Egg—EndoGlow, Rochester, New York, USA

Green Egg (Fig. 2.13) was developed as a transillumination device for use in minimally invasive and open surgical procedures. The device contains its own fluorescence polymer which emits NIR when excited by an FGS system. The device is 30 mm in diameter and can be inserted into target tissue areas such as the vagina or rectum. When fluorescence mode is activated on the desired system, transillumination of near-infrared images can be visualized. This device works in a similar manner to fluorophores

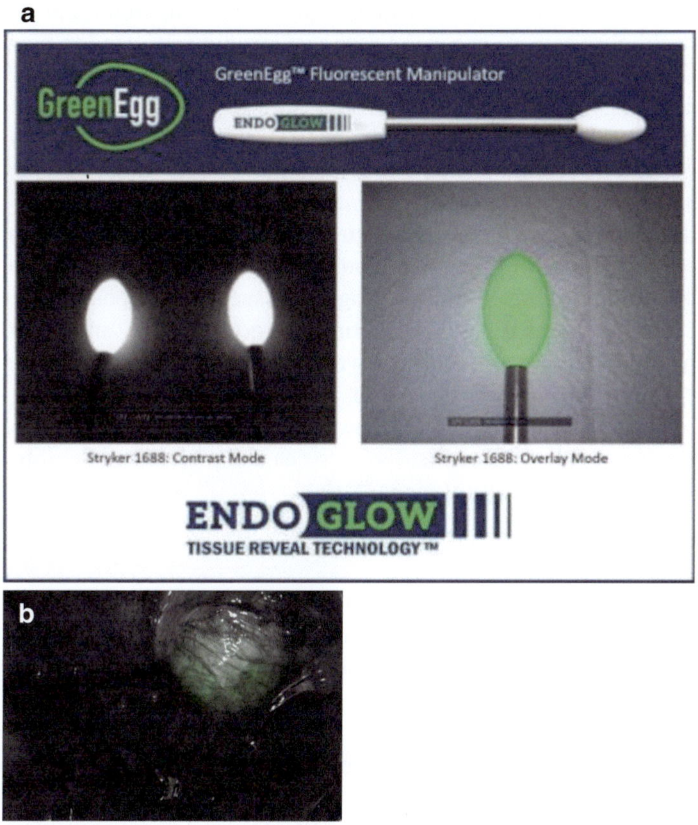

Fig. 2.13 (**a**) Green Egg—Image courtesy of EndoGlow. (**b**) Transillumination with use of Green Egg—Photo courtesy of EndoGlow

with emission of NIR light when activated. EndoGlow developed the device, which is pending FDA approval as of November 2021. It utilizes tissue reveal technology which is a fluorescent polymer device used in minimally invasive surgeries via transillumination. The indication for use of Green Egg is for transillumination of anatomic structures to assist in delineating tissue planes, depth, and anatomic borders. It has been used in gynecologic, urologic, and colorectal minimally invasive surgeries. The device has clinical use as a vaginal or rectal manipulator that can backlight tissue to enhance tissue visualization. Its use has been beneficial in the visualization and dissection of scarred tissue, reducing rectal injuries in prostatectomies, low anterior resections, and complex hysterectomies [93]. Pilot studies have demonstrated several benefits to the transillumination effect of using a fluorescent manipulator [94]. Surgeons were able to identify deep infiltrating rectal endometriosis, better recognize surgical planes in complex anatomy, and visualize relative tissue depth. The ability to transilluminate vaginal tissue aided in post-hysterectomy bladder dissections during sacrocolpopexies and rectopexies. An unexpected benefit was the increased communication between the attending surgeon and surgical learners (fellows/ residents) or surgical assists. The enhanced visualization allowed the surgical learner or first-assist to see and understand the intricacies of the dissection more easily.

Pearls and Pitfalls

- Autoclavable device that can be inserted directly into tissue areas (e.g., vagina and rectum).
- Sustainable autofluorescence device that obviates the need for dye injection.

Infrared Illuminating System (IRIS) Ureteral Kit—Stryker, Kalamazoo, Michigan, USA

Infrared Illuminating System (IRIS) Ureteral Kit (Fig. 2.14) is a transilluminating ureteral stent placed intraoperatively to assist in the identification of ureters during minimally invasive and open surgical procedures. This device connects to Stryker's LED light sources to provide transillumination of the ureter. The L11 LED light source is able to provide excitation at 830 nm transillumination [95, 96]. The device catheters are inserted sterilely via cystoscopy as a ureteral stent at the onset of the case. Catheters are advanced 20 cm in each ureter which is denoted by a double black line on the device. Once the catheters are in place, the emitting diodes are inserted into each catheter until the stopping mechanism on each diode is reached. The IRIS fiber prongs are inserted into

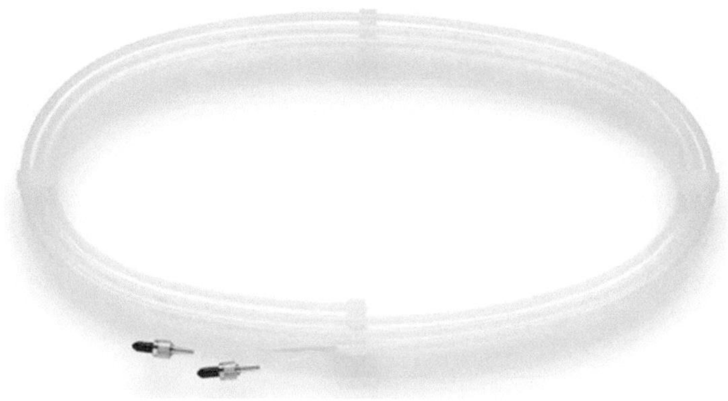

Fig. 2.14 Infrared Illuminating System Ureteral Kit—Image courtesy of Stryker

the Stryker light source on the far left of the unit. Once the light source is activated, the ureteral stents will illuminate and can be visible in any minimally invasive and open surgery. The indication for use of IRIS Ureteral Kit is for the transillumination of ureters to assist in delineating tissue planes during pelvic dissection in both minimally invasive and open surgery. It has been used in gynecologic, urologic, and colorectal surgeries to enhance tissue visualization to help reduce the risk of ureteral injuries [71, 97].

Pearls and Pitfalls

- Catheters compatible with guidewires up to 0.038 in.
- Catheters from kit can be left in place as needed for use as general use ureteral stents.
- IRIS menu on the Stryker's control unit can toggle IRIS illumination brightness, and the illumination can provide continuous transillumination or pulsating transillumination.

Endolumik Fluorescence-Guided Gastric Calibration Tube—Endolumik Inc., Morgantown, West Virginia, USA

The Endolumik Fluorescence-Guided Gastric Calibration Tube (Figs. 2.15 and 2.16) is a single-use, fluorescence-guided

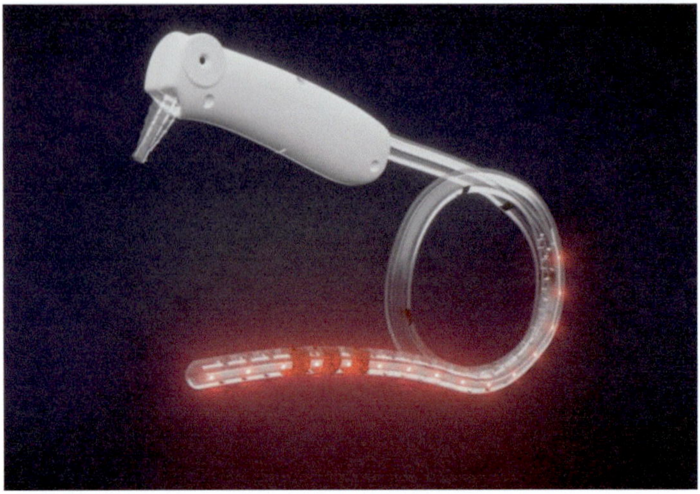

Fig. 2.15 The Endolumik Fluorescence-Guided Gastric Calibration Tube after turning on NIR lighting system, white light view

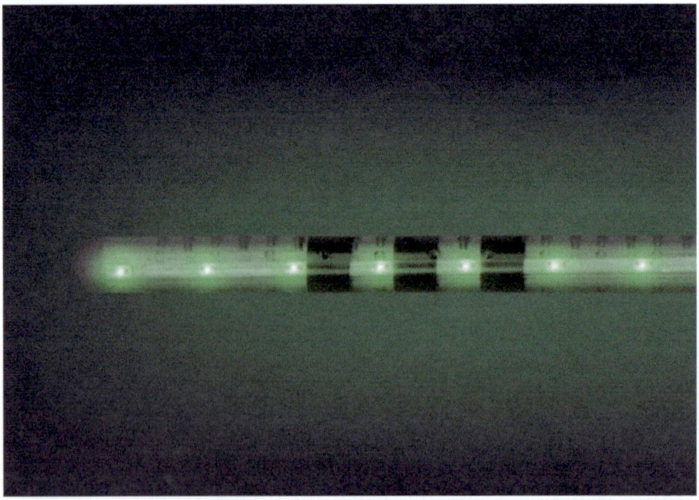

Fig. 2.16 The Endolumik Fluorescence-Guided Gastric Calibration Tube after turning on NIR lighting system, NIR light view

calibration tube indicated for use in bariatric, gastric, and esophageal surgery to improve visualization of tube position and to serve as a sizing and measurement guide, for the application of suction, gastric decompression/drainage of gastric fluids, and irrigation and leak testing [98]. This device combines the functionality of a nasogastric or orogastric tube, a calibration tube, and a leak testing system. The device was designed to improve intraoperative visualization and provide surgeons with additional visual cues to identify anatomic structures and delineate tissue planes with the goal of improving the precision of surgical dissection.

The Endolumik Gastric Calibration Tube is lit using NIR spectrum LEDs which enable transillumination through esophagogastric tissues. The tube is 80 cm long and is available in two different diameters: 36 and 40 French. It has a rounded tip and small side holes at the distal end to enable gastric decompression and/or irrigation. The proximal end includes a handle with an integral suction regulator. An additional squeeze bulb with pressure gauge may be attached to the end of the regulator to perform leak testing. Pilot studies have been completed using the device to improve visualization during laparoscopic sleeve gastrectomy and laparoscopic gastric bypass (Figs. 2.17, 2.18, and 2.19). The three black stripes at the distal end of the device enable fluorescence-guided measurement of up to 10 cm of length (Fig. 2.20).

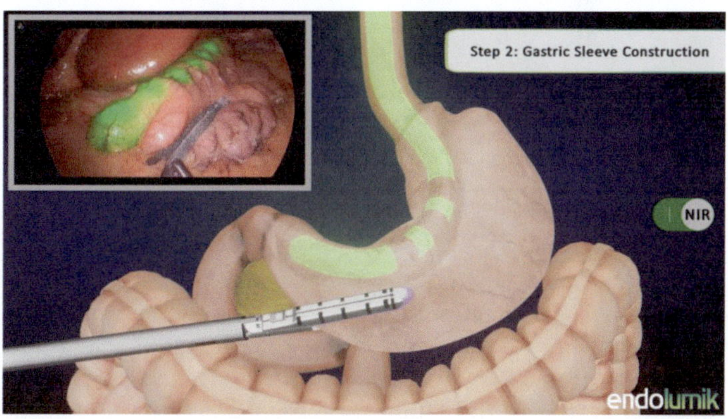

Fig. 2.17 Use of the Endolumik Fluorescence-Guided Gastric Calibration Tube during gastric sleeve construction

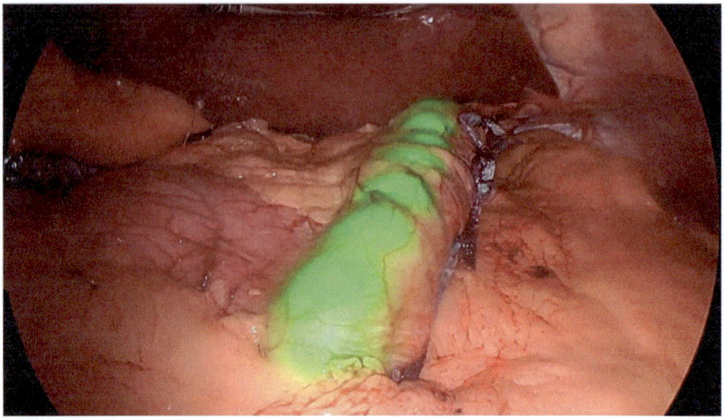

Fig. 2.18 Fluorescence-guided gastric sleeve construction during sleeve gastrectomy operation using the Endolumik calibration tube

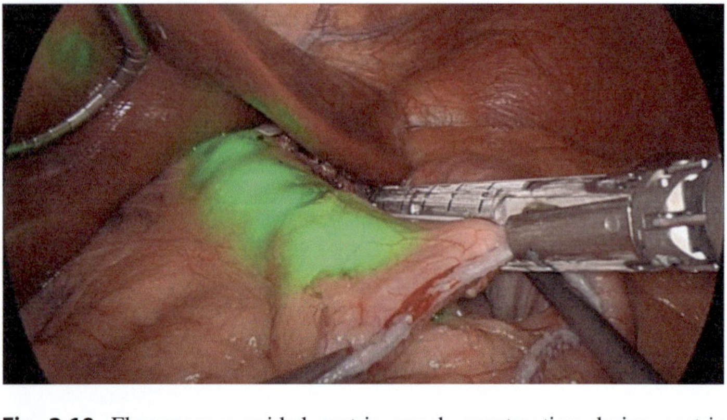

Fig. 2.19 Fluorescence-guided gastric pouch construction during gastric bypass operation using the Endolumik calibration tube

The device was FDA authorized on March 3, 2023, via the 510K pathway [99] and is also the first device to be authorized through the FDA Safer Technologies Program (STeP), a voluntary program for medical devices that are reasonably expected to significantly improve the safety of currently available treatments.

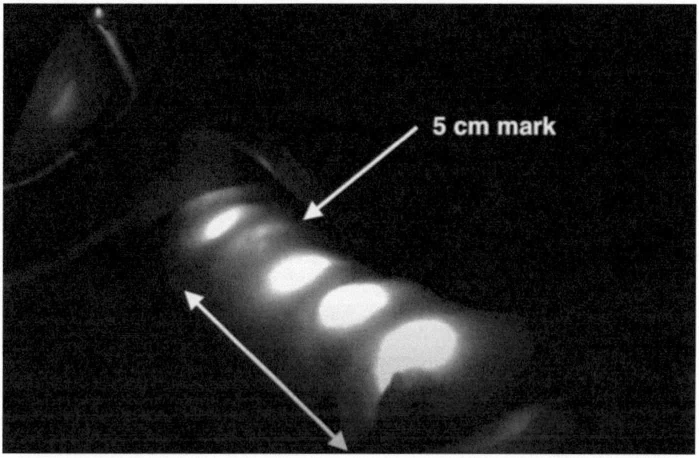

Fig. 2.20 Use of the Endolumik Fluorescence-Guided Gastric Calibration Tube to make fluorescence-guided measurements of gastric pouch length during gastric bypass

Pearls and Pitfalls

- LED-powered NIR device obviates the need for ICG dye injection.
- Compatible with all NIR surgical camera systems.
- Combines functionality of orogastric tube, calibration tube, and leak testing system.
- Provides fluorescence-guided intraoperative visualization to enable more precise positioning and surgical dissection.

References

1. Yang H, Kim J, Nam W, Kim HJ, Cha IH, Kim D. Handheld near-infrared fluorescence Imaging device using modified action cameras for perioperative guidance of microvascular flap surgery. J Clin Med. 2021;10(3):410. https://doi.org/10.3390/jcm10030410.
2. Frangioni JV. New technologies for human cancer imaging. J Clin Oncol Off J Am Soc Clin Oncol. 2008;26:4012–21. https://doi.org/10.1200/JCO.2007.14.3065.

3. Gioux S, Choi HS, Frangioni. Image-guided surgery using invisible near-infrared light: fundamentals of clinical translation. Mol Imaging. 2010;9(5):237–55. https://doi.org/10.2310/7290.2010.00034.
4. Goldstein S, Heaton T, Bondoc A, et al. Evolving applications of fluorescence guided surgery in pediatric surgical oncology: a practical guide for surgeons. J Pediatr Surg. 2021;56(2):215–23.
5. Nagaya T, Nakamura Y, Choyke P, et al. Fluorescence-guided surgery. Front Oncol. 2017;7:314. https://doi.org/10.3389/fonc.2017.00314.
6. DSouza AV, Lin H, Henderson ER, Samkoe KS, Pogue BW. Review of fluorescence guided surgery systems: identification of key performance capabilities beyond indocyanine green imaging. J Biomed Opt. 2016;21(8):80901.
7. Egloff-Juras C, Bezdetnaya L, Dolivet G, Lassalle HP. NIR fluorescence-guided tumor surgery: new strategies for the use of indocyanine green. Int J Nanomed. 2019;14:7823–38. https://doi.org/10.2147/IJN.S207486.
8. Nagaya T, Nakamura Y, Choyke P, Kobayashi H. Fluorescence guided surgery. Front Oncol. 2017;7:314.
9. Folli S, Wagnieres G, Pelegrin A. Immunophotodiagnosis of colon carcinomas in patients injected with fluoresceinated chimeric antibodies against carcinoembryonic antigen. Proc Natl Acad Sci U S A. 1992;89(17):7973–7.
10. Namikawa T, Sato T, Hanazaki K. Recent advances in near-infrared fluorescence-guided imaging surgery using indocyanine green. Surg Today. 2015;45(12):1467–74. https://doi.org/10.1007/s00595-015-1158-7. Epub 2015 Mar 29. PMID: 25820596.
11. Barth CW, Gibbs SL. Fluorescence image-guided surgery - a perspective on contrast agent development. Proc SPIE Int Soc Opt Eng. 2020;11222:112220J. https://doi.org/10.1117/12.2545292.
12. Mondal SB, Gao S, Zhu N, et al. Real-time fluorescence image-guided oncologic surgery. Adv Cancer Res. 2014;124:171–211.
13. Chi C, Du Y, Ye J, et al. Intraoperative imaging-guided cancer surgery. Teranostics. 2014;4(11):1072–84. https://doi.org/10.7150/thno.9899.
14. Troyan SL, et al. The FLARE intraoperative near-infrared fluorescence imaging system: a first-in-human clinical trial in breast cancer sentinel lymph node mapping. Ann Surg Oncol. 2009;16:2943–52.
15. National Center for Biotechnology Information. PubChem compound summary for CID 16850, Fluorescein. 2021. https://pubchem.ncbi.nlm.nih.gov/compound/Fluorescein. Accessed 27 Aug 2021.
16. Alander JT, Kaartinen I, Laakso A, Pätilä T, Spillmann T, Tuchin VV, Venermo M, Välisuo P. A review of indocyanine green fluorescent imaging in surgery. Int J Biomed Imaging. 2012;2012:940585. https://doi.org/10.1155/2012/940585.
17. van Manen L, Handgraaf HJM, Diana M, et al. A practical guide for the use of indocyanine green and methylene blue in fluorescence-guided abdominal surgery. Journal of Surg Oncol. 2018;118(2):283–300. https://doi.org/10.1002/jso.25105.

18. SPY Elite intraoperative perfusion assessment system - operator's manual. 2015. Accessed Oct 2021.
19. SPY Elite product brochure. 2018. Accessed Oct 2021.
20. SPY Elite intraoperative perfusion assessment system: K182907. 510K approval. 2018. Available: https://www.accessdata.fda.gov/cdrh_docs/pdf18/K182907.pdf. Accessed Oct 2021.
21. Gurtner GC, Jones GE, Neligan PC, et al. Intraoperative laser angiography using the SPY system: review of the literature and recommendations for use. Ann Surg Innov Res. 2013;7(1):1. https://doi.org/10.1186/1750-1164-7-1.
22. Venturi ML, Mesbahi AN, Copeland-Halperin LR, Suh VY, Yemc L. SPY Elite's ability to predict nipple necrosis in nipple-sparing mastectomy and immediate tissue expander reconstruction. Plast Reconstr Surg Glob Open. 2017;5(5):e1334. https://doi.org/10.1097/GOX.0000000000001334.
23. Kislevitz ML, Lu KB, Sanniec K, Amirlak B. Unique uses of SPY: high-risk facelift. Plast Reconstr Surg Glob Open. 2019;7(6):e2183. https://doi.org/10.1097/GOX.0000000000002183. PMID: 31624665; PMCID: PMC6635201.
24. Newman MI, Jack MC, Samson MC. SPY-Q analysis toolkit values potentially predict mastectomy flap necrosis. Ann Plast Surg. 2013;70(5):595–8. https://doi.org/10.1097/SAP.0b013e3182650b4e. PMID: 23542838.
25. Girard N, Delomenie M, et al. Innovative DIEP flap perfusion evaluation tool: qualitative and quantitative analysis of indocyanine green-based fluorescence angiography with the SPY-Q proprietary software. PLoS One. 2019;14:e0217698.
26. Heniford T. A clinical trial using spy Elite System in planning tissue advancement flaps after ventral hernia repair. ClinicalTrialsgov. 2016.
27. Foppa C, Denoya PI, Tarta C, Bergamaschi R. Indocyanine green fluorescent dye during bowel surgery: are the blood supply "guessing days" over? Tech Coloproctol. 2014;18(8):753–8. https://doi.org/10.1007/s10151-014-1130-3. Epub 2014 Feb 21. PMID: 24558047.
28. Phillips BT, Fourman MS, Rivara A, Dagum AB, Huston TL, Ganz JC, Bui DT, Khan SU. Comparing quantitative values of two generations of laser-assisted indocyanine green dye angiography systems: can we predict necrosis? Eplasty. 2014;14:e44. PMID: 25525483; PMCID: PMC4258931.
29. Protyniak B, Dinallo AM, Boyan WP Jr, Dressner RM, Arvanitis ML. Intraoperative indocyanine green fluorescence angiography--an objective evaluation of anastomotic perfusion in colorectal surgery. Am Surg. 2015;81(6):580–4. https://doi.org/10.1177/000313481508100621. PMID: 26031270.
30. Hajiran A, Zekan D, et al. Use of SPY Elite fluorescence imaging in creation of a continent urinary diversion. Case Rep Urol. 2019;2019:9069841.

31. Morozov AO, Alyaev YG, Rapoport LM, Tsarichenko DG, Bezrukov EA, Butnaru DV, Sirota ES. Near-infrared fluorescence with indocyanine green for diagnostics in urology: initial experience. Urologia. 2017;84(3):197–202. https://doi.org/10.5301/uj.5000235.
32. Takahashi M, Ishikawa T, Higashidani K, Katoh H. SPY™: an innovative intra-operative imaging system to evaluate graft patency during off-pump coronary artery bypass grafting. Interact Cardiovasc Thorac Surg. 2004;3(33):479–83.
33. Korn JM, Tellez-Diaz A, Bartz-Kurycki M, Gastman B. Indocyanine green SPY elite-assisted sentinel lymph node biopsy in cutaneous melanoma. Plast Reconstr Surg. 2014;133(4):914–22. https://doi.org/10.1097/PRS.0000000000000006.
34. Vahabzadeh-Hagh AM, Blackwell KE, Abemayor E, St John MA. Sentinel lymph node biopsy in cutaneous melanoma of the head and neck using the indocyanine green SPY Elite system. Am J Otolaryngol. 2018;39(5):485–8. https://doi.org/10.1016/j.amjoto.2018.05.006.
35. SPY PHI - operator's manual. 2020. Accessed Oct 2021.
36. SPY PHI_SPY-QP booklet supplied by Stryker. 2020. Accessed Oct 2021.
37. SPY PHI system with SPY-PHI fluorescence assessment software: K202244. 510K Approval 2020. Available https://www.accessdata.fda.gov/cdrh_docs/pdf20/K202244.pdf. Accessed Oct 2021.
38. Jakubietz RG, Schmidt K, Bernuth S, Meffert RH, Jakubietz MG. Evaluation of the intraoperative blood flow of pedicled perforator flaps using indocyanine green-fluorescence angiography. Plast Reconstr Surg Glob Open. 2019;7(8):2462. https://doi.org/10.1097/GOX.0000000000002462.
39. Nguyen JMV, Hogen L, Laframboise S, Bouchard-Fortier G, Ferguson SE, Bernardini MQ, May T. The use of indocyanine green fluorescence angiography to assess anastomotic perfusion following bowel resection in surgery for gynecologic malignancies - a report of 100 consecutive anastomoses. Gynecol Oncol. 2020;158(2):402–6. https://doi.org/10.1016/j.ygyno.2020.05.008. Epub 2020 May 15. PMID: 32423604.
40. pde-neoII (C10935) - operator's manual. 2016. Accessed Oct 2021.
41. Hamamatsu. PDE-neoII brochure. Available: https://www.hamamatsu.com/resources/pdf/sys/SMES0034E_C10935-400.pdf. Accessed Oct 2021.
42. Ped-neo: K133719. 510K approval 2014. Available: https://www.accessdata.fda.gov/cdrh_docs/pdf13/K133719.pdf. Accessed Oct 2021.
43. Shikayama T. Characteristics of the photodynamic eye camera. In: Kusano M, Kokudo N, Toi M, et al., editors. ICG fluorescence imaging and navigation surgery. Tokyo: Springer; 2016. p. 21–7.
44. Tagaya N, Aoyagi H, Nakagawa A, Abe A, Iwasaki Y, Tachibana M, Kubota K. A novel approach for sentinel lymph node identification

using fluorescence imaging and image overlay navigation surgery in patients with breast cancer. World J Surg. 2011;35(1):154–8. https://doi.org/10.1007/s00268-010-0811-y. PMID: 20931198
45. Funai K, Kawase A, Shimizu K, Sekihara K, Yamashita T, Shiiya N. Fluorescence navigation with indocyanine green for identification of intersegmental planes using a photodynamic eye camera. J Thorac Dis. 2020;12(9):4817–24. https://doi.org/10.21037/jtd-20-1448.
46. Kobayashi K, Kawaguchi Y, Kobayashi Y, Matsumura M, Ishizawa T, Akamatsu N, Kaneko J, Arita J, Sakamoto Y, Kokudo N, Hasegawa K. Identification of liver lesions using fluorescence imaging: comparison of methods for administering indocyanine green. HPB (Oxford). 2021;23(2):262–9. https://doi.org/10.1016/j.hpb.2020.06.006.
47. Chakedis J, Shirley LA, Terando AM, Skoracki R, Phay JE. Identification of the thoracic duct using indocyanine green during cervical lymphadenectomy. Ann Surg Oncol. 2018;25(12):3711–7. https://doi.org/10.1245/s10434-018-6690-4. Epub 2018 Aug 3. PMID: 30076554; PMCID: PMC6181776.
48. Suzuki Y, Sakuma H, Yamazaki S. Comparison of patency rates of lymphaticovenous anastomosis at different sites for lower extremity lymphedema. J Vasc Surg Venous Lymphat Disord. 2019;7(2):222–7. https://doi.org/10.1016/j.jvsv.2018.10.022.
49. Fluoptics: Fluobeam LX brochure Supplied by Fluoptics. 2021. Available https://fluoptics.us/wp-content/uploads/2019/10/Fluoptics-FluobeamLX-EN-web.pdf. Accessed Oct 2021.
50. Fluobeam LX: K190891. 510K approval. 2019. Available. https://www.accessdata.fda.gov/cdrh_docs/pdf19/K190891.pdf. Accessed Oct 2021.
51. Pruimboom T, van Kuijk SMJ, Qiu SS, van den Bos J, Wieringa FP, van der Hulst RRWJ, Schols RM. Optimizing indocyanine green fluorescence angiography in reconstructive flap surgery: a systematic review and ex vivo experiments. Surg Innov. 2020;27(1):103–19. https://doi.org/10.1177/1553350619862097.
52. Louges MA, Bellaiche J, Correia N, Chiriac S, François C. Relevance of intraoperative indocyanine green injection in breast reconstruction using DIEP procedure for abdominal scars. Ann Chir Plast Esthet. 2016;61(3):231–4. https://doi.org/10.1016/j.anplas.2016.03.002.
53. Hirche C, Engel H, Kolios L, Cognie J, Hünerbein M, Lehnhardt M, Kremer T. An experimental study to evaluate the Fluobeam 800 imaging system for fluorescence-guided lymphatic imaging and sentinel node biopsy. Surg Innov. 2013;20(5):516–23. https://doi.org/10.1177/1553350612468962. Epub 2012 Dec 27. PMID: 23275469.
54. Demarchi MS, Seeliger B, Lifante J-C, Alesina PF, Triponez F. Fluorescence image-guided surgery for thyroid cancer: utility for preventing hypoparathyroidism. Cancers. 2021;13(15):3792. https://doi.org/10.3390/cancers13153792.
55. Kose E, Kahramangil B, Aydin H, Donmez M, Berber E. Heterogeneous and low-intensity parathyroid autofluorescence: patterns suggesting

hyperfunction at parathyroid exploration. Surgery. 2019;165(2):431–7. https://doi.org/10.1016/j.surg.2018.08.006.
56. Demarchi MS, Karenovics W, Bédat B, De Vito C, Triponez F. Autofluorescence pattern of parathyroid adenomas. BJS Open. 2021;5(1):zraa047. https://doi.org/10.1093/bjsopen/zraa047.
57. Jafari MD, Wexner SD, Martz JE, McLemore EC, Margolin DA, Sherwinter DA, Lee SW, Senagore AJ, Phelan MJ, Stamos MJ. Perfusion assessment in laparoscopic left-sided/anterior resection (PILLAR II): a multi-institutional study. J Am Coll Surg. 2015;220(1):82–92.e1.
58. David G, Mangano A, Dionigi G, Rausei S, Spampatti S, Cassinotti E, Fingerhut A. Clinical applications of indocyanine green (ICG) enhanced fluorescence in laparoscopic surgery. Surg Endosc. 2015;29(7):2046–55. https://doi.org/10.1007/s00464-014-3895-x.
59. Pinpoint: endoscopic fluorescence imaging system brochure. Supplied by Novadaq. Available. https://www.mirabellmed.at/resources/media/pinpoint.pdf. Accessed Oct 2021.
60. Pinpoint endoscopic fluorescence imaging system: K182606 510K approval. 2018. Available. https://www.accessdata.fda.gov/cdrh_docs/pdf18/K182606.pdf. Accessed Oct 2021.
61. Tsutsui N, Yoshida M, Kitajima M, Suzuki Y. Laparoscopic cholecystectomy using the PINPOINT endoscopic fluorescence imaging system with intraoperative fluorescent imaging: a case report. Int J Surg Case Rep. 2016;21:129–32. https://doi.org/10.1016/j.ijscr.2016.02.036.
62. Arthrex SynergyID system instruction for use manual. 2020. Available. https://www.manualslib.com/manual/1868210/Arthrex-Synergyid-Ar-3200-0025.html. Accessed Oct 2021.
63. Synergy ID IR1-000394-en-US_A_IR1-000394 CCU and camera head playsheet Rev2. Supplied by Arthrex. Accessed Oct 2021.
64. Synergy ID FL2-000319-en-US_C_SynergyID_Flyer_210x297mm_web. Supplied by Arthrex. Accessed Oct 2021.
65. Synergy ID IR1-000390_SynergyID augmented reality Playsheet rev 2. Supplied by Arthrex Accessed Oct 2021.
66. Arthrex SynergyID endoscopic imaging system: K202582. 510K approval. 2021. Available https://www.accessdata.fda.gov/cdrh_docs/pdf20/K202582.pdf. Accessed Oct 2021.
67. Visera Elite II VEII_Borchure_A4_297x210mm_EN_v20 publically available on Olympus. Accessed Oct 2021.
68. Visera Elite II Xenon Light Source. K200542. 510K approval. 2020. Available at https://www.accessdata.fda.gov/cdrh_docs/pdf20/K200542.pdf. Accessed Oct 2021.
69. 1688 4K camera system with advanced imaging modality user manual. Available at https://5.imimg.com/data5/SELLER/Doc/2021/5/AY/MU/PK/24888028/stryker-1688-endoscopic-camera.pdf. Accessed Oct 2021.
70. 1688 AIM - 1588 to 1688 AIM 4K platform justification packet. Supplied by Stryker. Accessed Oct 2021.

71. Nitta T, Tanaka K, Kataoka J, et al. Novel technique with the IRIS U kit to prevent urethral injury in patients undergoing transanal total mesorectal excision. Ann Med Surg (Lond). 2019;46:1–3. https://doi.org/10.1016/j.amsu.2019.08.002.
72. Storz Image I user manual PDF. Accessed Oct 2021.
73. Image 1S Rubina Brochure. Available. https://www.karlstorz.com/cps/rde/xbcr/karlstorz_assets/ASSETS/3623282.pdf. Accessed Oct 2021.
74. Rubina: K201399. 510K approval. 2020. Available at https://www.accessdata.fda.gov/cdrh_docs/pdf20/K201399.pdf. Accessed Oct 2021.
75. Image 1S Rubina application in colorectal surgery - supplied by Karl Storz. Available at https://www.karlstorz.com/cps/rde/xbcr/karlstorz_assets/ASSETS/3646673.pdf. Accessed Oct 2021.
76. Image 1S Rubina application in cholecystectomy - supplied by Karl Storz. Available at https://www.karlstorz.com/cps/rde/xbcr/karlstorz_assets/ASSETS/3646675.pdf. Accessed Oct 2021.
77. VS3-Iridium - guide. Available at https://www.medtronic.com/content/dam/covidien/library/us/en/product/visualisation-systems/elevision-ir-platform-ibrochure.pdf. Accessed Oct 2021.
78. Elevision IR brochure. Available at http://www.medtronic.me/content/dam/covidien/library/us/en/product/visualisation-systems/elevision-ir-platform-mis-brochure.pdf. Accessed Oct 2021.
79. VS3-IR. 510K approval. 2019. Available at https://www.accessdata.fda.gov/cdrh_docs/pdf19/K191851.pdf. Accessed Oct 2021.
80. Hoveling R. Quest medical imaging. Brochure available at https://dutchphotonicsevent.nl/wp-content/uploads/2019/09/Richelle-Hoveling-Making-the-invisible-visible.pdf. Accessed Oct 2021.
81. Artemis handheld imaging system. K191851. 510K approval. 2015. Available https://www.accessdata.fda.gov/cdrh_docs/pdf14/K143474.pdf. Accessed Oct 2021.
82. van Driel PB, van de Giessen M, Boonstra MC, et al. Characterization and evaluation of the artemis camera for fluorescence-guided cancer surgery. Mol Imaging Biol. 2015;17(3):413–23. https://doi.org/10.1007/s11307-014-0799-z.
83. Wu G. Fluorescence image-guided robotic surgery. In: Liao J, Su LM, editors. Advances in image-guided urologic surgery. New York, NY: Springer; 2015. https://doi.org/10.1007/978-1-4939-1450-0_5.
84. DaVinci Xi system user manual - supplied by intuitive. Accessed 2021.
85. DaVinci Firefly imaging system. K141077. 510K approval. 2014. Available at https://www.accessdata.fda.gov/cdrh_docs/pdf14/K141077.pdf. Accessed 2021.
86. Intuitive; fluorescence imaging for da Vinci X and da Vinci Xi surgical systems provided by intuitive. 2021.
87. Kim J, Ferguson J, Shrand J, Pitt E, et al. Integrating Firefly fluorescence into image guidance for the da Vinci Robot. SPIE Digital Library; 2021.

88. Spinoglio G, Marano A, Formisano G. Robotic surgery using firefly system. In: Dip F, Ishizawa T, Kokudo N, Rosenthal R, editors. Fluorescence imaging for surgeons. Cham: Springer; 2015. https://doi.org/10.1007/978-3-319-15,678-1_6.
89. Heeman W, Steenbergen W, van Dam GM, Boerma EC. Clinical applications of laser speckle contrast imaging: a review. J Biomed Opt. 2019;24:1. https://doi.org/10.1117/1.jbo.24.8.080901.
90. Richards LM, Towle EL, Fox DJ, Dunn AK. Intraoperative laser speckle contrast imaging with retrospective motion correction for quantitative assessment of cerebral blood flow. Neurophotonics. 2014;1:1. https://doi.org/10.1117/1.nph.1.1.015006.
91. Lertsakdadet B, Yang BY, Dunn CE, Ponticorvo A, Crouzet C, Bernal N, Durkin AJ, Choi B. Correcting for motion artifact in handheld laser speckle images. J Biomed Opt. 2018;23:1. https://doi.org/10.1117/1.jbo.23.3.03600.
92. Haller M, Akbulut C, Brechtelsbauer H, Fett W, Briegel J, Finsterer U, Peter K. Determination of plasma volume with indocyanine green in man. Life Sci. 1993;53:1597–604. https://doi.org/10.1016/0024--3205(93)90183-4.
93. Doyle P. Endoglow tissue reveal technology. Available https://www.endoglow.com/aboutendoglow. Accessed Oct 2021.
94. Panza J, Hernandez D, Gubbels A, Byrnes J. Near infrared fluorescence during minimally invasive sacrocolpopexy: a pilot study. San Antonio, TX: Society of Gynecologic Surgery Video; 2022.
95. AIM (Advanced Imaging Modality) system K 210088. 510K approval 2021. Available at https://www.accessdata.fda.gov/cdrh_docs/pdf21/K210088.pdf. Accessed Oct 2021.
96. Stryker Infrared Illumination System (IRIS) [AIM light source and ureteral kit]. K151243. 510K approval. 2015. Available at https://www.accessdata.fda.gov/cdrh_docs/pdf15/K151243.pdf. Accessed Oct 2021.
97. Song C, Lee S, Chung H, et al. Case report…using lighted ureteral stent. World J Surg and Surg Res. 2020;3:1262.

Towle EL, Richards LM, Kazmi SMS, Fox DJ, Dunn AK. Comparison of indocyanine green angiography and laser speckle contrast imaging for the assessment of vasculature perfusion. Neurosurgery. 2012;71:1023–30. https://doi.org/10.1227/NEU.0b013e31826adf88.

98. https://www.accessdata.fda.gov/cdrh_docs/pdf22/K222880.pdf.

Use of Fluorescence Guidance in Colorectal Surgery

3

Michael R. Freund, Anna Duprée, and Steven D. Wexner

Anastomotic Leak

Introduction

One of the most significant persistent challenges of colorectal surgery is trying to reduce or eliminate the rate of anastomotic leaks (AL). Despite recent advances in technology and surgical technique, AL rates remain between 1% and 19% contingent on the location of anastomosis. The more distal the anastomosis, the

M. R. Freund
Ellen Leifer Shulman and Steven Shulman Digestive Disease Center, Cleveland Clinic Florida, Weston, FL, USA

Department of General Surgery, Shaare Zedek Medical Center, Faculty of Medicine, Hebrew University of Jerusalem, Jerusalem, Israel

A. Duprée
Department of General, Visceral and Thoracic Surgery, University Medical Center Hamburg-Eppendorf, Hamburg, Germany
e-mail: adupree@uke.de

S. D. Wexner (✉)
Ellen Leifer Shulman and Steven Shulman Digestive Disease Center, Cleveland Clinic Florida, Weston, FL, USA
e-mail: wexners@ccf.org

N. Szoka et al. (eds.), *The SAGES Manual of Fluorescence-Guided Surgery*, https://doi.org/10.1007/978-3-031-40685-0_3

higher the leak rate: ileocolic (1–8%), colocolonic (2–3%), ileorectal (3–7%), colorectal, or coloanal (5–19%) [1–3]. The anastomosis most prone to AL is a distal pelvic anastomosis, usually performed for low anterior resection (LAR) in patients who were previously treated with neoadjuvant chemoradiotherapy [4]. In these high-risk patients, AL rates can range between 10% and 20% and therefore these patients have been traditionally preemptively diverted with a loop ileostomy. Table 3.1 presents AL rates and reoperation rates for colorectal anastomoses.

In addition to the short-term postoperative morbidity, AL is also associated with suboptimal long-term function and oncologic outcomes including increased local recurrence rates and reduced 5-year survival rates [4, 15, 16]. Stormark et al. [4] reviewed 22,985 patients from the Swedish, Norwegian, and Danish colorectal cancer registries and showed that five-year relative survival in patients with anastomotic leak was 64.7% compared with 87% for patients with no leak ($P < 0.001$). The clinical and economic outcomes of AL were assessed by Hammond et al. [17] using the Premier Perspective™ database. In their study 6174 patients with colorectal AL were propensity-score matched to patients who did not suffer an AL, and the leak rate was approximately 6%. The authors showed that patients with AL had a 1.3 higher 30-day readmission rate and 0.8–1.9 times higher rate of postoperative infection compared to patients without AL ($P < 0.001$). They also showed that AL was associated with additional length of stay and hospital cost of 7.3 days and $24,129, respectively, per patient, within the index hospitalization (Table 3.1).

A variety of risk factors for AL have been recognized and have been generally classified as modifiable and non-modifiable risk factors. Well-known non-modifiable risk include male gender and increasing age, previous pelvic radiation, diabetes, emergency surgery, and tumor-related factors such as a rectal tumor necessitating a distal anastomosis [18–20].

One of the more important intraoperative considerations for forming an anastomosis is ensuring adequate vascularity to the anastomosis. Previous studies have shown that the surgeon's intraoperative evaluation and judgment is subjective and that pre-

Table 3.1 Colorectal anastomosis leak rate and re-operative rate in selected series

Author/year	Journal	Location	Sample size	Leak rate (%)	Reoperation rate (%)
Karliczek et al. (2009) [5]	Int J Colorect Dis	Netherlands	191 colorectal anastomoses	14	NR
Ashraf et al. (2013) [6]	Colorectal Dis	UK	285 LAR	10	5.6
Caulfied et al. (2013) [7]	JAMA Surg	USA	198 LAR	15	NR
Senagore et al. (2014) [8]	Dis. Colon Rectum	USA	258 colorectal anastomoses	12	7.4
Mongin et al. (2014) [9]	Int J Colorect Dis	France	171 LAR	12	7.6
Leahy et al. (2014) [10]	J Gastroinest. Surg	USA	245 colorectal anastomoses	14	NR
Shiomi et al. (2015) [11]	JACS	Japan	936 LAR	13	4.7
Borstlap et al. (2017) [12]	Ann Surg	Netherlands	998 LAR	13 (<30 d) 20 (>30 d)	NR
Detering et al. (2019) [13]	JACS	Netherlands	396 LAP	12.2	NR
			396 TatME	16.5	NR
Furnee et al. (2019) [14]	J Gastroinest. Surg	Netherlands	746 LAR	14.2	NR

LAR low anterior resection, *NR* not reported, *UK* United Kingdom, *USA* United States of America, *taTME* transanal total mesorectal excision, *LAP* laparoscopic diction of postoperative AL, based on traditional methods such as tissue color or palpable mesenteric pulses, is fairly limited [21, 22]. In recent years, indocyanine green (ICG) fluorescence had been increasingly employed for intraoperative perfusion evaluation to try to reduce the incidence of AL [23–26]. Its application and use in colorectal surgery are hereby explained and discussed.

Use of ICG to Evaluate Anastomotic Perfusion: Technical Aspects

All patients are preoperatively screened for allergy to shellfish or any prior hypersensitivity reaction to ICG. Immediately prior to bowel resection, after the surgeon decides on the intended location of the resection margins, an intravenous injection of 3.5 ml ICG is administered followed by a 10 mL intravenous saline flush. The recommended ICG dose in assessing bowel perfusion should be in the range of 0.1–0.3 mg/Kg. This dose is usually achieved by dilution of the ICG vial containing 25 mg of ICG powder with 10 ml of sterile water prior to administration, resulting in a concentration of 2.5 mg per 1 ml of reconstituted solution. Using a laparoscope equipped with a near-infrared (NIR) camera and filter, visual assessment of tissue perfusion is performed. This assessment can be achieved by switching the camera from white light mode (Fig. 3.1a) to contrast (spy) or overlay fluorescence mode (Fig. 3.1b). At this point, the proximal margin may be modified based on fluorescence perfusion assessment findings.

After extracorporeal extraction and after placing the EEA or stapler but prior to firing, ICG perfusion assessment may be again performed by injecting a second bolus of 3.5 ml of ICG, again followed by a 10 ml flush of saline solution (Fig. 3.2). For intracorporal anastomosis, an NIR-equipped laparoscope is used to assess the serosal aspects of both ends of the intended anastomosis (Fig. 3.3). For pelvic anastomosis, it is our practice to also ascertain mucosal perfusion using a custom-designed rigid proctoscope equipped with an NIR camera. A third bolus of 3.5 ml of ICG is administered, again followed by a 10 ml flush, and the

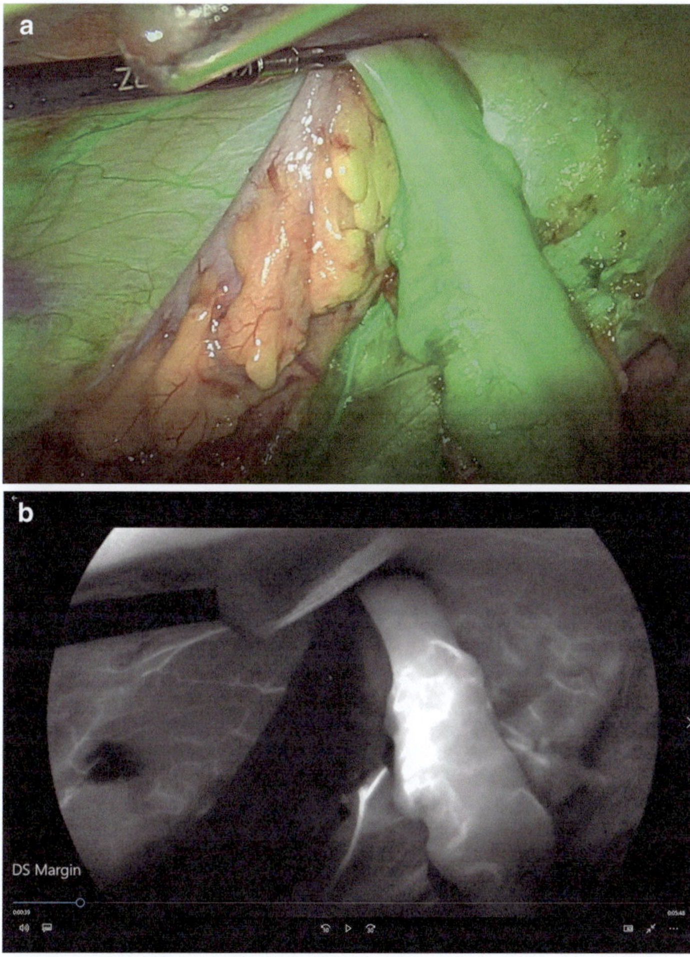

Fig. 3.1 (**a**) White light, (**b**) Fluorescence mode

mucosal appearance of both proximal and distal mucosal aspects of the anastomosis is visually assessed.

For extracorporeal anastomosis, following mobilization and division of the mesentery, 3.5 mL of ICG followed by 10 mL of saline is administrated (Fig. 3.4a). Using ICG fluorescence angiog-

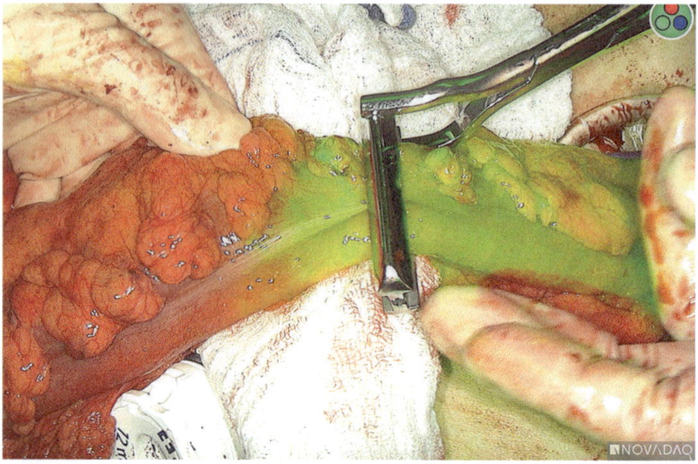

Fig. 3.2 For extracorporeal anastomosis, indocyanine green (ICG) perfusion assessment performed by injecting a second bolus of 3.5 ml of ICG, followed by a 10 ml flush of saline solution

raphy guidance, each end of the bowel is divided with a standard linear stapler (Fig. 3.4b). The anastomosis is then formed with a stapler in a side-to-side functional end-to-end manner. Once the anastomosis is completed, ICG perfusion assessment is performed using a 0-degree NIR camera-equipped laparoscope (Fig. 3.5). Prior to fluorescence assessment, an additional standard dose of 3.5 mL of ICG followed by 10 mL of saline is injected. For accurate assessment, all room lighting is turned off to minimize artifacts for extracorporeal fluorescence perfusion assessment.

Pearls and Pitfalls

Timing ICG fluorescence perfusion assessment is time dependent. The ingress phase takes approximately 20–30 s for ICG to become visible on NIR camera depending on different patient-related factors [27]. The optimal time to assess perfusion is approximately 30–120 s from ICG administration, when ICG fluorescence is at its peak. After 2 min, ICG fluorescence will start

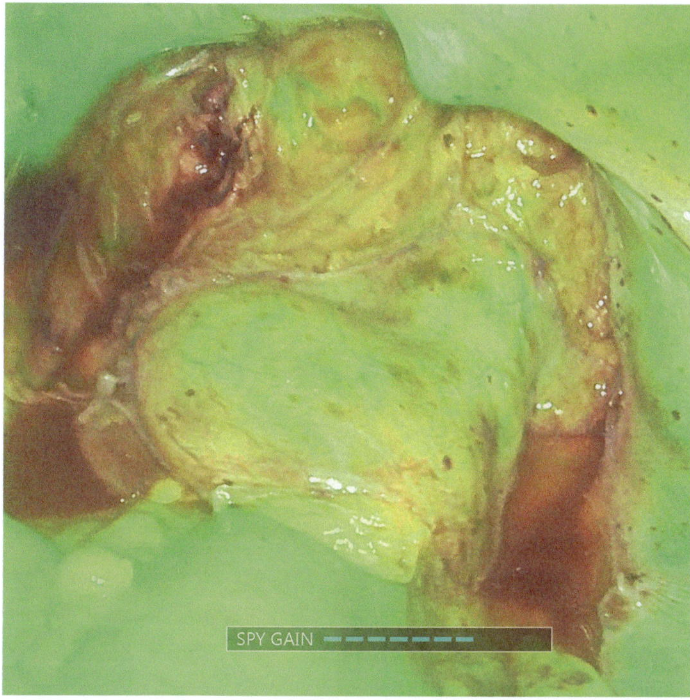

Fig. 3.3 For intracorporal anastomosis, a near-infrared (NIR) equipped laparoscope is used to assess the serosal aspects of both ends of the intended anastomosis

to decrease, although some degree of ICG fluorescence may still be visible up until 15–17 min from initial administration.

Initially, the circular stapler line is compressed by the stapler and therefore does not fluoresce as well as the rest of the tissue at first. After the circular stapler is fired and removed, the tissue surrounding the staple line is able to decompress and appropriately fluoresces after a few seconds.

Gain When utilizing fluorescence for bowel perfusion assessment, we generally recommend establishing set gain of 5 or 6 bars

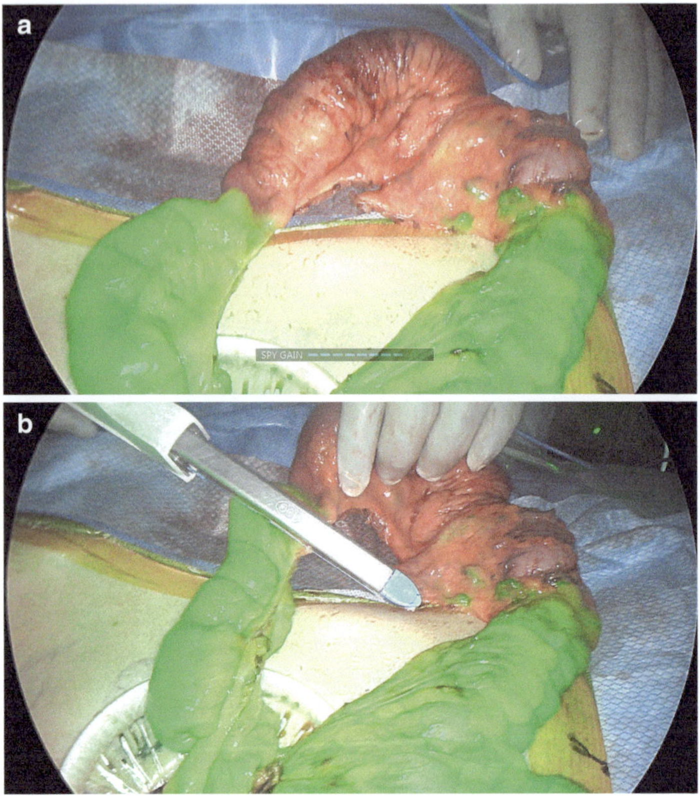

Fig. 3.4 (**a**) For extracorporeal anastomosis, following mobilization and division of the mesentery, 3.5 mL of indocyanine green (ICG) followed by 10 mL of saline is administrated. (**b**) Using ICG fluorescence angiography guidance, each end of the bowel is divided with a standard linear stapler

as a baseline. We find it useful in setting a standard for comparison and to reduce subjective assessment bias.

Ureters ICG fluorescence imaging of the ureters can be quite helpful during colorectal surgery [28]. The same dilution method

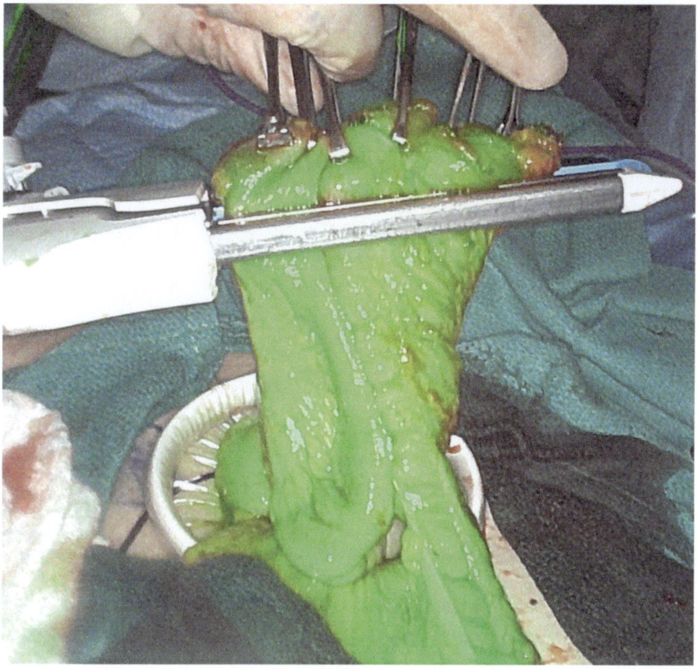

Fig. 3.5 Once the anastomosis is completed, indocyanine green (ICG) perfusion assessment is performed using a 0-degree near-infrared (NIR) camera-equipped laparoscope

can be used (dilution of the ICG vile containing 25 mg of ICG powder with 10 ml of sterile water), and after ureteral stents are placed under cystoscopy, a 5 ml of reconstituted solution can be injected in each ureter. To insure long-standing visualization during surgery, the ureteral stent can be occluded for approximately 30 s to allow the ICG to bind to the protein molecules in the urine (Fig. 3.6). Recent data also suggest that ICG injection alone is faster than with indwelling ureteral catheter placement and equally reliable at intraoperative ureteral identification [29]. Either way, injecting ICG will stain the urine green for the remain-

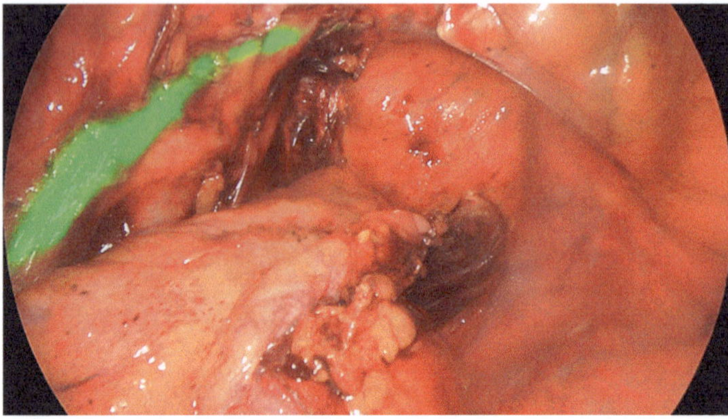

Fig. 3.6 To ensure long-standing visualization during surgery, the ureteral stent can be occluded for approximately 30 s to allow the indocyanine green (ICG) to bind to the protein molecules in the urine

der of the procedure, a fact of which nursing and anesthesia team should be aware.

Literature Review of Use of Fluorescence Guidance in Colorectal Surgery

In recent years, there have been an increasing number of publications regarding use of ICG fluorescence perfusion assessment in colorectal surgery and its effect on reducing anastomotic leak complications [30]. We will succinctly review the most significant and relevant articles (Table 3.2).

The earliest and one of the largest studies exploring the effect of ICG fluorescence perfusion assessment on anastomotic leak came from Germany by Kudzos et al. [38]. The ICG perfusion assessment study group, after matching, included 201 patients undergoing surgery for colorectal cancer between 2003 and 2008. The control group contained a similar number of patients operated between 1998 and 2003. The study included laparoscopic as well as open surgery and right colectomies, left colectomies, and low anterior resection (LAR). The study looked at clinically apparent

Table 3.2 Literature review of use of fluorescence guidance in colorectal surgery

Author/year	Study type	System used	No. of patients	Operations	Endpoint	Conclusions
Jafari (2015) [31]	PILLAR II—Prospective multicenter clinical trial, 11 centers	POINPOINT—Novadaq	139 assessed with ICG	Left-sided colectomy and anterior resection	*Primary:* Feasibility and safety; intraoperative decision-making *Secondary:* Clinical outcomes including anastomotic leak	8% change in surgical plan. Overall leak rate 1.4%. 0% leak rate in patients with revised anastomosis based on inadequate fluorescence
Ris (2018) [27]	Prospective phase II study, 3 centers	POINPOINT—Novadaq	504 assessed with ICG	Right hemicolectomy, high and low anterior resection, reversal of Hartmann's, ileoanal K pouch, and ileorectal anastomosis	*Primary:* Intraoperative decision-making *Secondary:* Anastomotic leak.	5.8% change in surgical plan. No anastomotic leaks in group with change in surgical plan. Overall leak rate for colorectal procedures 2.6%. Overall leak rate for low anterior resection 3%.

(continued)

Table 3.2 (continued)

Author/year	Study type	System used	No. of patients	Operations	Endpoint	Conclusions
Starker (2018) [32]	Retrospective, single center	PINPOINT—Novadaq	347 (238 ICG, 109 control)	Colectomy, anterior resection, reversal of Hartmann's	Anastomotic leakage or stricture	Non-PINPOINT group 5.5% anastomotic failure. PINPOINT group 0.84% anastomotic failure, 4.6% had change in resection margin based on fluorescence; none had anastomotic failure
De Nardi (2020) [33]	Multicenter	Karl Storz	240 (118 ICG, 122 control)	Left-sided and rectal resections	*Primary:* Anastomotic leak *Secondary:* Intraoperative decision-making	Anastomotic leak 9% in control group vs 5% in ICG group
Watanabe (2020_ [34]	Retrospective study, 3 centers	Karl Storz	422 (211 in each group, ICG vs control, propensity score matched)	Laparoscopic low anterior resections for rectal cancer	*Primary:* Anastomotic leak *Secondary:* Intraoperative change of surgical plan	For Clavien-Dindo grade ≥3 anastomotic leaks, leak rate 9.5% in control group and 2.8% in ICG group. OR 0.280 ($p = 0.007$)

Impellizzeri (2020) [26]	Retrospective study, 1 center	Karl Storz	196 (98 ICG, 98 control)	Left hemicolectomy, sigmoid colectomy, anterior resection	*Primary:* Anastomotic leak	Anastomotic leak 6% in control group, 0% in ICG group
Marquardt (2020) [35]	Retrospective study, 1 center	SPY—Novadaq/ Firefly for robotic	296 assessed with ICG	Right and left colectomy, anterior resection, Hartmann's reversal	*Primary:* Intraoperative decision-making *Secondary:* Anastomotic leak	Overall anastomotic leak rate 5.4%. For patients with low anterior resection, leak rate 4.5% compared to 13.6% in control group
Hasegawa (2020) [36]	Retrospective study, 1 center	Karl Storz/ Mizuho medical SPY—Stryker	420 (141 ICG, 279 control, propensity score matched)	Laparoscopic anterior resection or intersphincteric resection for rectal cancer	*Primary:* Anastomotic leak	Anastomotic leak 13.6% in control, 2.8% in ICG group
Yanagita (2021) [37]	Prospective collected data, retrospective analyzed study, 1 center	Karl Storz/ Mizuho Medical	384 (197 ICG, 187 control)	Left colectomy, anterior resection	*Primary:* Anastomotic leak	Anastomotic leak 10.7% in control group, 3.3% in ICG group

RCT randomized controlled trial, *ICG* indocyanine green, *OR* odds ratio. Reused with permission.

AL requiring surgical intervention and showed that this rate was lower in the ICG study group (3.5% vs 7.5%). Although this difference did not reach statistical significance, subgroup analysis revealed that in elective resections the rate of revision was 3.1% in the ICG study group compared to 7.7% in the control group ($p = 0.04$), amounting to a reduced risk of revision by 60%. This study is classified as level of evidence IV as it is a well-designed case-control study.

The first large-scale clinical trial that investigated the use of ICG fluorescence perfusion assessment and its impact on AL rate was the PILLAR II trial study [31]. This was a prospective, multicenter, open-label trial consisting of 139 patients who underwent intraoperative ICG perfusion assessment during left-sided colectomy and anterior resection. The most common indications were diverticulitis (44%), rectal cancer (25%), and colon cancer (21%). ICG perfusion assessment was successful in 99% of patients and dictated a change in the operative plan in 7.9%, with the majority of changes related to the transection of the proximal margin (7%). Overall anastomotic leak rate was quite low (1.4%), and there were no anastomotic leaks in those patients in which ICG dictated a change in surgical plan. This study is considered level of evidence III as it lacked randomization and included both left-sided resections and anterior resections, as well as laparoscopic and robotic procedures in its analysis.

Ris et al. [27] published a prospective phase II study which included 504 patients from three European referral centers who underwent elective colorectal surgery with anastomosis using ICG perfusion assessment over a 3-year interval. Indications for surgery included 330 patients with rectal cancer and 174 patients with benign pathology. ICG perfusion assessment was successful in all patients and dictated a change in the site of bowel resection margins in 5.8% of patients with no anastomotic leaks detected in this group of patients. Overall leak rates were again quite low (2.4%) including 2.6% for colorectal anastomosis and 3% for LAR anastomoses. When comparing this data to over 1000 similar procedures performed in the participating centers without ICG, they showed a reduced overall leak rate for colorectal procedures from 5.8 to 2.6%, and reduced the leak rate for LAR from 10.7 to 3%. This study is also considered level of evidence III as it lacked randomization and consisted of a relatively low proportion of low anterior resections (only 17.9% of the study group).

Starker et al. [32] described a retrospective single institution experience of 347 patients undergoing colectomy with primary anastomosis. Two hundred thirty-eight patients underwent intraoperative ICG perfusion assessment and 109 patients were in the control group. ICG perfusion assessment dictated a change in resection margin in 4.6% of patients, and none of these patients developed AL. Anastomotic leak rate was 0.84% in the ICG group and 5.5% in the control group. Since this publication was a retrospective descriptive study from a single center, it is assigned the level of evidence VI.

A more recent multicentered randomized controlled trial from Italy by De Nardi et al. [33] focused on patients undergoing laparoscopic left-sided colon resections and LAR for rectal cancer. After randomization, a total of 240 patients were included in the analysis, 118 in the ICG perfusion assessment study group and 122 in the control group. ICG perfusion assessment dictated a change in proximal resection margin in 11% of patients. AL rates were lower in the study group (5%) than in the control group (9%), but this difference was not statistically significant due to this study having been underpowered. This large multi-site randomized controlled trial is considered level II evidence.

Another larger multicenter retrospective study from Japan by Watanabe et al. [34] focused on the effect of ICG fluorescence perfusion assessment on reducing the risk of AL in LAR for rectal cancer. A total of 211 patients from three institutions were matched into the ICG study and the control group by propensity score. ICG perfusion assessment dictated a change in proximal resection margin in 5.7% of patients. The reported clinical leak rate was 9.5% in the control group and 2.8% in the ICG group. This well-designed case-control study is classified as level of evidence IV.

Four additional retrospective single center studies by Impellizzeri et al. [26], Yanagita et al. [37], Marquardt et al. [35], and Hasegawa et al. [36] looked at the effect of ICG fluorescence perfusion assessment in patients undergoing colon and rectal resections (summarized in Table 3.1). They all reported statistically significant reduced anastomotic leak rates in the ICG group compared to the control group. Since they were all single center descriptive non-randomized studies, they are classified as level of evidence VI.

A consensus conference statement on the general use of near-infrared fluorescence imaging and ICG-guided surgery showed the result of a modified Delphi study [39]. Experts from five continents reached consensus on 41 of 44 statements, including strong consensus that near-infrared fluorescence-guided surgery is both effective and safe across a broad variety of clinical settings, including the assessment of tissue perfusion and anastomotic leaks. This report of an expert committee is assigned a level of evidence VII. More recently, the results of an intercontinental Delphi survey including 35 experts from five continents regarding the use of fluorescence imaging and ICG during colorectal surgery were published [40]. At least 70% consensus was reached on 60 statements and all seven statements regarding ICG being used to assess anastomoses reached a consensus. There was a 100% consensus regarding that statement that confirming adequate perfusion of the anastomosis is a reason for ICG use during colorectal surgery. There was also a 96% consensus regarding the statement that use of ICG potentially decreases the risk of anastomotic leakage. Some of the statements also included a recommendation for using ICG to also assess right-sided anastomoses when there is indecision regarding adequate or optimal anastomosis perfusion or when there is significant atherosclerosis and mesenteric occlusion. This report of an expert committee is also assigned a level of evidence VII.

The most recently debated randomized controlled trial focusing on perfusion assessment in left-sided resections and LAR was the PILLAR III trial [41]. This multicenter study planned to recruit 450 to 1000 patients and randomize them with a 1:1 ratio. This study was concluded early because of decreasing accrual rates. A total of 25 centers recruited 347 patients, of whom 178 were randomly assigned to the ICG perfusion group and 169 to the control group. Anastomotic leak rate was 9.0% in the study group compared with 9.6% of standard ($p = 0.37$). Unfortunately, this trial was heavily underpowered as it was originally designed to enroll up to 1000 patients. Nevertheless, the level of evidence assigned for this well-designed albeit vastly underpowered RCT is level II.

Treatment of Metastatic Colorectal Cancer

Indocyanine green fluorescence imaging (ICG-FI) has recently emerged as a tool for the detection of metastatic lesions, primary tumors, and lymph nodes in several entities. In the following section, the opportunities for tumor detection in colorectal carcinoma (CRC) is reviewed.

Peritoneal Carcinomatosis

Cytoreductive surgery (CRS) combined with hyperthermic intraperitoneal chemotherapy (HIPEC) remains an important therapeutic option that prolongs overall survival (OS) in select patients with peritoneal carcinomatosis (PC) from colorectal carcinoma (CRC). To clinically quantify and classify PC, Paul Sugarbaker established the peritoneal carcinomatosis index (PCI) in 1966 [42]. The main goal of CRS is complete macroscopic resection of all peritoneal metastatic lesions [43–45].

Preoperative computed tomography (CT) and positron-emission tomography CT (PET-CT) scans to determine the extent of PC are unreliable. Sensitivities range between 30% to 47% for CT and 20% to 57% for PET-CT scans [46–49].

To achieve complete macroscopic resection, the intraoperative visualization of peritoneal metastatic lesions using ICG-FI has been investigated. Liberale and colleagues performed one of the first studies, including 17 patients in a prospective evaluation. In a pilot case, ICG was administered 24 h prior to surgery, analogous to the ICG administration procedure for hepatic lesions. In this study, there were no fluorescent signals from peritoneal lesions. The following patients received an intravenous dose of 0.25 mg/kg of body weight after initial exploration of the abdominal cavity. As a result, additional lesions that could not be detected under white light and manual palpation were identified in 4 out of 14 patients (29%) with non-mucinous colorectal cancer. Because of the associated hypervascularization of these lesions, they appeared to be isofluorescent or hyperfluorescent. Sensitivity and specificity were 87.5% and 100%, respectively. In contrast to the detection of lesions from non-mucinous tumors, sensitivity was 0% for mucinous tumors [50].

Likewise, Lieto et al. report an increased intraoperative detection sensitivity using ICG-FI in patients with PC from CRC. A total of 65 peritoneal lesions could be identified in the seven included patients. Sixteen lesions (25%) could not be identified by surgical exploration alone. The same dosage was used as in the previously described study. Analysis occurred at a median of 50 min after administration. Compared to the preoperative CT scan and the clinical evaluation, ICG-FI showed the highest sensitivity (43.1%, 76.9%, and 96.9%, respectively) [51].

Barabino et al. also reported the use of ICG-FI in patients with PC from CRC. They administered 0.25 mg of ICG per kg of body weight 24 h prior to surgery. The authors were unable to identify additional lesions, the sensitivity of ICG-FI was 72.4%, and the specificity was 60.0% [52].

In summary, there is currently little data with level V evidence on the intraoperative use of ICG-FI to detect peritoneal metastatic lesions from CRC [53], and the sensitivity and specificity vary greatly between studies. However, there is an overall benefit due to the potentially increased detection rate of PC lesions.

Taking these findings into consideration, we propose the intraoperative administration of ICG with a dose of 0.25 mg/kg of body weight before abdominal exploration. Injection after adhesiolysis or intrabdominal bleeding (associated with excretion of ICG) can make the subsequent detection of the PC impossible. Detection should be performed within 60 min after administration. The current literature suggests that ICG-FI might lead to the detection of additional lesions, especially in non-mucinous CRCs. Thus, the use of ICG-FI may result in a more accurate identification and resection of peritoneal metastatic lesions.

Liver Metastasis

The liver is the most common site of CRC metastasis [54, 55]. The recommended therapeutic approach for patients with synchronous or metachronous liver metastasis in the absence of extrahepatic metastatic lesions is an R0 resection if technically possible. There are several approaches including portal vein ligation, perioperative chemotherapy to downsize the lesions for resectability, and step-up approaches with sequential resections of bilobar metastasis. Preoperative high-resolution magnetic resonance imaging (MRI) and CT scans are recommended to determine the extent of metastasis [56–58]. Surgical resection of colorectal liver metastasis (CRLM) is associated with a prolonged 5-year OS (40%) and 10-year OS (25%) [56, 59].

Regarding preoperative imaging of CRLM, MRI is preferable to a CT scan. A recently published meta-analysis on the detection rate of CRLM with MRI showed a sensitivity and specificity of 90% and 88%, respectively [60]. For additional detection, intraoperative ultrasound (IOUS) is recommended, especially for lesions smaller than 10 mm in diameter, which are detected much more frequently using IOUS when compared to CT and MRI [61].

Fluorescence Pattern of CRLM

To understand the fluorescent appearance of CRLM after ICG injection, the mechanism of ICG metabolism in the liver parenchyma must be explained. ICG is physiologically excreted via the biliary tract starting several minutes after injection [62]. Due to this fact, there are different fluorescence patterns depending on the tumor entity. A study published in 2009 by Ishizawa and colleagues investigated the real-time identification of liver cancers using ICG-FI. A dose of 0.5 mg ICG per kg of body weight was administered between 1 and 7 days before surgical resection. A total of 91 resected hepatic lesions were analyzed and three different fluorescence patterns could be identified: a total fluorescent type with a homogeneous hyperfluorescence pattern, a partial fluorescent type with inhomogeneous fluorescence pattern, and a rim fluorescent type.

The last type shows no fluorescence in the lesion itself but rather surrounding fluorescence. In addition, the fluorescent type depended on the histopathological entity of the cancer. Well-differentiated hepatocellular carcinomas (HCC) showed a total fluorescence, while poorly differentiated HCCs and all 28 analyzed CRLMs showed a rim fluorescence [63].

This characteristic rim is a consequence of the biliary drainage obstruction due to the metastasis in the surrounding hepatocytes. On the other hand, well-differentiated HCCs show a dysfunction of biliary excretion [63, 64]. The fluorescence in the surrounding hepatocytes could be detected using a fluorescence microscope [65].

Dosage and Timing of Administration

ICG may be administered via a central or peripheral venous catheter; there is no need for a bolus prior to liver surgery. Different approaches regarding the administration timing of ICG range from 14 days to 24 h before the operation as the optimal timing remains unclear. The dosage recommendations also vary between a body weight-adapted dose of 0.1 mg/kg up to individual doses of 50 mg of ICG [46]. Van der Vorst et al. investigated different dosages and timings for the detection of CRLM with ICG-FI. They were not able to report a statistically significant difference between a dosage of 10 and 20 mg. There was also no significant difference between application 24 and 48 h prior to surgery [64].

We prefer the administration of 0.1 mg/kg 24 h prior to surgery via a peripheral venous catheter. This also has organizational rea-

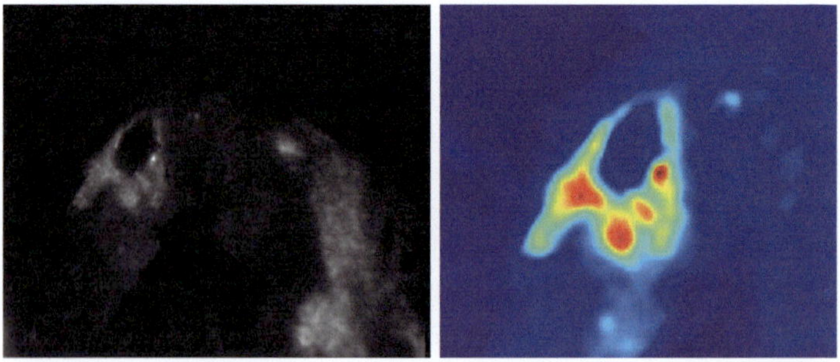

Fig. 3.7 Liver metastasis of colorectal cancer with typical fluorescent rim. Application of 0.02 mg/kg was performed 12 h before surgery

sons since most patients are admitted 1 day prior to surgery. The administration of the dye should take place at least 24 h prior to surgery to avoid interferences due to the biliary secretion of ICG. If the dye is applicated less than 24 h, we chose a dosage of 0.02 mg/kg 24 (Fig. 3.7).

Detection of Additional Metastatic Lesions

A lesion <10 mm is currently difficult to detect using preoperative diagnostics. Thus, additional diagnostic modalities, e.g., IOUS and ICG-FI, are becoming increasingly important in the surgical treatment of metastatic CRC.

Liberale and colleagues reviewed the available literature regarding ICG-FI for the intraoperative detection of CRLM. Ten publications published between 2009 and 2016 were included. Their results showed the smallest detectable lesions ranged from 1 to 5 mm in diameter. In 20 of the 130 patients, additional CRLM could be identified that were not detected preoperatively.

The detection sensitivity ranged between 69% and 100%. However, the sensitivity is limited by the depth, ranging from 5 to 10 mm below the liver capsule. The authors concluded that ICG-FI could be used as a diagnostic tool to detect additional lesions, especially combined with IOUS for lesions located deeper within the liver parenchyma [46].

Determination of Resection Margins Using ICG-FI

The resection margin is one of the most important factors influencing local recurrence and disease-free survival. Several studies have investigated ways to improve resection technique using ICG-FI. New systems, including robotic devices, enable real-time intraoperative navigation through combined ICG and white light images.

In a retrospective analysis of 86 patients undergoing ICG-FI-assisted surgery for CRLM compared to a control group of 87 patients, the ICG-FI group showed a 4-year liver-specific relapse-free survival of 47%, while the control group showed 39%. However, these results were not statistically significant due to an underpowered cohort size [66].

Nevertheless, in a pilot study on real-time surgical margin assessment using the previously described fluorescent rim as guidance, whole resection including the fluorescent area resulted in an improved rate of negative resection margins [67]. Aoki and colleagues also presented similar results. Twenty-five patients undergoing laparoscopic liver resection received ICG with a dose of 0.5 mg/kg of body weight 2–14 days before surgery. Seventeen of the 25 patients had CRLM. In comparison to the control group (72 patients from retrospective data), there were no R1 resection margins in the ICG group, indicating an advantage [68].

The reliability of the fluorescence resection margin was also investigated using a fluorescence microscope. In 72 cases of CRLM, the fluorescent rim could be microscopically identified in 50% of all cases. There were no malignant findings in the fluorescent rim. In conclusion, the fluorescent rim represents a reliable oncologic CRLM resection border [69].

Pulmonary Metastasis

The second most common CRC metastasis location is the lung [54, 55]. Limited pulmonary colorectal metastasis resection is a widely accepted surgical approach. However, the detection of pulmonary metastatic lesions remains challenging, especially during video-assisted thoracoscopic surgery (VATS).

There are very limited data on ICG-FI for pulmonary CRC metastasis. In a case series of eight patients, Keating and colleagues transferred results from previous experiments on mice to an in vivo study. A dose of 5 mg of ICG per kg of body weight was administered 24 h before surgery via a peripheral vein. Previously described pulmonary metastases presented as hyperfluorescent lesions. Furthermore, additional lesions could be identified in some cases [70]. As a limitation of the technology in terms of detectability, lesions deeper than 2 cm could not be displayed [65].

Lymphatic Mapping in Colorectal Cancer

Regional and distant lymph node status is one of the most important prognostic factors in malignant disease.

Sentinel lymph node (SLN) mapping is an important validated diagnostic marker for breast cancer and melanoma [71]. The diagnostic reliability in gastrointestinal cancers is still unclear and controversially discussed. Analogous to the total mesorectal excision (TME) for rectal cancers, the complete mesocolic excision (CME) technique for colonic cancers has become an increasingly popular practice in colorectal surgery. A key part of this technique is central vascular ligation with consecutive radical lymphadenectomy. Thus, the usefulness of SLN mapping in CRC remains unclear.

Morton et al. defined the sentinel lymph node as “the first lymph node that receives afferent lymphatic drainage from a primary tumor” [72]. The first benefit of SLN detection in CRC is to recognize aberrant lymphatic drainage, which has been reported in 2–29% of cases [71]. Second, complex lymphatic drainages may be mapped in flexure cancers, most likely leading to better surgical and oncological outcomes. Various methods have been reported for intraoperative SLN mapping. Methylene blue is the most common agent used to detect the SLN.

A randomized controlled trial highlighted that using indocyanine green instead of methylene blue in endometrial cancer significantly increased the lymph node detection rate per hemipelvis after intracervical injection of 2 ml ICG (1.25 mg/ml) [73]. This gave way to the first international guideline recommending the use of ICG for SLN mapping, in this case for endometrial cancer (Level II, A) [74].

Few studies exist describing an SLN mapping technique for CRC. Most studies are prospective case series with a low number of included patients. Currently, there is one level V meta-analysis published by Emile et al. in 2017 which discusses the topic in a well-founded manner.

They included 12 level VI case studies with a total of 248 patients [75]. The technical aspects of ICG administration in the included studies were found to be heterogenous. The authors of the underlying case studies used different ICG concentrations (0.5, 2.5, 5 mg/ml), doses (0.2–5 ml), injection sites (intravenous, submucosal, subserosal, a combination), and injection times (preoperative, intraoperative, preoperative, and intraoperative). Moreover, the time of detection differed from study to study (intraoperative, ex vivo, intraoperative and ex vivo). To determine the sensitivity, specificity, and accuracy of ICG-guided lymph node mapping, Emile et al. included the 1175 lymph nodes which were found to be metastatic. Of those included, 73% were fluorescent positive (n = 895) and 26% fluorescent negative (n = 315). This resulted in a median sensitivity of 73.7% and specificity of 100%. The positive predictive value was 100%, while the negative predictive value was 96.7%. The accuracy was found to be 75.7% (range 0–100%) [75]. Due to the variability of the underlying studies, these results must be interpretated carefully. To minimize the publication bias, the authors worked out pooled parameters. Pooled sensitivity was 71% (95% CI: 68.3–73.3%), while specificity was 84.6% (95% CI: 83.2–86%). A subgroup analysis by Emile et al. found that a weight-based dosage of 0.25 mg/kg had the highest sensitivity (89%) and accuracy rates (88%). Combined injection into the submucosa and subserosa achieved 100% rates of sensitivity, specificity, and accuracy. The optimal dosage timing is still unclear. In a second subgroup analysis, Emile and colleagues showed the characteristics of the CRC to be an important factor in diagnostic accuracy. ICG lymphatic mapping in early-stage cancers (stages I–II) shows a better diagnostic accuracy than in advanced stages [33]. Van der Zaag et al. showed similar findings in a meta-analysis discussing SLN mapping for CRC (without ICG) [76]. These findings are supported by Cahill et al., where in a meta-analysis, they described that 5% of stage T1/T2 CRCs showed false-negative SLNs, while stage T3/T4 CRCs showed 17% [77]. An explanation for this issue might be the tumor-associated obstruction of lymphatic vessels and nodes in advanced stages. The two included studies dealing with ICG lymphatic mapping in rectal cancers showed divergent results. Handgraaf et al. described a sensitivity of 0% [78], while Noura et al. had a sensitivity of 100% [79]. An explanation might be that none of the patients in the latter study received chemoradiotherapy or radiotherapy, while 90% in the first study did. This leads to the theory that neoadjuvant therapy in rectal cancer highly affects the diagnostic viability of ICG lymphatic mapping. Ultimately, there is little data and further investigations are needed.

A proof-of-concept study by Liberale et al. reported a detection of lymph nodes as small as 6 mm using 0.25 mg per kg of body weight intravenous ICG. The dye was injected directly after abdominal incision [80]. The authors confirmed these results in a retrospective study showing malignant lymph nodes to be more fluorescent than benign ones [81]. However, a sensitivity of only 63% was reached. Next, Liberale and coworkers published a feasibility study to evaluate the hypothesis that intravenous ICG injection allows for the detection and a pathological prognosis of metastatic lymph nodes [82].

Although local injection yields the best results according to the meta-analysis by Emile et al. [75], intravenous injection seems to be a more viable option. Accurate local injection requires experience and expertise, and the targeted structure might be missed. These two application techniques are principally different. Local administration gives an accurate picture of the lymphatic route. Intravenous injection works by ICG accumulation in tumor tissues due to the compromised endothelial barriers, which most likely leads to a better detection of malignant lymph nodes [80].

Based on these results, Cao and associates recently published a study using ICG-FI to evaluate the localization of and determine the tumor margin, map lymph nodes, and detect malignant lymph nodes [83]. They intravenously injected a bolus of 25 mg of ICG and took measurements at different points in time (0.5, 1, 2, 4, and 24 h). The tumor boundaries were found to be apparent 1 h after injection, but clearest after 2–4 h. According to the tumor signal-to-background ratio (SBR), optimal visualization occurred 2 h after injection. In the same study, the authors mapped a total of 40 lymph nodes. All lymph nodes were detected by ICG from 0.5 up to 5 h after injection. A minimum SBR of 1.13 showed a detection rate of 95% for any lymph node (38/40). The optimal SBR threshold for metastatic lymph nodes was found to be 2.5 according to the Youden Index (sensitivity 80.0%, specificity 48.6%). They concluded that it was not possible to differentiate between meta-

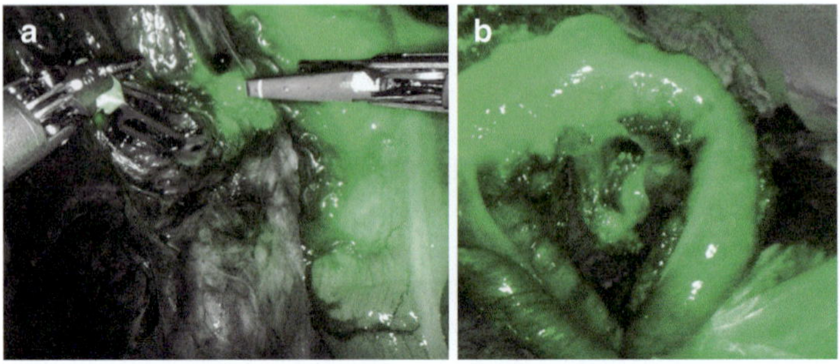

Fig. 3.8 (**a**) Sentinel lymph node after submucosal application of 1 mg indocyanine green (ICG) in a case of colonic cancer. Injection is performed endoscopically 24 h before surgery If the tumor can be passed, four spots are injected around the tumor (two oral, two aboral). (**b**) ICG application used for tumor and sentinel lymph node detection

static and nonmetastatic lymph nodes using the SBR technique. Unfortunately, the authors did not further investigate the correlation between injection timing and lymph node detection accuracy. According to these studies, using this technique accurately detects the tumor as well as most of the lymph nodes.

All in all, the existing studies are too inhomogeneous with few cases and low evidence, leading to a low reliability. Thus, the results must be interpreted carefully. Data suggests that a dosage of 0.25 mg/kg of body weight results in the highest sensitivity, specificity, and accuracy. Preoperative injection into both the subserosa and submucosa showed the best detection rates (Fig. 3.8), followed by intravenous injection [75]. However, intravenous injection prior to surgery is more easily standardized and reliable. The data also suggest that after intravenous ICG injection, the fluorescence may be used for tumor detection and lymphatic mapping without additional doses. The timing of injection remains unclear and depends strongly on which form of application is used. Further studies are needed to confirm these preliminary data and to establish a standardized technique for CRC lymphatic mapping. To that extent, in a recently published intercontinental Delphi survey, no consensus was reached on the value of ICG use for mapping of sentinel node, and the only consensus achieved for lymph node assessment was that two to four injection points are required [40].

Future Perspectives: Fluorescence-Guided Tumor Targeting

The current detection of sentinel or additional lymph nodes and colorectal metastasis is based on fluorescence patterns. However, although there are data that fluorescence intensity correlates with pathologic findings, it remains unspecific. Lately, there have been innovative approaches to identify additional lesions in a more targeted manner. Overall, there are multiple different molecular targets that can be addressed [84].

Regarding the more specific detection of additional colorectal lesions, SGM-101 should be mentioned. SGM-101 is a fluorescent dye-conjugated antibody against carcinoembryonic antigen (CEA) [85]. In a recently published clinical trial on the detection of colorectal and pancreatic liver metastasis, SGM-101 was administered 2 to 4 days prior to surgery. Nineteen lesions were detected, 17 of which were histopathologically confirmed malignant lesions [86]. In a similar approach, Harlaar and co-authors investigated a fluorescent dye conjugated to bevacizumab in patients with PC from CRC. The idea behind the study is the hyperexpression of vascular epithelial growth factor (VEGF) in PC from CRC. Bevacizumab is a monoclonal antibody against VEGF, and therefore, after conjugation of the fluorescent dye to bevacizumab, PC fluorescence may be achieved. The study showed that lesions without fluorescence were benign; however, lesions with hyperfluorescence were false-positive in 47% of cases [87].

Conclusion

Although there is still an ongoing debate, it appears that ICG fluorescence perfusion assessment may be beneficial in lowering the risk for AL. This technology has been proven to be safe, cost-effective, easy to implement, readily available, and effective in the evaluation of bowel perfusion. The data also suggest that preoperative ICG injection may be used for tumor detection and lymphatic mapping. ICG may also be used to detect additional CRLM and its fluorescent rim represents a reliable oncologic CRLM resection border. Targeted fluorescence is a promising approach and future goal of ICG-FI in oncological surgery. Additional study results are necessary for further evaluation of this technology.

References

1. 2015 European Society of Coloproctology Collaborating Group. The relationship between method of anastomosis and anastomotic failure after right hemicolectomy and ileo-caecal resection: an international snapshot audit. Color Dis. 2017;19(8):e296–311.
2. Phitayakorn R, Delaney ACP, Reynolds AHL, Champagne ABJ, Heriot AAG, Neary AP, et al. Standardized algorithms for management of anastomotic leaks and related abdominal and pelvic abscesses after colorectal surgery. World J Surg. 2008;32(6):1147–56.
3. McDermott FD, Heeney A, Kelly ME, Steele RJ, Carlson GL, Winter DC. Systematic review of preoperative, intraoperative and postoperative risk factors for colorectal anastomotic leaks. Br J Surg. 2015;102(5):462–79.
4. Branagan G, Finnis D, Wessex Colorectal Cancer Audit Working Group. Prognosis after anastomotic leakage in colorectal surgery. Dis Colon Rectum. 2005;48(5):1021–6.
5. Karliczek A, Benaron DA, Baas PC, Zeebregts CJ, Wiggers T, van Dam GM. Intraoperative assessment of microperfusion with visible light spectroscopy for prediction of anastomotic leakage in colorectal anastomoses. Color Dis. 2010;12(10):1018–25.
6. Ashraf SQ, Burns EM, Jani A, Altman S, Young JD, Cunningham C, Faiz O, Mortensen NJ. The economic impact of anastomotic leakage after anterior resections in English NHS hospitals: are we adequately remunerating them? Color Dis. 2013;15(4):e190–8.
7. Caulfield H, Hyman NH. Anastomotic leak after low anterior resection: a spectrum of clinical entities. JAMA Surg. 2013;148(2):177–82.
8. Senagore A, Lane FR, Lee E, Wexner S, Dujovny N, Sklow B, Rider P, Bonello J, Bioabsorbable Staple Line Reinforcement Study Group. Bioabsorbable staple line reinforcement in restorative proctectomy and

anterior resection: a randomized study. Dis Colon Rectum. 2014;57(3):324–30.
9. Mongin C, Maggiori L, Agostini J, Ferron M, Panis Y. Does anastomotic leakage impair functional results and quality of life after laparoscopic sphincter-saving total mesorectal excision for rectal cancer? A case-matched study. Int J Color Dis. 2014;29(4):459–67.
10. Leahy J, Schoetz D, Marcello P, Read T, Hall J, Roberts P, Ricciardi R. What is the risk of clinical anastomotic leak in the diverted colorectal anastomosis? J Gastrointest Surg. 2014;18(10):1812–6.
11. Shiomi A, Ito M, Maeda K, Kinugasa Y, Ota M, Yamaue H, Shiozawa M, Horie H, Kuriu Y, Saito N. Effects of a diverting stoma on symptomatic anastomotic leakage after low anterior resection for rectal cancer: a propensity score matching analysis of 1,014 consecutive patients. J Am Coll Surg. 2015;220(2):186–94.
12. Borstlap WAA, Westerduin E, Aukema TS, Bemelman WA, Tanis PJ, Dutch Snapshot Research Group. Anastomotic leakage and chronic presacral sinus formation after Low anterior resection: results from a large cross-sectional study. Ann Surg. 2017;266(5):870–7.
13. Detering R, Roodbeen SX, van Oostendorp SE, Dekker JT, Sietses C, Bemelman WA, Tanis PJ, Hompes R, Tuynman JB, Dutch ColoRectal Cancer Audit Group. Three-year nationwide experience with transanal total mesorectal excision for rectal cancer in the Netherlands: a propensity score-matched comparison with conventional laparoscopic total mesorectal excision. J Am Coll Surg. 2019, 228;(3):235–244.e1.
14. Furnée EJB, Aukema TS, Oosterling SJ, Borstlap WAA, Bemelman WA, Tanis PJ, Dutch Snapshot Research Group. Influence of conversion and anastomotic leakage on survival in rectal cancer surgery; retrospective cross-sectional study. J Gastrointest Surg. 2019;23(10):2007–18.
15. McArdle CS, McMillan DC, Hole DJ. Impact of anastomotic leakage on long-term survival of patients undergoing curative resection for colorectal cancer. Br J Surg. 2005;92(9):1150–4.
16. Nesbakken A, Nygaard K, Lunde OC. Outcome and late functional results after anastomotic leakage following mesorectal excision for rectal cancer. Br J Surg. 2001;88(3):400–4.
17. Hammond J, Lim S, Wan Y, Gao X, Patkar A. The burden of gastrointestinal anastomotic leaks: an evaluation of clinical and economic outcomes. J Gastrointest Surg. 2014;18(6):1176–85.
18. Bertelsen CA, Andreasen AH, Jørgensen T, Harling H, Danish Colorectal Cancer Group. Anastomotic leakage after anterior resection for rectal cancer: risk factors. Color Dis. 2010;12(1):37–43.
19. Park JS, Choi GS, Kim SH, Kim HR, Kim NK, Lee KY, Kang SB, Kim JY, Lee KY, Kim BC, Bae BN, Son GM, Lee SI, Kang H. Multicenter analysis of risk factors for anastomotic leakage after laparoscopic rectal cancer excision: the Korean laparoscopic colorectal surgery study group. Ann Surg. 2013;257(4):665–71.

20. Trencheva K, Morrissey KP, Wells M, Mancuso CA, Lee SW, Sonoda T, Michelassi F, Charlson ME, Milsom JW. Identifying important predictors for anastomotic leak after colon and rectal resection: prospective study on 616 patients. Ann Surg. 2013;257(1):108–13.
21. Markus PM, Martell J, Leister I, Horstmann O, Brinker J, Becker H. Predicting postoperative morbidity by clinical assessment. Br J Surg. 2005;92(1):101–6.
22. Karliczek A, Harlaar NJ, Zeebregts CJ, Wiggers T, Baas PC, van Dam GM. Surgeons lack predictive accuracy for anastomotic leakage in gastrointestinal surgery. Int J Color Dis. 2009;24(5):569–76.
23. Boni L, David G, Mangano A, Dionigi G, Rausei S, Spampatti S, et al. Clinical applications of indocyanine green (ICG) enhanced fluorescence in laparoscopic surgery. Surg Endosc. 2015;29(7):2046–55.
24. Boni L, David G, Dionigi G, Rausei S, Cassinotti E, Fingerhut A. Indocyanine green-enhanced fluorescence to assess bowel perfusion during laparoscopic colorectal resection. Surg Endosc. 2016;30(7):2736–42.
25. Mizrahi I, Abu-Gazala M, Rickles AS, Fernandez LM, Petrucci A, Wolf J, et al. Indocyanine green fluorescence angiography during low anterior resection for low rectal cancer: results of a comparative cohort study. Tech Coloproctol. 2018;22(7):535–40.
26. Impellizzeri HG, Pulvirenti A, Inama M, Bacchion M, Marrano E, Creciun M, Casaril A, Moretto G. Near-infrared fluorescence angiography for colorectal surgery is associated with a reduction of anastomotic leak rate. Updat Surg. 2020;72(4):991–8.
27. Ris F, Liot E, Buchs NC, Kraus R, Ismael G, Belfontali V, Douissard J, Cunningham C, Lindsey I, Guy R, Jones O, George B, Morel P, Mortensen NJ, Hompes R, Cahill RA, Near-Infrared Anastomotic Perfusion Assessment Network VOIR. Multicentre phase II trial of near-infrared imaging in elective colorectal surgery. Br J Surg. 2018;105(10):1359–67.
28. Siddighi S, Yune JJ, Hardesty J. Indocyanine green for intraoperative localization of ureter. Am J Obstet Gynecol. 2014;211(4):436.e1–2.
29. Soriano CR, Cheng RR, Corman JM, Moonka R, Simianu VV, Kaplan JA. Feasibility of injected indocyanine green for ureteral identification during robotic left-sided colorectal resections. Am J Surg. 2021:S0002-9610(21)00392-5.
30. Yeung TM. Fluorescence imaging in colorectal surgery. Surg Endosc. 2021;35(9):4956–63.
31. Jafari MD, Wexner SD, Martz JE, McLemore EC, Margolin DA, Sherwinter DA, Lee SW, Senagore AJ, Phelan MJ, Stamos MJ. Perfusion assessment in laparoscopic left-sided/anterior resection (PILLAR II): a multi-institutional study. J Am Coll Surg. 2015;220(1):82–92.e1.
32. Starker PM, Chinn B. Using outcomes data to justify instituting new technology: a single institution's experience. Surg Endosc. 2018;32(3):1586–92.

33. De Nardi P, Elmore U, Maggi G, Maggiore R, Boni L, Cassinotti E, Fumagalli U, Gardani M, De Pascale S, Parise P, Vignali A, Rosati R. Intraoperative angiography with indocyanine green to assess anastomosis perfusion in patients undergoing laparoscopic colorectal resection: results of a multicenter randomized controlled trial. Surg Endosc. 2020;34(1):53–60.
34. Watanabe J, Ishibe A, Suwa Y, Suwa H, Ota M, Kunisaki C, Endo I. Indocyanine green fluorescence imaging to reduce the risk of anastomotic leakage in laparoscopic low anterior resection for rectal cancer: a propensity score-matched cohort study. Surg Endosc. 2020;34(1):202–8.
35. Marquardt C, Kalev G, Schiedeck T. Intraoperative fluorescence angiography with indocyanine green: retrospective evaluation and detailed analysis of our single-center 5-year experience focused on colorectal surgery. Innov Surg Sci. 2020;5(1–2):35–42.
36. Hasegawa H, Tsukada Y, Wakabayashi M, Nomura S, Sasaki T, Nishizawa Y, Ikeda K, Akimoto T, Ito M. Impact of intraoperative indocyanine green fluorescence angiography on anastomotic leakage after laparoscopic sphincter-sparing surgery for malignant rectal tumors. Int J Color Dis. 2020;35(3):471–80.
37. Yanagita T, Hara M, Osaga S, Nakai N, Maeda Y, Shiga K, Hirokawa T, Matsuo Y, Takahashi H, Takiguchi S. Efficacy of intraoperative ICG fluorescence imaging evaluation for preventing anastomotic leakage after left-sided colon or rectal cancer surgery: a propensity score-matched analysis. Surg Endosc. 2021;35(5):2373–85.
38. Kudszus S, Roesel C, Schachtrupp A, Höer JJ. Intraoperative laser fluorescence angiography in colorectal surgery: a noninvasive analysis to reduce the rate of anastomotic leakage. Langenbeck's Arch Surg. 2010;395(8):1025–30.
39. Dip F, Boni L, Bouvet M, Carus T, Diana M, Falco J, Gurtner GC, Ishizawa T, Kokudo N, Lo Menzo E, Low PS, Masia J, Muehrcke D, Papay FA, Pulitano C, Schneider-Koraith S, Sherwinter D, Spinoglio G, Stassen L, Urano Y, Vahrmeijer A, Vibert E, Warram J, Wexner SD, White K, Rosenthal RJ. Consensus conference statement on the general use of near-infrared fluorescence imaging and indocyanine green guided surgery: results of a modified Delphi study. Ann Surg. 2022;275(4):685–91.
40. Wexner S, Abu-Gazala M, Boni L, et al. Use of fluorescence imaging and indocyanine green during colorectal surgery: results of an intercontinental Delphi survey. Surgery. 2022;172(6S):S38–45.
41. Jafari MD, Pigazzi A, McLemore EC, Mutch MG, Haas E, Rasheid SH, Wait AD, Paquette IM, Bardakcioglu O, Safar B, Landmann RG, Varma MG, Maron DJ, Martz J, Bauer JJ, George VV, Fleshman JW Jr, Steele SR, Stamos MJ. Perfusion assessment in left-sided/Low anterior resection (PILLAR III): a randomized, controlled, parallel, multicenter study assessing perfusion outcomes with PINPOINT near-infrared fluorescence

imaging in low anterior resection. Dis Colon Rectum. 2021;64(8):995–1002.
42. Jacquet P, Sugarbaker PH. Clinical research methodologies in diagnosis and staging of patients with peritoneal carcinomatosis. Cancer Treat Res. 1996;82:359–74.
43. Quenet F, Elias D, Roca L, Goere D, Ghouti L, Pocard M, et al. Cytoreductive surgery plus hyperthermic intraperitoneal chemotherapy versus cytoreductive surgery alone for colorectal peritoneal metastases (PRODIGE 7): a multicentre, randomised, open-label, phase 3 trial. Lancet Oncol. 2021;22(2):256–66.
44. Esquivel J. Cytoreductive surgery and hyperthermic intraperitoneal chemotherapy for colorectal cancer: survival outcomes and patient selection. J Gastrointest Oncol. 2016;7(1):72–8.
45. Vassos N, Piso P. Metastatic colorectal cancer to the peritoneum: current treatment options. Curr Treat Options in Oncol. 2018;19(10):49.
46. Liberale G, Bourgeois P, Larsimont D, Moreau M, Donckier V, Ishizawa T. Indocyanine green fluorescence-guided surgery after IV injection in metastatic colorectal cancer: a systematic review. Eur J Surg Oncol. 2017;43(9):1656–67.
47. De Vos N, Goethals I, Ceelen W. Clinical value of (18)F-FDG- PET-CT in the preoperative staging of peritoneal carcinomatosis from colorectal origin. Acta Chir Belg. 2014;114(6):370–5.
48. Dromain C, Leboulleux S, Auperin A, Goere D, Malka D, Lumbroso J, et al. Staging of peritoneal carcinomatosis: enhanced CT vs. PET/CT Abdom Imaging. 2008;33(1):87–93.
49. Pasqual EM, Bertozzi S, Bacchetti S, Londero AP, Basso SM, Santeufemia DA, et al. Preoperative assessment of peritoneal carcinomatosis in patients undergoing hyperthermic intraperitoneal chemotherapy following cytoreductive surgery. Anticancer Res. 2014;34(5):2363–8.
50. Liberale G, Vankerckhove S, Caldon MG, Ahmed B, Moreau M, Nakadi IE, et al. Fluorescence imaging after indocyanine green injection for detection of peritoneal metastases in patients undergoing cytoreductive surgery for peritoneal carcinomatosis from colorectal cancer: a pilot study. Ann Surg. 2016;264(6):1110–5.
51. Lieto E, Auricchio A, Cardella F, Mabilia A, Basile N, Castellano P, et al. Fluorescence-guided surgery in the combined treatment of peritoneal carcinomatosis from colorectal cancer: preliminary results and considerations. World J Surg. 2018;42(4):1154–60.
52. Barabino G, Klein JP, Porcheron J, Grichine A, Coll JL, Cottier M. Intraoperative near-infrared fluorescence imaging using indocyanine green in colorectal carcinomatosis surgery: proof of concept. Eur J Surg Oncol. 2016;42(12):1931–7.
53. Baiocchi GL, Gheza F, Molfino S, Arru L, Vaira M, Giacopuzzi S. Indocyanine green fluorescence-guided intraoperative detection of peritoneal carcinomatosis: systematic review. BMC Surg. 2020;20(1):158.

54. Robinson JR, Newcomb PA, Hardikar S, Cohen SA, Phipps AI. Stage IV colorectal cancer primary site and patterns of distant metastasis. Cancer Epidemiol. 2017;48:92–5.
55. van Gestel YR, de Hingh IH, van Herk-Sukel MP, van Erning FN, Beerepoot LV, Wijsman JH, et al. Patterns of metachronous metastases after curative treatment of colorectal cancer. Cancer Epidemiol. 2014;38(4):448–54.
56. Fong Y, Fortner J, Sun RL, Brennan MF, Blumgart LH. Clinical score for predicting recurrence after hepatic resection for metastatic colorectal cancer: analysis of 1001 consecutive cases. Ann Surg. 1999;230(3):309–18; discussion 18–21.
57. Van Cutsem E, Cervantes A, Adam R, Sobrero A, Van Krieken JH, Aderka D, et al. ESMO consensus guidelines for the management of patients with metastatic colorectal cancer. Ann Oncol. 2016;27(8):1386–422.
58. Adam R, De Gramont A, Figueras J, Guthrie A, Kokudo N, Kunstlinger F, et al. The oncosurgery approach to managing liver metastases from colorectal cancer: a multidisciplinary international consensus. Oncologist. 2012;17(10):1225–39.
59. Rees M, Tekkis PP, Welsh FK, O'Rourke T, John TG. Evaluation of long-term survival after hepatic resection for metastatic colorectal cancer: a multifactorial model of 929 patients. Ann Surg. 2008;247(1):125–35.
60. Mao Y, Chen B, Wang H, Zhang Y, Yi X, Liao W, et al. Diagnostic performance of magnetic resonance imaging for colorectal liver metastasis: a systematic review and meta-analysis. Sci Rep. 2020;10(1):1969.
61. Ellebaek SB, Fristrup CW, Mortensen MB. Intraoperative ultrasound as a screening modality for the detection of liver metastases during resection of primary colorectal cancer - a systematic review. Ultrasound Int Open. 2017;3(2):E60–E8.
62. Reinhart MB, Huntington CR, Blair LJ, Heniford BT, Augenstein VA. Indocyanine green: historical context, current applications, and future considerations. Surg Innov. 2016;23(2):166–75.
63. Ishizawa T, Fukushima N, Shibahara J, Masuda K, Tamura S, Aoki T, et al. Real-time identification of liver cancers by using indocyanine green fluorescent imaging. Cancer. 2009;115(11):2491–504.
64. van der Vorst JR, Schaafsma BE, Hutteman M, Verbeek FP, Liefers GJ, Hartgrink HH, et al. Near-infrared fluorescence-guided resection of colorectal liver metastases. Cancer. 2013;119(18):3411–8.
65. Okusanya OT, Holt D, Heitjan D, Deshpande C, Venegas O, Jiang J, et al. Intraoperative near-infrared imaging can identify pulmonary nodules. Ann Thorac Surg. 2014;98(4):1223–30.
66. Handgraaf HJM, Boogerd LSF, Hoppener DJ, Peloso A, Sibinga Mulder BG, Hoogstins CES, et al. Long-term follow-up after near-infrared fluorescence-guided resection of colorectal liver metastases: a retrospective multicenter analysis. Eur J Surg Oncol. 2017;43(8):1463–71.

67. Achterberg FB, Sibinga Mulder BG, Meijer RPJ, Bonsing BA, Hartgrink HH, Mieog JSD, et al. Real-time surgical margin assessment using ICG-fluorescence during laparoscopic and robot-assisted resections of colorectal liver metastases. Ann Transl Med. 2020;8(21):1448.
68. Aoki T, Murakami M, Koizumi T, Matsuda K, Fujimori A, Kusano T, et al. Determination of the surgical margin in laparoscopic liver resections using infrared indocyanine green fluorescence. Langenbeck's Arch Surg. 2018;403(5):671–80.
69. Tashiro Y, Aoki T, Hirai T, Koizumi T, Mansou DA, Kusano T, et al. Pathological validity of using near-infrared fluorescence imaging for securing surgical margins during liver resection. Anticancer Res. 2020;40(7):3873–82.
70. Keating J, Newton A, Venegas O, Nims S, Zeh R, Predina J, et al. Near-infrared intraoperative molecular imaging can locate metastases to the lung. Ann Thorac Surg. 2017;103(2):390–8.
71. Tuech JJ, Pessaux P, Regenet N, Bergamaschi R, Colson A. Sentinel lymph node mapping in colon cancer. Surg Endosc. 2004;18(12):1721–9.
72. Morton DL, Wen DR, Wong JH, Economou JS, Cagle LA, Storm FK, et al. Technical details of intraoperative lymphatic mapping for early stage melanoma. Arch Surg. 1992;127(4):392–9.
73. Rozenholc A, Samouelian V, Warkus T, Gauthier P, Provencher D, Sauthier P, et al. Green versus blue: randomized controlled trial comparing indocyanine green with methylene blue for sentinel lymph node detection in endometrial cancer. Gynecol Oncol. 2019;153(3):500–4.
74. Concin N, Matias-Guiu X, Vergote I, Cibula D, Mirza MR, Marnitz S, et al. ESGO/ESTRO/ESP guidelines for the management of patients with endometrial carcinoma. Int J Gynecol Cancer. 2020;31(1):12–39.
75. Emile SH, Elfeki H, Shalaby M, Sakr A, Sileri P, Laurberg S, et al. Sensitivity and specificity of indocyanine green near-infrared fluorescence imaging in detection of metastatic lymph nodes in colorectal cancer: systematic review and meta-analysis. J Surg Oncol. 2017;116(6):730–40.
76. van der Zaag ES, Bouma WH, Tanis PJ, Ubbink DT, Bemelman WA, Buskens CJ. Systematic review of sentinel lymph node mapping procedure in colorectal cancer. Ann Surg Oncol. 2012;19(11):3449–59.
77. Cahill RA, Bembenek A, Sirop S, Waterhouse DF, Schneider W, Leroy J, et al. Sentinel node biopsy for the individualization of surgical strategy for cure of early-stage colon cancer. Ann Surg Oncol. 2009;16(8):2170–80.
78. Handgraaf HJ, Boogerd LS, Verbeek FP, Tummers QR, Hardwick JC, Baeten CI, et al. Intraoperative fluorescence imaging to localize tumors and sentinel lymph nodes in rectal cancer. Minim Invasive Ther Allied Technol. 2016;25(1):48–53.
79. Noura S, Ohue M, Seki Y, Tanaka K, Motoori M, Kishi K, et al. Feasibility of a lateral region sentinel node biopsy of lower rectal cancer guided by

indocyanine green using a near-infrared camera system. Ann Surg Oncol. 2010;17(1):144–51.
80. Liberale G, Vankerckhove S, Galdon MG, Donckier V, Larsimont D, Bourgeois P. Fluorescence imaging after intraoperative intravenous injection of indocyanine green for detection of lymph node metastases in colorectal cancer. Eur J Surg Oncol. 2015;41(9):1256–60.
81. Liberale G, Galdon MG, Moreau M, Vankerckhove S, El Nakadi I, Larsimont D, et al. Ex vivo detection of tumoral lymph nodes of colorectal origin with fluorescence imaging after intraoperative intravenous injection of indocyanine green. J Surg Oncol. 2016;114(3):348–53.
82. Liberale G, Vankerckhove S, Bouazza F, Gomez Galdon M, Larsimont D, Moreau M, et al. Systemic sentinel lymph node detection using fluorescence imaging after Indocyanine green intravenous injection in colorectal cancer: protocol for a feasibility study. JMIR Res Protoc. 2020;9(8):e17976.
83. Cao Y, Wang P, Wang Z, Zhang W, Lu Q, Butch CJ, et al. A pilot study of near-infrared fluorescence guided surgery for primary tumor localization and lymph node mapping in colorectal cancer. Ann Transl Med. 2021;9(16):1342.
84. Hernot S, van Manen L, Debie P, Mieog JSD, Vahrmeijer AL. Latest developments in molecular tracers for fluorescence image-guided cancer surgery. Lancet Oncol. 2019;20(7):e354–e67.
85. Gutowski M, Framery B, Boonstra MC, Garambois V, Quenet F, Dumas K, et al. SGM-101: an innovative near-infrared dye-antibody conjugate that targets CEA for fluorescence-guided surgery. Surg Oncol. 2017;26(2):153–62.
86. Meijer RPJ, de Valk KS, Deken MM, Boogerd LSF, Hoogstins CES, Bhairosingh SS, et al. Intraoperative detection of colorectal and pancreatic liver metastases using SGM-101, a fluorescent antibody targeting CEA. Eur J Surg Oncol. 2021;47(3 Pt B):667–73.
87. Harlaar NJ, Koller M, de Jongh SJ, van Leeuwen BL, Hemmer PH, Kruijff S, et al. Molecular fluorescence-guided surgery of peritoneal carcinomatosis of colorectal origin: a single-centre feasibility study. Lancet Gastroenterol Hepatol. 2016;1(4):283–90.

Use of Fluorescence Guidance in Cholecystectomy

4

Ryan C. Broderick, David Renton, and Santiago Horgan

Introduction

Laparoscopic cholecystectomy (LC) is widely accepted as the standard of care for cholecystectomy. It is currently the most commonly performed procedure performed by general surgeons in the United States. Bile duct injuries in the era of laparoscopic cholecystectomy range from 0.03% to 0.5% [1–4]. While infrequent, they represent a significant patient and healthcare burden when these injuries occur. Cost of treating bile duct injuries can be 4.5 to 26 times the cost of an uncomplicated procedure with an average 32-day hospitalization and significant mortality rate [5].

Supplementary Information The online version contains supplementary material available at https://doi.org/10.1007/978-3-031-40685-0_4.

R. C. Broderick (✉) · S. Horgan
Division of Minimally Invasive Surgery, Department of Surgery, University of California San Diego, La Jolla, CA, USA
e-mail: rbroderick@health.ucsd.edu; shorgan@health.ucsd.edu

D. Renton
Center for Minimally Invasive Surgery, The Ohio State University Wexner Medical Center, Columbus, OH, USA
e-mail: david.renton@osumc.edu

N. Szoka et al. (eds.), *The SAGES Manual of Fluorescence-Guided Surgery*, https://doi.org/10.1007/978-3-031-40685-0_4

Indocyanine green (ICG) dye is a water-soluble dye with spectral absorption at 800 nm. It has been described visualizing the biliary tree since 2008 [6]. When injected intravenously, ICG binds plasma proteins before being rapidly metabolized by hepatocytes and excreted exclusively into the bile; protein-bound ICG fluoresces green when illuminated with near-infrared (NIR) light [6–9]. The excretion of ICG into the biliary tree peaks at 2–4 h after intravenous injection [10]. Dynamic, real-time NIR light capability is built-in to many modern laparoscopic and robotic cameras. As described elsewhere in this manual, there are also cameras designed to image ICG in open surgery. These cameras are able to toggle between white-light and NIR light with the push of a button, allowing real-time imaging without disrupting surgical workflow, especially in the case of laparoscopic or robotic surgery (Figs. 4.1, 4.2, and 4.3; video clip attached for video chapter). The technology incorporates smoothly into the operation without increased need for staffing or additional supplies in the operative theater.

Through constant reassessment of the anatomy with NIR imaging, surgeons may continuously identify the position of critical biliary structures; these structures are often identifiable prior to dissection of peritoneal layer of the gallbladder, providing a safe dissection starting point as well as areas of critical importance. FC offers the potential detailed anatomical mapping of extrahepatic biliary structures and can be a useful adjunct to the critical view of safety [6–14]. FC allows for surgeons to identify either normal anatomy or anatomic variation prior to dissection

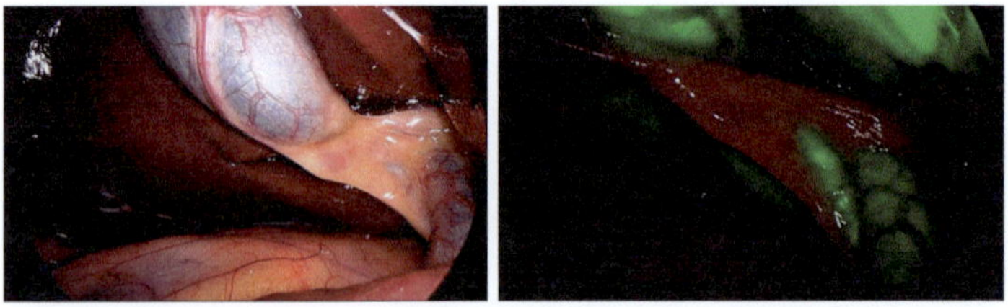

Fig. 4.1 Top panel: white-light laparoscopic view of gallbladder during cholecystectomy. Bottom panel: "overlay mode" ICG view of same patient showing cystic duct and common bile duct junction

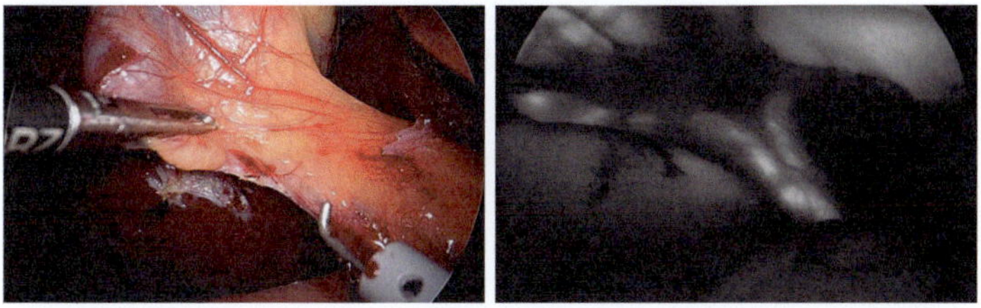

Fig. 4.2 Top panel: white-light laparoscopic view of gallbladder during cholecystectomy prior to peritoneal dissection. Bottom panel: "gray mode" ICG view of same image showing cystic duct, common bile duct, and junction

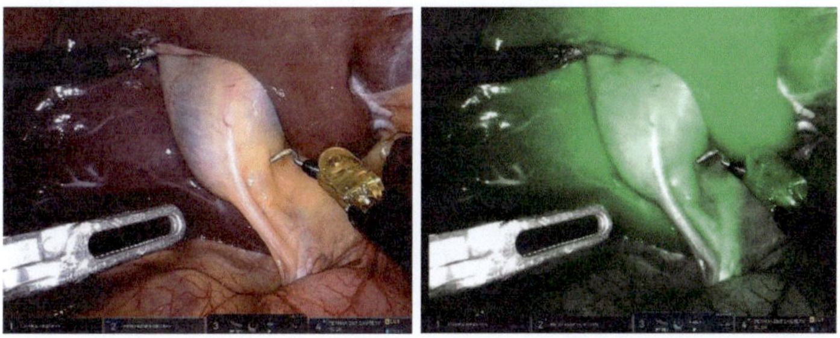

Fig. 4.3 Use of fluorescence cholangiography in robotic surgery. Left panel is traditional bright light view. Right panel is ICG mode highlighting cystic duct, CBD, and CD-CBD junction

and during active dissection. In contrast, IOC can be time consuming and involves exposure of the patient and ancillary staff to radiation, with associated increases in cost [15].

Literature Review

Ishizawa et al. described their laparoscopic experience with preoperative ICG injection for cholangiography during cholecystectomy, demonstrating a 100% visualization of the cystic duct and 96% visualization of the common hepatic duct prior to any dissection, which improved to 100% visualization of both structures with dissection [7]. Several other groups have demonstrated simi-

Table 4.1 Fluorescence cholangiography in laparoscopic cholecystectomy in literature. Reported common bile duct injuries and level of evidence for each study

First author (year)	Total patients	Bile duct injuries	Adverse reactions	Conversions to open	Level of evidence
Ishizawa (2010)	52	0	0	–	IV
Boni (2015)	52	0	0		IV
Dip (2015)	45	0	0		IV
Osayi (2015)	82	0	0		IV
van Dam (2015)	37	0	0		IV
Dip (2016)	70	0	0	0	IV
Dip (2019)	318	0	0	1	II
Hiwatashi (2018)	65	0	0	7	IV
Broderick (2022)	828	0	0	6	III

lar findings during laparoscopic cholecystectomy, as well as during robotic-assisted laparoscopic cholecystectomy, including in obese individuals [6–21]. With a growing body of literature, some surgeons have advocated for FC to become the standard of care in laparoscopic cholecystectomy in both elective and emergent cholecystectomy.

The highest level evidence confirming fluorescent visualization of extrahepatic biliary anatomy was shown in two studies. Dip et al. in 2019 published a single-blind randomized controlled trial comparing FC ($n = 312$) vs LC ($n = 318$) demonstrating that FC was statistically superior in identifying extrahepatic biliary structures [13]. Bile duct injury was zero in FC and two patients in LC; operative times and other complications were not reported. Lim et al. performed a meta-analysis of seven studies comparing biliary anatomy visualization with IOC versus FC. Rates of extrahepatic biliary anatomy identification included cystic duct, common bile duct, CD-CBD junction, and common hepatic duct. FC was safe and effective [14].

Tables 4.1 and 4.2 feature studies evaluating fluorescence cholangiography (FC) during cholecystectomy to evaluate common bile duct injury and operative times. The studies listed are mostly

Table 4.2 Fluorescence use in laparoscopic cholecystectomy with reported decreases in operative times

First author (year)	Number of patients (n)	Operative duration (FC)	Operative duration (LC)	Difference in duration
Ambe (2019)	29	53	54	−1
Bleszynski (2019)	108	70	80	−10
Quaresima (2019)	44	86.9	118	−31.1
Yoshiya (2019)	39	129	150	−21
Esposito (2019)	15	52	69	−17
Broderick (2022)	828	68	99	−31

cohort or case series studies. Currently, there are no reported bile duct injuries for FC in literature.

Broderick et al. performed a clinical review of their institutional experience with adopting ICG as standard of care. FC with ICG reduced operative time by 26.47 min per case compared to traditional LC without IOC ($p < 0.0001$) [16]. For patients with BMI ≥ 30 kg/m^2, operative duration for ICG vs non-ICG groups was 75.57 vs 104.9 min, respectively ($p < 0.0001$). ICG required conversion to open at a rate of 1.5%, while non-ICG converted at a rate of 8.5% ($p < 0.0001$). Conversion rate remained significant with multivariable analysis (OR 0.212, $p = 0.001$). Bile leaks (classified as Strasberg A injuries) were more common in the non-ICG group, with nine patients in the non-ICG group and two in the ICG group. One CBDI occurred in the non-ICG group, although this was not clinically significant. There was no significant difference in 30-day complication rates between groups [16]. Follow-up of this study and expansion on the cohort was published in 2022, confirming the above findings with further reduction in operative times [17].

Osayi et al. reported that significant improvements in patient outcomes are in decreased operative time and reduced rates of conversion to open surgery when comparing FC with white-light cholecystectomy. There is also a significant reduction in operative time when compared to IOC (1.9 ± 1.7 min vs 11.8 ± 5.2 min, $p < 0.001$) [11]. In this study, IOC was unobtainable in 24.4% of patients, while ICG did not visualize biliary structures in 4.9% of patients. After complete dissection, the rates of visualization of the cystic duct, common bile duct, and common hepatic duct using ICG were 95.1, 76.8, and 69.5%, respectively, compared to 72.0, 75.6, and 74.3% for IOC. In patients where IOC could not be obtained, FC successfully identified biliary structures in 80% of the cases. Higher BMI was not a deterrent to visualization of anatomy with ICG.

Reeves et al. utilized a Markov model to shows that use of ICG during cholecystectomy is cost-effective and improves quality of care with $1235 cost reduction per case and 0.09 quality-adjusted life years (QALY) compared to standard white-light cholecystectomy [22]. These improvements were demonstrated due to a reduction in operating time of 20 minutes and decreased conversion to open rate from 6.7% to 1.2% in averaged over available literature [22]. Recommendations in their manuscript are limited by the nature of the predictive model and should be studied prospectively to verify findings. The manuscript also reviewed all published reports of FC in literature to determine the parameters of the predictive model; improvements in operative time and outcomes were in multiple retrospective studies [16–21].

Best evidence is Level III–IV from these studies as well as designed controlled trials or cohorts. No randomized trials evaluating conversion to open surgery, operative times, and common bile duct injuries have been published to date. There is early Level II evidence showing better visualization of extrahepatic biliary structures with FC compared to IOC and white light alone.

Advantages of Indocyanine Green Fluorescence Cholangiography

Fluorescence cholangiography has multiple advantages. Compared to IOC, FC can save time and operative costs associated with traditional radiographic IOC with respect to cannula insertion and contrast injection for biliary imaging [23, 24]. FC is viewed as quite versatile, as a single preoperative injection allows the surgeon to obtain fluorescent imaging at any point during the procedure without the added personnel and equipment needed for

IOC. The fluorescent images can be viewed from several angles, in real time with real-time tissue manipulation, to better understand anatomic relationships. In centers for education, it can be a good adjunct to assist surgical trainees in understanding anatomy and CVS in real time. Additionally, repeated imaging with repeat intravenous ICG injections is possible throughout the surgical procedure to help delineate vascular anatomy. Unlike arguments around routine versus selective IOC, routine use of ICG is supported by the above benefits without additional cost, equipment, or time. Lastly, the use of fluorescence cholangiography is safe and does not involve radiation exposure; it has been used safely in patient with traditional iodine allergies (e.g., rash). Each of these benefits may translate to improved patient outcomes, especially with respect to decreased operative time, overall cost, and conversion to open surgery. [16, 17, 22]

The most significant improvements in patient outcomes are in decreased operative time and reduced rates of conversion to open surgery when comparing FC with white-light cholecystectomy. There is also a significant reduction in operative time when compared to IOC (1.9 ± 1.7 min vs 11.8 ± 5.2 min, $p < 0.001$) [11].

The topic of cost always plays an important role in adopting new technologies or techniques. As described above, comparing FC to traditional white-light LC (without use of IOC), Reeves et al. utilized a Markov model to show that use of ICG during cholecystectomy is cost-effective and improves quality of care with $1235 cost reduction per case and 0.09 quality-adjusted life years (QALY) compared to standard white-light cholecystectomy [22]. Thus, ICG use can be viewed as a cost-effective surgical strategy which improves healthcare outcomes and suggests this should be considered as standard of care for laparoscopic cholecystectomy.

Although current firm recommendations are limited by published sample size, early data suggest both reduced operative time and conversion to open surgery in FC cases for both inflamed and non-inflamed pathology as well as obese patients. Whether FC significantly moves the needle on reducing major common bile duct injury remains to be confirmed with further collation of data and use in practice, although this will take hundreds of thousands of cases due to the low rate of CBD injury.

Limitations of Indocyanine Green Fluorescence Cholangiography

Despite the above advantages, FC with ICG has some limitations. In institutions where there is no NIR camera capability, an up-front cost for purchasing new equipment would be needed to implement FC. There would also be the need to protocol pre-op ordering, reconstitution, and administration of intravenous ICG. Nurse education is often necessary to relay the importance of appropriate dose timing and standardize seamlessly into practice. The cost of ICG alone is inexpensive ($17–130/bottle), and the up-front equipment cost can be recouped if reduced operative time and conversion to open data holds true.

Fluorescence cholangiography cannot visualize deep structures. While Dip et al. note that there is increased visualization of CHD, CBD, and cystic duct in FC, the penetration of the NIR light can still be limited in cases of thick surrounding fat or inflamed tissue in the porta hepatis. The ability to detect bile duct stones with fluorescence cholangiography is also questionable. FC cannot be used as a replacement to IOC in the setting of identifying and treating choledocholithiasis; however, it can be used simultaneously with IOC for identifying overall anatomy and safe cannulation of the cystic duct.

Conclusion

Fluorescence cholangiography with ICG appears to be a promising technology that is safe and cost-effective and improves patient outcomes. The ability to visualize biliary anatomy can have a great benefit to the surgeon and may help prevent complications in the surgical patient.

References

1. Deziel DJ, Millikan KW, Economou SG, Doolas A, Ko ST, Airan MC. Complications of laparoscopic cholecystectomy: a national survey of 4,292 hospitals and an analysis of 77,604 cases. Am J Surg. 1993;165(1):9–14. https://doi.org/10.1016/S0002-9610(05)80397-6.

2. Flum DR, Cheadle A, Prela C, Dellinger EP, Chan L. Bile duct injury during cholecystectomy and survival in Medicare beneficiaries. J Am Med Assoc. 2003;290(16):2168–73. https://doi.org/10.1001/jama.290.16.2168.
3. Dolan JP, Diggs BS, Sheppard BC, Hunter JG. Ten-year trend in the national volume of bile duct injuries requiring operative repair. Surg Endosc Other Interv Tech. 2005;19(7):967–73. https://doi.org/10.1007/s00464-004-8942-6.
4. Halbert C, Pagkratis S, Yang J, et al. Beyond the learning curve: incidence of bile duct injuries following laparoscopic cholecystectomy normalize to open in the modern era. Surg Endosc. 2016;30(6):2239–43. https://doi.org/10.1007/s00464-015-4485-2.
5. Savader SJ, Lillemoe KD, Prescott CA, Winick AB, Venbrux AC, Lund GB, Mitchell SE, Cameron JL, Osterman FA Jr. Laparoscopic cholecystectomy-related bile duct injuries: a health and financial disaster. Ann Surg. 1997;225(3):268–73. https://doi.org/10.1097/00000658-199703000-00005. PMID: 9060582; PMCID: PMC1190676.
6. Ishizawa T, Tamura S, Masuda K, Aoki T, Hasegawa K, Imamura H, Beck Y, Kokudo N. Intraoperative fluorescent cholangiography using indocyanine green: a biliary road map for safe surgery. J Am Coll Surg. 2009;208(1):e1–4. https://doi.org/10.1016/j.jamcollsurg.2008.09.024. Epub 2008 Oct 31. PMID: 19228492.
7. Ishizawa T, Bandai Y, Ijichi M, Kaneko J, Hasegawa K, Kokudo N. Fluorescent cholangiography illuminating the biliary tree during laparoscopic cholecystectomy. Br J Surg. 2010;97:1369. https://doi.org/10.1002/bjs.7125.
8. Boni L, David G, Mangano A, Dionigi G, Rausei S, Spampatti S, Cassinotti E, Fingerhut A. Clinical applications of indocyanine green (ICG) enhanced fluorescence in laparoscopic surgery. Surg Endosc. 2015;29(7):2046–55. https://doi.org/10.1007/s00464-014-3895-x. Epub 2014 Oct 11. PMID: 25303914; PMCID: PMC4471386.9.
9. Oddi A, Di Nicola V, Panzini A, et al. The intraoperative visualization of the bile ducts by the use of fluorescent substances. A feasibility study. G Chir. 1996;17(11–12):620–3.
10. Sandler BJ. Immunofluorescence in the operating room for biliary visualization and perfusion assessment - a SAGES Technology and Value Assessment [Internet]. SAGES. 2019 [cited 2022 May 1]. Available from: https://www.sages.org/publications/tavac/immunofluorescence-operating-room-biliary-visualization-perfusion-assessment/.
11. Osayi SN, Wendling MR, Drosdeck JM, Chaudhry UI, Perry KA, Noria SF, Mikami DJ, Needleman BJ, Muscarella P 2nd, Abdel-Rasoul M, Renton DB, Melvin WS, Hazey JW, Narula VK. Near-infrared fluorescent cholangiography facilitates identification of biliary anatomy during laparoscopic cholecystectomy. Surg Endosc. 2015;29(2):368–75. https://doi.org/10.1007/s00464-014-3677-5. Epub 2014 Jul 2. PMID: 24986018; PMCID: PMC4415528.

12. Dip F, Nguyen D, Montorfano L, et al. Accuracy of near infrared-guided surgery in morbidly obese subjects undergoing laparoscopic cholecystectomy. Obes Surg. 2016;26(3):525–30. https://doi.org/10.1007/s11695-015-1781-9.
13. Spinoglio G, P.F. Real-time near-infrared (NIR) fluorescent cholangiography in single site robotic cholecystectomy (SSRC): a single institutional study. Surg Endosc. 2013;27:2156–62.
14. Dip F, LoMenzo E, Sarotto L, et al. Randomized trial of near-infrared incisionless fluorescent cholangiography. Ann Surg. 2019;270(6):992–9. https://doi.org/10.1097/SLA.0000000000003178.
15. Lim SH, Tan HTA, Shelat VG. Comparison of indocyanine green dye fluorescent cholangiography with intra-operative cholangiography in laparoscopic cholecystectomy: a meta-analysis. Surg Endosc. 2021;35(4):1511–20. https://doi.org/10.1007/s00464-020-08164-5. Epub 2021 Jan 4. PMID: 33398590.
16. Broderick RC, Lee AM, Cheverie JN, et al. Fluorescent cholangiography significantly improves patient outcomes for laparoscopic cholecystectomy. Surg Endosc. 2021;35(10):5729–39. https://doi.org/10.1007/S00464-020-08045-X.
17. Broderick RC, Li JZ, Huang EY, Blitzer RR, Lee AM, Serra JL, Bouvet M, Sandler BJ, Jacobsen GR, Horgan S. Lighting the way with fluorescent cholangiography in laparoscopic cholecystectomy: reviewing 7 years of experience. J Am Coll Surg. 2022;235(5):713–23. https://doi.org/10.1097/XCS.0000000000000314. Epub 2022 Oct 17. PMID: 36102574.
18. Ambe PC, Plambeck J, Fernandez-Jesberg V, Zarras K. The role of indocyanine green fluoroscopy for intraoperative bile duct visualization during laparoscopic cholecystectomy: an observational cohort study in 70 patients. Patient Saf Surg. 2019;13:2. https://doi.org/10.1186/s13037-019-0182-8. PMID: 30651756; PMCID: PMC6330420.
19. Bleszynski MS, DeGirolamo KM, Meneghetti AT, Chiu CJ, Panton ON. Fluorescent cholangiography in laparoscopic cholecystectomy: an updated Canadian experience. Surg Innov. 2020;27(1):38–43. https://doi.org/10.1177/1553350619885792. Epub 2019 Nov 19. PMID: 31744398.
20. Yoshiya S, Minagawa R, Kamo K, Kasai M, Taketani K, Yukaya T, Kimura Y, Koga T, Kai M, Kajiyama K, Yoshizumi T. Usability of intraoperative fluorescence imaging with indocyanine green during laparoscopic cholecystectomy after percutaneous transhepatic gallbladder drainage. World J Surg. 2019;43(1):127–33. https://doi.org/10.1007/s00268-018-4760-1. PMID: 30105635.
21. Esposito C, Corcione F, Settimi A, Farina A, Centonze A, Esposito G, Spagnuolo MI, Escolino M. Twenty-five year experience with laparoscopic cholecystectomy in the pediatric population-from 10 mm clips to indocyanine green fluorescence technology: long-term results and technical considerations. J Laparoendosc Adv Surg Tech A. 2019;29(9):1185–91. https://doi.org/10.1089/lap.2019.0254. Epub 2019 Jun 14. PMID: 31199700.

22. Reeves JJ, Broderick RC, Lee AM, et al. The price is right: routine fluorescent cholangiography during laparoscopic cholecystectomy. Surgery. 2021;171(5):1168–76. https://doi.org/10.1016/j.surg.2021.09.027.
23. Hiwatashi K, Okumura H, Setoyama T, et al. Evaluation of laparoscopic cholecystectomy using indocyanine green cholangiography including cholecystitis. Medicine. 2018;97(30):e11654. https://doi.org/10.1097/MD.0000000000011654.
24. Dip FD, Asbun D, Rosales-Velderrain A, et al. Cost analysis and effectiveness comparing the routine use of intraoperative fluorescent cholangiography with fluoroscopic cholangiogram in patients undergoing laparoscopic cholecystectomy. Surg Endosc. 2014;28(6):1838–43. https://doi.org/10.1007/s00464-013-3394-5.

Use of Fluorescence Guidance in Hepatic Surgery

5

Iswanto Sucandy, Emanuel Shapera,
and Takeaki Ishizawa

Introduction

Hepatobiliary operations are complex with varying degrees of anatomical and technical challenges. Attention must be paid to the small and often variant details of intra- and extrahepatic anatomy, as these details dictate the operative approach and can affect post-operative outcomes. The rise in fluorescent technology has armed hepatobiliary surgeons with an additional tool to delineate bilio-vascular anatomy and tackle these demanding operations. By far, the most successful and well-studied application of fluorescent-guided surgery involves the use of indocyanine green (ICG), a

Supplementary Information The online version contains supplementary material available at https://doi.org/10.1007/978-3-031-40685-0_5.

I. Sucandy (✉)
Department of Surgery, Advent Health Tampa, Tampa, FL, USA
e-mail: Iswanto.Sucandy.MD@adventhealth.com

E. Shapera
Department of Surgery, SHARP Grossmont Hospital, La Mesa, CA, USA

T. Ishizawa
Department of Hepatobiliary-Pancreatic Surgery, Graduate School of Medicine, Osaka Metropolitan University, Abeno-ku, Osaka, Japan

N. Szoka et al. (eds.), *The SAGES Manual of Fluorescence-Guided Surgery*, https://doi.org/10.1007/978-3-031-40685-0_5

nontoxic chemical that fluoresces at near-infrared wavelengths [1]. This chapter will therefore focus predominantly on the application of this particular fluorescent agent in hepatobiliary surgery. We have included the level of the evidence (I–VII) for each of the recommendations in the use of ICG fluorescence based on the available published literature.

In the clinical setting, ICG can be injected intravenously (Level IV) and is albumin bound, permitting angiography [2]. Within minutes, the fluorescent angiogram dissipates as the chemical is taken up by the hepatocytes and excreted into the biliary system, reaching a maximum concentration in bile within 2 h and lasting for another couple of hours [3, 4]. ICG is therefore useful in visualizing both vascular (including portal venous, hepatic arterial, and hepatic venous vessels) and biliary structures within the liver. These two mediums (blood and bile) by which ICG traverses allow for four distinct, but related, functions in ICG fluorescent (ICGF)-guided hepatobiliary operations: angiography, identification of the extrahepatic biliary system (fluorescence cholangiography), localization of hepatic malignancies, and visualization of hepatic (sub)segments to be resected or preserved (hepatic segmentation).

Identification of Biliary Ductal Anatomy (Fluorescence Cholangiography)

The first application of ICG in clinical practice is for the identification of biliary ductal anatomy. Originally, fluorescent images of the extrahepatic bile ducts were obtained by intrabiliary [5] or intravenous [6] administration of ICG in the setting of open surgery. Since the first report in 2009 of its clinical application in laparoscopic surgery [7], fluorescence cholangiography by intravenous ICG has widely been used as a radiation-free and incisionless cholangiography technique during laparoscopic cholecystectomy [8, 9] (Level IV). Recently, the advantage of fluorescence cholangiography over white-light imaging in identifying the extrahepatic biliary anatomy during laparoscopic cholecystectomy was demonstrated by a multicenter international randomized clinical trial (RCT) [10] (Level II).

Another RCT in Denmark also confirmed non-inferiority of fluorescence imaging over conventional radiographic cholangiography in terms of visualizing the critical junction between the cystic duct and the common hepatic/bile duct [11] (Level II). The hepatobiliary surgeon can identify bile leaks from a transected liver parenchymal surface under ICG fluorescence and subsequently apply suture ligation or place clips to areas actively exuding fluorescent bile. This is a critical step, preventing postoperative bile leaks and further significant postoperative morbidity to the patient [12, 13] (Level III). Based on this collective evidence, fluorescence cholangiography has recently been recommended as a technique to avoid bile duct injury in the current recommendations of multiple societies for safe laparoscopic cholecystectomy [14] (Level VII).

More recently in the United States, general surgeons are adopting the robotic platform, particularly the da Vinci Xi system with incorporated ICG fluorescence camera capability, which can generate a real-time cholangiogram via biliary excretion of ICG. This integrated functionality of the robotic system provides a fluorescent map of the extrahepatic biliary tree. In these circumstances, the common hepatic duct is identified in 83% and the cystic duct in 97%, preventing conversion to open operation or injury to the common bile duct [15] (Level IV). Since cholecystectomies are short cases, surgeons must ensure preoperative ICG injection prior to anesthetic induction to allow adequate time for hepatic uptake and biliary excretion. Additionally, circumvention of this timing has been described in the literature by directly injecting ICG into the gallbladder, thereby bypassing hepatic uptake and proceeding straight to biliary fluorescence [16] (Level IV).

At our tertiary hepatobiliary institution, the vast majority (~90%) of our hepatectomies are approached in a minimally invasive robotic fashion. We utilize the Intuitive da Vinci Xi® platform with its built-in Firefly ™ camera system, which can be activated by a pedal at the console, allowing rapid alternation with the white-light camera. We also utilize ICG fluorescence as an adjunct during our bile duct dissection. For this purpose of application, the anesthesia team administers 0.5 mL of a diluted ICG solution injected intravenously approximately 45 min prior to its anticipated need. Although some data suggests that fluorescent identification can occur as early as 20 min after injection, we have found identification of biliary anatomy during hepatectomy to occur much later than 20 min, particularly in patients with liver cirrhosis. This is caused by the delay in uptake and secretion by the hepatocytes. Correct timing and dosage is critical in patients with liver cirrhosis, as they are less tolerant of perioperative complications such as bile leak and intra-abdominal infection; therefore, they benefit the most from an accurate anatomical delineation during hepatobiliary resections.

The ICG is mixed so that one ampule (25 mg) dissolves in 20 mL of 0.9% normal saline. In our experience, a higher concentration or dose results in difficulty discriminating biliary and nonbiliary structures. This is particularly true when the patient has an obstructive malignancy or stricture, which dilates smaller bile ducts, resulting in ICG accumulation and an increase in background fluorescent "noise." It is possible to attenuate the intensity of the fluorescent image on the robotic console at the expense of sensitivity, should this problem arise.

When performing an anatomical left or right hepatectomy, we do not routinely dissect the common hepatic duct bifurcation at the porta hepatis prior to liver parenchymal transection, except for extrahepatic cholangiocarcinoma or tumor located near the hilum, in order to preserve the collateral blood supply to the remnant hepatic duct. Instead, after committing to hemihepatic vascular inflow (portal venous, hepatic arterial) ligation, we initiate the parenchymal transection. The corresponding right or left hepatic duct is identified intraparenchymal at the level of the hilar place, isolated, and ligated. By utilizing a combination of preoperative imaging and ICG fluorescence and appreciating the relationship between the glissonean pedicles, we are able to complete an anatomical hepatectomy while avoiding encroachment and injury to the fragile blood supply of the remnant hepatic duct. Our technique is demonstrated here in Figs. 5.1, 5.2 and 5.3, in Video 5.1, and has been previously reported in the literature [17–19]. This technique can also be used to identify the biliary anatomy on the hepatic hilum during minimally invasive donor hepatectomy [20].

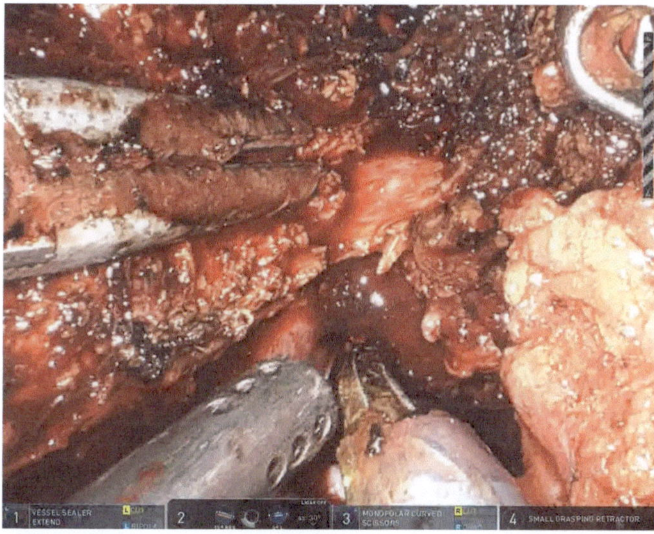

Fig. 5.1 Left hepatic duct identified within the parenchyma during left hepatectomy prior to transection under white light

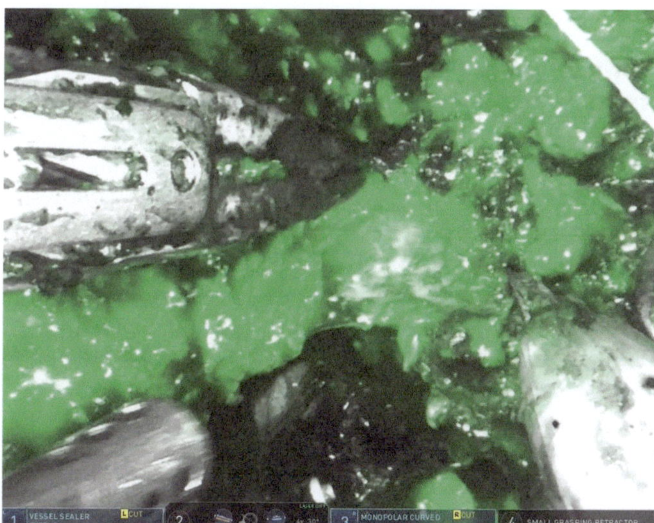

Fig. 5.2 Left hepatic duct identified within the parenchyma during left hepatectomy prior to transection under ICG fluorescence

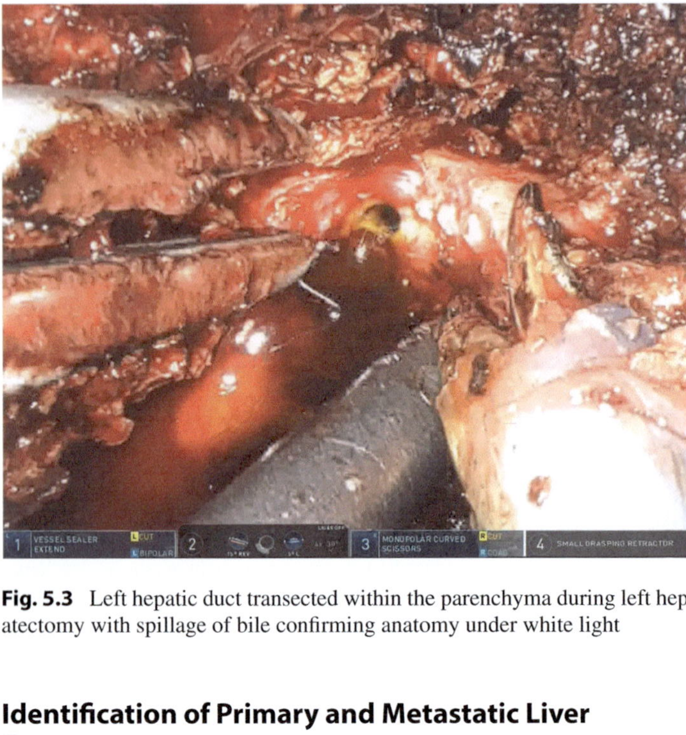

Fig. 5.3 Left hepatic duct transected within the parenchyma during left hepatectomy with spillage of bile confirming anatomy under white light

Identification of Primary and Metastatic Liver Tumors

The second application of ICG fluorescence imaging is localization of liver cancers in real time during hepatectomy. This technique is based on the fact that ICG injected IV before surgery is acquired and retained by HCC and other cancerous tissues with significant differentiation and retention vs. normal hepatocytes, due to washout from surrounding noncancerous hepatic parenchyma (Fig. 5.4a, b) [21–23]. In poorly differentiated HCC and metastatic liver cancers, portal uptake of ICG into cancerous tissues is difficult to observe. However, biliary stasis surrounding these cancers results in a rim of ICG retention and fluorescence in the noncancerous hepatic parenchyma surrounding the tumor, possibly due to compression [23, 24] or immature hepatocyte function, resulting in decreased biliary

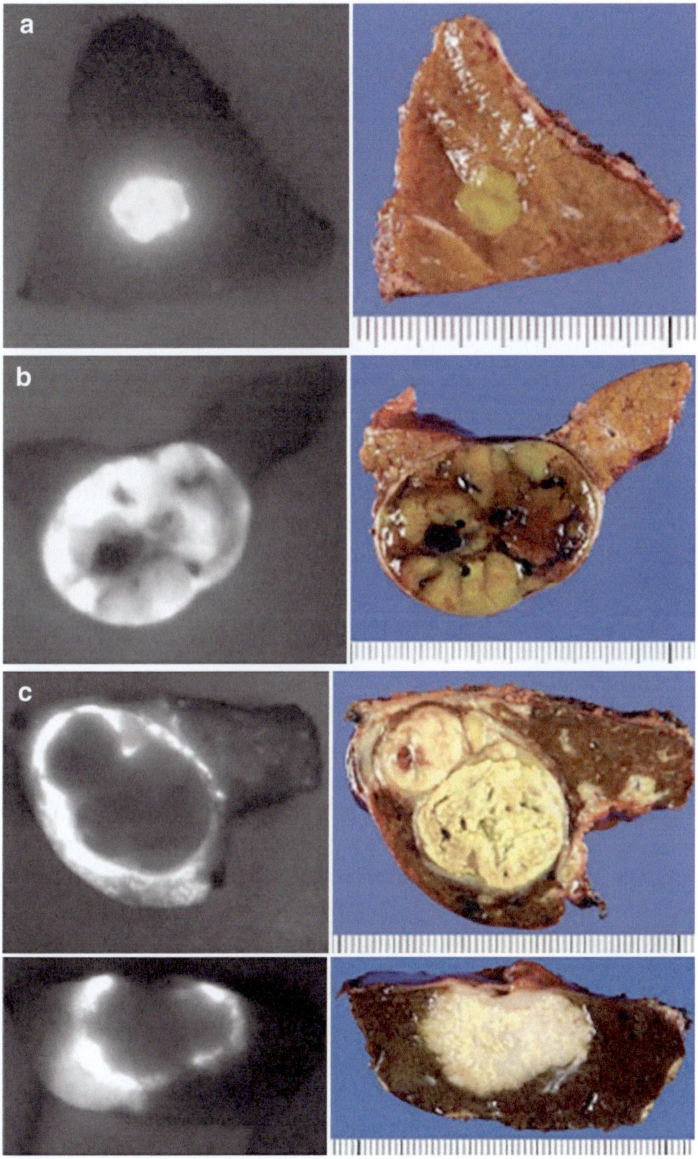

Fig. 5.4 Fluorescence images of hepatic malignancies on cut surfaces of resected specimen after preoperative intravenous injection of ICG (Fig. X). (**a**) Well-differentiated HCC. (**b**) Moderately differentiated HCC. (**c**) Poorly differentiated HCC (upper) and colorectal liver metastasis (below)

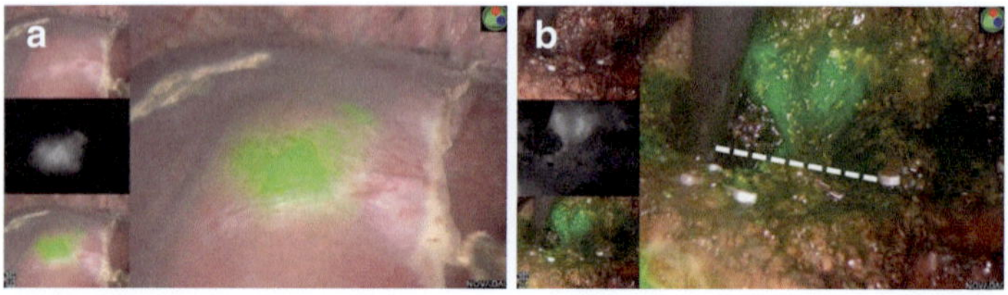

Fig. 5.5 Tumor localization during laparoscopic hepatectomy for colorectal liver metastasis (Fig. Y). (**a**) A subcapsular tumor is identified by fluorescence imaging on the surface of hepatic segment 4 prior to hepatic transection. (**b**) Fluorescence imaging during hepatic transection identified fluorescence signals emitted from noncancerous hepatic parenchyma surrounding the tumor, suggesting the optimal transection plane (dotted line)

excretion [25] and rim-enhancing fluorescence (Fig. 5.4c). Regardless of the fluorescence patterns, surgeons can utilize the above mechanism of ICG accumulation for intraoperative identification of subcapsular liver cancers by near-infrared fluorescence imaging [21, 26] (Level IV), especially in the setting of minimally invasive hepatectomy [27, 28] (Level IV) where surgeons cannot palpate hepatic surfaces directly for intraoperative diagnosis (Fig. 5.5a).

The utility of ICG in hepatic retention as a measure of liver function (described in more detail below) led to its use for intraoperative cancer localization [28, 29]. As a consequence, the most commonly administered dose and timing of ICG is similar for both modalities, notably at 0.5 mg/kg, usually 1–14 days prior to surgery [21]. Alternatively, intravenous ICG injection at a dose of 10 mg 24 h before surgery [30] or 0.05–0.1 mg/kg 24–72 h before surgery [31] works for intraoperative fluorescence imaging of hepatic malignancies. Administration of ICG on the day before surgery should be avoided to achieve sufficient tumor-to-background contrast at the time of surgery [23] (Level IV), particularly in instances of decreased liver function due to cirrhosis or preoperative chemotherapy.

This strategy may not be practical in many countries, where patient transportation to and from the hospital is sociogeographically challenging. Additionally, HCC even when well-differentiated will vary in tumor biology not only from patient to patient but also among multiple tumors in the same given patient [32]. Cirrhotic but noncancerous liver parenchyma will vary in ICG excretion from patient to patient, depending on the level of parenchymal fibrosis and other factors (evidence: Level IV) [33]. As a consequence of all these variabilities, the timing between preoperative administration and operative resection is not exact, and it is difficult to standardize between patients. The ICG administration must be long enough to allow the often dysfunctional liver parenchyma to completely excrete the ICG while not permitting too much time to pass for the malignancy to excrete it as well.

The advantages of tumor localization by ICG fluorescence imaging lie in its feasibility and high sensitivity (around 90% or higher [23, 27, 30], Level IV) for subcapsular tumors. On the other hand, this technique has limitations in tissue permeability (5–8 mm from hepatic surfaces) and a relatively high false-positive rate [23] (Level IV). Surgeons still need intraoperative ultrasonography for identification of deeply located tumors and its spatial relationships with intrahepatic vasculature. Any additional resection for newly detected lesions by ICG fluorescence imaging, and not part of the preoperative plan, should only be considered when malignancy is suggested by other modalities such as palpation, ultrasonography, or re-evaluation of preoperative imaging studies.

In experienced hands, the high sensitivity and specificity of liver tumor detection associated with IOUS approaches 95% [34] (Level IV). Many high-volume liver surgery centers therefore do not feel that a 1–2-week delay for ICGF tumor identification is warranted.

Oftentimes, before proceeding to liver resection, a tissue diagnosis is required via percutaneous liver biopsy to confirm the type of liver cancer. While this can worsen oncologic outcomes via tumor cell seeding, the biopsy can also alter the dynamic of ICG absorption and excretion at the local level [35] (Level III). As a result, the surgeon cannot always be sure as to whether they are looking for a fluorescent HCC or a rim-enhancing non-HCC malignancy at the time of diagnostic laparoscopy prior to the intended liver resection.

Despite these limitations and pitfalls, however, liver cancer imaging by ICG fluorescence retains a critical role in detecting tiny tumors after effective neoadjuvant therapy or residual tumors from prior resection [23, 27] (Level IV) and improves acquisition of appropriate surgical margins (Fig. 5.5b) [27, 36, 37] (Level IV). Some authors have demonstrated a reduction in operative duration and recurrence risk with ICG [38, 39] (Level III). Prospective trials demonstrating clinical efficacy of ICG in generating superior outcomes for liver cancer localization are required to justify further development and dissemination of this modality, particularly for hepatobiliary centers that do not routinely evaluate preoperative liver function with ICG.

Identification of Vascular Structures and Hepatic Segmentation by Fluorescence Angiography

The third application of ICG is based on its albumin-bound status, where it can freely circulate in the blood before being taken up by hepatocytes for biliary excretion. This permits generation of a rapid fluorescent angiogram while performing hepatobiliary resections. Dissipation of ICG and the angiogram is fairly rapid, although the biliary excretion requires some time; therefore, multiple fluorescent angiograms can be obtained in the same operation. This permits test clamping of multiple candidate pedicles prior to transection followed by ICGF angiography to ensure correct anatomical identification of inflow vessels to ultimately preserve the perfusion of the future liver remnant. A finer dissection of segmental pedicle anatomy can permit highly accurate segmentectomy and subsegmentectomy, which has been described extensively in the literature to be associated with significantly less blood loss and blood transfusions—relevant factors in achieving superior oncological outcomes [40, 41] (Level III).

Since the 2008 landmark paper on the use of ICG fluorescence imaging in the field of hepatobiliary surgery [42] (Level IV), this modality has been used for hepatic segmental boundary visualization (hepatic segmentation). In 2012, Ishizawa and Gayet [43] first

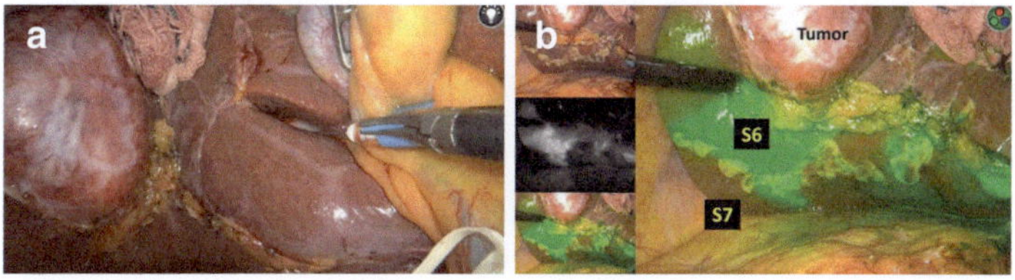

Fig. 5.6 Hepatic segmentation with positive staining technique (Fig. X/Z). (**a**) ICG solution (0.25 mg/5 mg) is injected into the tumor (HCC)-bearing hepatic segment (segment 6) following intracorporal puncture of the root of corresponding portal branch. (**b**) Fluorescence imaging clearly visualizes boundaries between hepatic segments 6 and 7

applied fluorescence-guided hepatic segmentation to laparoscopic hepatectomy utilizing a "positive staining technique" (injection of ICG solution directly into the corresponding portal branch under ultrasound guidance, following conventional dye-staining technique [44]) and "negative staining technique" (intravenous ICG injection following closure of the corresponding portal pedicle at its root, not unlike a conventional Glissonian approach [45]). The positive staining technique (Fig. 5.6) has the advantage in omitting unnecessary dissection at the hepatic hilum; however, puncture of the portal pedicle from the skin surface of the abdominal wall is technically demanding, despite some described technical tricks [46, 47], especially in the setting of minimally invasive surgery. Robotic-assisted surgery may facilitate needle manipulation to puncture the portal venous branch in the patient's abdominal cavity [48] (Level III). In contrast, a negative staining technique is suitable when the root of the target Glissonian sheath is easy to access (e.c. Couinaud's segment 2 to 6), as suggested by the current consensus guidelines [49] (Level VII).

Hepatic segmentation by ICG fluorescence imaging enables clear identification of intersegmental planes not only from the hepatic surface but also on raw surfaces during parenchymal dissection throughout the hepatectomy procedure [27], enhancing the accuracy of anatomical hepatectomy [50] (Level IV) and improving operative outcomes. Liver remnant ischemia, prevented by ICG fluorescence-guided hepatectomy, is known to result in higher postoperative bile leaks, bilomas, and abscesses [51] (Level IV). This is also associated with inferior long-term oncological survival, especially in the case of hepatectomy for primary liver cancer [52] (Level III).

In the growing field of partial liver donation in hepatic transplantation, graft viability can be accurately assessed by ICG fluorescence angiography. The caveat to ICG fluorescence angiography is that repeat application will be hindered 20–40 min later following the initial injection when biliary uptake and excretion occurs so that any functional liver will fluoresce and will continue to do so for a few hours regardless of ischemic clamping. Therefore, if the surgeon wishes to perform repeated angiograms, they must do so before significant biliary uptake renders background noise too great to differentiate ischemic and perfused tissue.

At our tertiary hepatobiliary institution, we isolate and visually test clamp the candidate specimen portal and hepatic arterial pedicle during minimally invasive robotic hepatectomy to compensate for the absence of palpation. A bedside assistant, usually a board-certified general surgeon who participates as a hepatobiliary surgery fellow, laparoscopically inserts a bulldog clamp through a right lower quadrant GelPort®. The console surgeon will then apply the clamp at the candidate pedicle. The anesthesia team will then administer 0.5 mL of our aforementioned ICG mixture (25 mg in 20 mL of 0.9% normal saline) through a venous access. After 1–2 min, the console surgeon activates the Firefly ™ camera system and can switch back and forth between white light and ICG fluorescence camera visualization. The surgeon can also continue the operation in ICG fluorescence mode, allowing a robotic monopolar cautery to be used to mark the transection plane along the visualized fluorescent demarcation. Upon confirmation of devascularization of the specimen side and perfusion of the future liver remnant side, the bulldog clamp is released under white light, the pedicle is ligated, and the hepatectomy proceeds. Our technique is demonstrated in Figs. 5.7, 5.8, 5.9 and 5.10 and Video 5.2. Very little-to-no ischemic-appearing tissue should remain on the transected liver edge (Fig. 5.11).

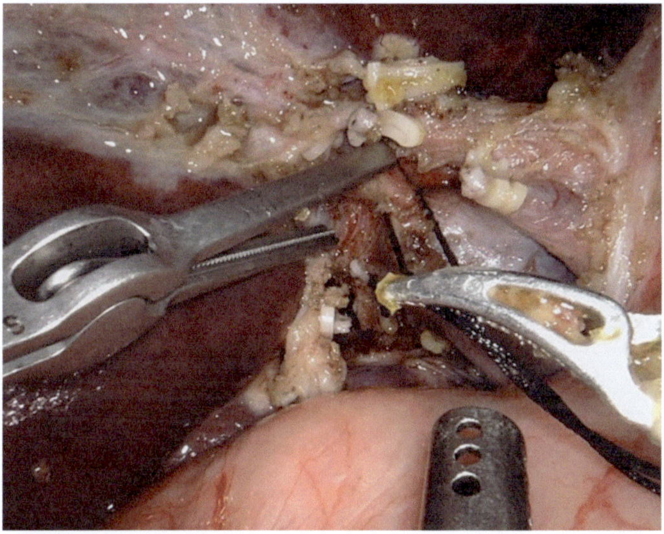

Fig. 5.7 Right hepatic artery identified at the hepatic hilum prior to clamping during a right hepatectomy under white light

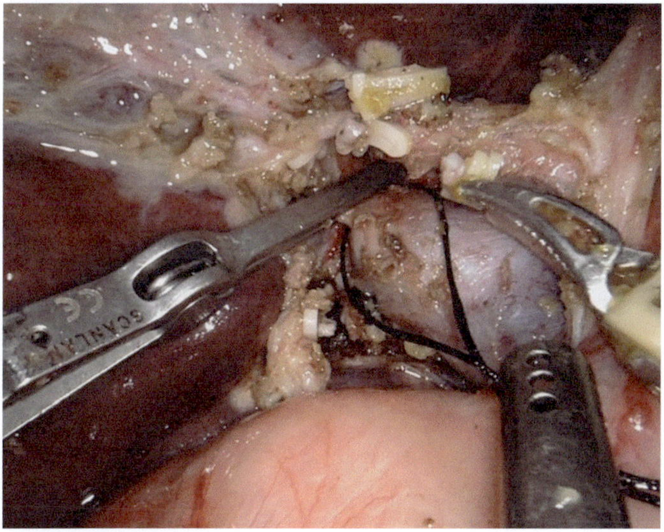

Fig. 5.8 Right hepatic artery identified at the hepatic hilum with bulldog clamp applied during a right hepatectomy under white light

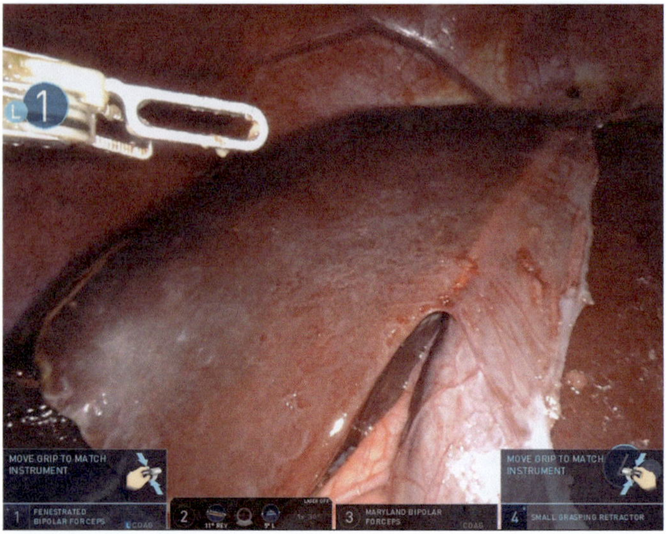

Fig. 5.9 Ischemic demarcation of the right lobe of the liver following bulldog clamp application to the right hepatic artery under white light

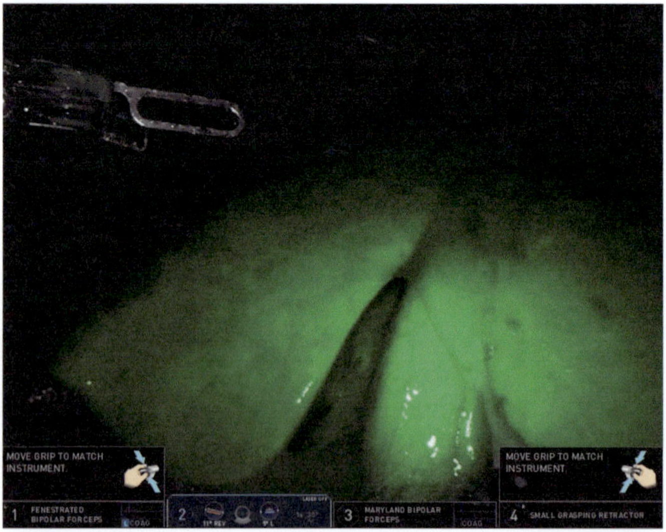

Fig. 5.10 Ischemic demarcation of the right lobe of the liver following bulldog clamp application to the right hepatic artery under ICG fluorescence

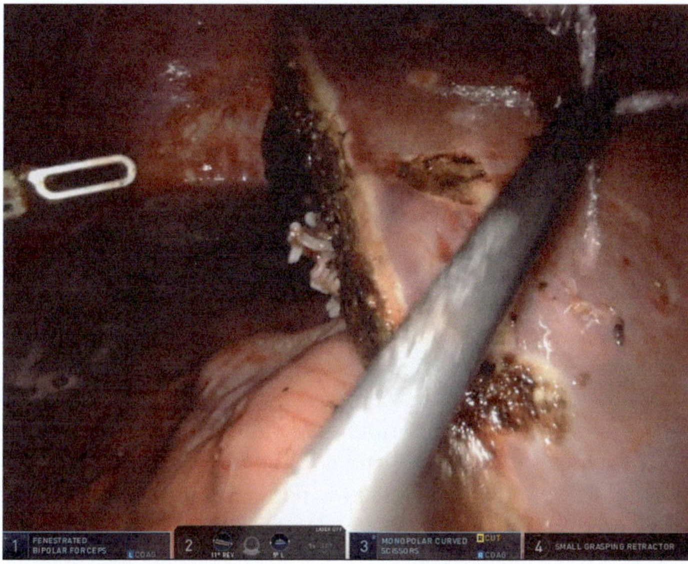

Fig. 5.11 Left lobe of the liver status post right hepatectomy with no significant ischemic tissue left behind under white light

Prediction of Posthepatectomy Liver Failure

The fourth application of ICG relates to its application in predicting posthepatectomy liver failure (PHLF). The details, consequences, and ultimate outcomes of this unfortunate condition require its own textbook, let alone chapter. Nonetheless, based on the International Study Group of Liver Surgeries definition, we may define it as an acquired failure of hepatic synthetic, excretionary, and detoxifying functions after liver resection as reflected by rises in bilirubin and international normalized ratio (INR) [53] (Level V). ICG clearance is an attractive predictor of PHLF [29] (Level IV), which enables curative anatomic segmentectomies of the liver even in patients with portal hypertension [54] (Level IV). Its clearance depends on hepatic synthetic and biliary excretion function as mentioned previously, which can be quantified by its fluorescence; more fluorescent liver parenchyma is indicative of greater parenchymal dysfunction.

In a study involving 284 major hepatectomies for bile duct cancer, an ICG retention of >11.8% was predictive of a life-threatening complication (Clavien-Dindo Classification ≥ IV complication) [55] (Level IV). A more novel approach utilizes future liver remnant ICG clearance; intraoperative ICG retention >13.8% by the future remnant liver during specimen pedicle clamping was 79.7% accurate in predicting PHLF in a study of 35 major liver resections [56] (Level IV). If retention >13.8% is noted, the surgeon can unclamp the specimen pedicle and abort the operation.

At our tertiary hepatobiliary institution, we do not routinely utilize ICG clearance preoperatively nor intraoperatively for selecting candidates for hepatectomy. Along the lines of Makuuchi's decisional algorithm, we are hesitant to offer major liver resection to patients with total bilirubin greater than 1 mg/dL in the absence of biliary obstruction nor in the presence of uncontrolled or significant ascites. We also are hesitant to offer major resection if the platelet count is less than 100,000 per microliter or in the presence of significant varices as this reflects significant portal hypertension and an inability of the future liver remnant to accommodate further increases in portal venous flow. In candidates with borderline features, we will attempt medical optimization or initiate a referral to a transplant center.

Finally, there are a few other functions that are deserving of mention. HCC has an affinity for ICG beyond mere degradation and excretion [21]. It is possible that photodynamic therapy and other targeted regimens based on the affinity for ICG can be implemented in the near future, which will expand anatomical treatment options for nonsurgical candidates who are unable to attain a liver transplant [57, 58]. Newer technologies have been developed to increase the accuracy of fluorescence imaging in distinguishing malignancies from benign dysfunctional liver parenchyma based on cancer-specific enzymatic activities [59] and biomarkers [60], molecular targeting, and single photon emission computed tomography [61]. Clinical trials to enroll patients in real-time ICG-guided liver surgery are underway [62].

Conclusion

In conclusion, the liver is an anatomically complex organ, consisting of varying vascular and biliary structures. Precise hepatic tumor localization and surgical margin assessment adds further technical difficulty, particularly in parenchyma-sparing hepatectomy. Application of ICG permits biliary and vascular identification and selective manipulation. Hepatic synthesis and biliary excretion permits functional assessment of candidate patients prior to major hepatic resection, while the degraded ability of cancerous or dysfunctional liver to metabolize ICG permits its utilization in hepatic malignant lesion targeting. Careful timing, dosage, and application of ICG can increase sensitivity and specificity of cancer imaging, which may enhance curability after hepatobiliary operations. While the current expert panels have reached consensus on intraoperative fluorescence imaging utilization [31, 63], continued research elucidating the impact of fluorescence guidance imaging on clinical outcomes is required to generate higher level of evidence.

References

1. Shapera E, Hsiung RW. Assessment of anastomotic perfusion in left-sided robotic assisted colorectal resection by Indocyanine green fluorescence angiography. Minim Invasive Surg. 2019;2019:3267217.
2. Reinhart MB, Huntington CR, Blair LJ, Heniford BT, Augenstein VA. Indocyanine green: historical context, current applications, and future considerations. Surg Innov. 2016;23:166–75.
3. Cherrick GR, Stein SW, Leevy CM, Davidson CS. Indocyanine green: observations on its physical properties, plasma decay, and hepatic extraction. J Clin Invest. 1960;39:592–600.
4. Chijiiwa K, Watanabe M, Nakano K, Noshiro H, Tanaka M. Biliary indocyanine green excretion as a predictor of hepatic adenosine triphosphate levels in patients with obstructive jaundice. Am J Surg. 2000;179:161–6.
5. Ishizawa T, Tamura S, Masuda K, Aoki T, Hasegawa K, Imamura H, Beck Y, Kokudo N. Intraoperative fluorescent cholangiography using indocyanine green: a biliary road map for safe surgery. J Am Coll Surg. 2009;208:e1–4.

6. Mitsuhashi N, Kimura F, Shimizu H, Imamaki M, Yoshidome H, Ohtsuka M, Kato A, Yoshitomi H, Nozawa S, Furukawa K, Takeuchi D, Takayashiki T, Suda K, Igarashi T, Miyazaki M. Usefulness of intraoperative fluorescence imaging to evaluate local anatomy in hepatobiliary surgery. J Hepatobiliary Pancreat Surg. 2008;15:508–14.
7. Ishizawa T, Bandai Y, Kokudo N. Fluorescent cholangiography using indocyanine green for laparoscopic cholecystectomy: an initial experience. Arch Surg. 2009;144:381–2.
8. Ishizawa T, Bandai Y, Ijichi M, Kaneko J, Hasegawa K, Kokudo N. Fluorescent cholangiography illuminating the biliary tree during laparoscopic cholecystectomy. Br J Surg. 2010 Sep;97(9):1369–77.
9. Agnus V, Pesce A, Boni L, Van Den Bos J, Morales-Conde S, Paganini AM, Quaresima S, Balla A, La Greca G, Plaudis H, Moretto G, Castagnola M, Santi C, Casali L, Tartamella L, Saadi A, Picchetto A, Arezzo A, Marescaux J, Diana M. Fluorescence-based cholangiography: preliminary results from the IHU-IRCAD-EAES EURO-FIGS registry. Surg Endosc. 2020;34(9):3888–96.
10. Dip F, LoMenzo E, Sarotto L, Phillips E, Todeschini H, Nahmod M, Alle L, Schneider S, Kaja L, Boni L, Ferraina P, Carus T, Kokudo N, Ishizawa T, Walsh M, Simpfendorfer C, Mayank R, White K, Rosenthal RJ. Randomized trial of near-infrared incisionless fluorescent cholangiography. Ann Surg. 2019;270(6):992–9.
11. Lehrskov LL, Westen M, Larsen SS, Jensen AB, Kristensen BB, Bisgaard T. Fluorescence or X-ray cholangiography in elective laparoscopic cholecystectomy: a randomized clinical trial. Br J Surg. 2020;107:655–61.
12. Kaibori M, Ishizaki M, Matsui K, Kwon AH. Intraoperative indocyanine green fluorescent imaging for prevention of bile leakage after hepatic resection. Surgery. 2011;150:91–8.
13. Marino MV, Builes Ramirez S, Gomez Ruiz M. The application of Indocyanine green (ICG) staining technique during robotic-assisted right hepatectomy: with video. J Gastrointest Surg. 2019;23:2312–3.
14. Brunt LM, Deziel DJ, Telem DA, Strasberg SM, Aggarwal R, Asbun H, Bonjer J, McDonald M, Alseidi A, Ujiki M, Riall TS, Hammill C, Moulton CA, Pucher PH, Parks RW, Ansari MT, Connor S, Dirks RC, Anderson B, Altieri MS, Tsamalaidze L, Stefanidis D, The Prevention of Bile Duct Injury Consensus Work Group. Safe cholecystectomy multi-society practice guideline and state of the art consensus conference on prevention of bile duct injury during cholecystectomy. Ann Surg. 2020;272:3–23.
15. Schols RM, Bouvy ND, van Dam RM, Masclee AAM, Dejong CHC, Stassen LPS. Combined vascular and biliary fluorescence imaging in laparoscopic cholecystectomy. Surg Endosc. 2013;27:4511–7.
16. Gené Škrabec C, Pardo Aranda F, Espín F, Cremades M, Navinés J, Zárate A, Cugat E. Fluorescent cholangiography with direct injection of

indocyanine green (ICG) into the gallbladder: a safety method to outline biliary anatomy. Langenbecks Arch Surg. 2020;405:827–32.
17. Sucandy I, Luberice K, Lippert T, Castro M, Krill E, Ross S, Rosemurgy A. Robotic major hepatectomy: an institutional experience and clinical outcomes. Ann Surg Oncol. 2020;27:4970–9.
18. Sucandy I, Giovannetti A, Ross S, Rosemurgy A. Institutional first 100 case experience and outcomes of robotic hepatectomy for liver tumors. Am Surg. 2020;86:200–7.
19. Sucandy I, Schlosser S, Bourdeau T, Spence J, Attili A, Ross S, Rosemurgy A. Robotic hepatectomy for benign and malignant liver tumors. J Robot Surg. 2020;14:75–80.
20. Kim J, Hong SK, Lim J, Lee JM, Cho JH, Choi Y, Yi NJ, Lee KW, Suh KS. Demarcating the exact midplane of the liver using Indocyanine green near-infrared fluorescence imaging during laparoscopic donor hepatectomy. Liver Transpl. 2021;27(6):830–9.
21. Ishizawa T, Fukushima N, Shibahara J, Masuda K, Tamura S, Aoki T, Hasegawa K, Beck Y, Fukayama M, Kokudo N. Real-time identification of liver cancers by using indocyanine green fluorescent imaging. Cancer. 2009;115:2491–504.
22. Lim C, Vibert E, Azoulay D, et al. Indocyanine green fluorescence imaging in the surgical management of liver cancers: current facts and future implications. J Visc Surg. 2014;151:117–24.
23. Ishizawa T, Masuda K, Urano Y, et al. Mechanistic background and clinical applications of indocyanine green-fluorescence imaging of hepatocellular carcinoma. Ann Surg Oncol. 2014;21:440–8.
24. Achterberg FB, Sibinga Mulder BG, Meijer RPJ, et al. Real-time surgical margin assessment using ICG-fluorescence during laparoscopic and robot-assisted resections of colorectal liver metastases. Ann Transl Med. 2020;8:1448.
25. van der Vorst JR, Schaafsma BE, Hutteman M, et al. Near-infrared fluorescence-guided resection of colorectal liver metastases. Cancer. 2013;119:3411–8.
26. Gotoh K, Yamada T, Ishikawa O, Takahashi H, Eguchi H, Yano M, Ohigashi H, Tomita Y, Miyamoto Y, Imaoka S. A novel image-guided surgery of hepatocellular carcinoma by indocyanine green fluorescence imaging navigation. J Surg Oncol. 2009;100:75–9.
27. Terasawa M, Ishizawa T, Saiura A, et al. Applications of fusion fluorescence imaging using indocyanine green in laparoscopic hepatectomy. Surg Endosc. 2017;31:5111–8.
28. Kudo H, Ishizawa T, Tani K, et al. Visualization of subcapsular hepatic malignancy by indocyanine-green fluorescence imaging during laparoscopic hepatectomy. Surg Endosc. 2014;28:2504–8.
29. Makuuchi M, Kosuge T, Takayama T, et al. Surgery for small liver cancers. Semin Surg Oncol. 1993;9:298–304.

30. Achterberg FB, Sibinga Mulder BG, Meijer RPJ, Bonsing BA, Hartgrink HH, Mieog JSD, Zlitni A, Park SM, Farina Sarasqueta A, Vahrmeijer AL, Swijnenburg RJ. Real-time surgical margin assessment using ICG-fluorescence during laparoscopic and robot-assisted resections of colorectal liver metastases. Ann Transl Med. 2020;8(21):1448.
31. Zhang P, Luo H, Zhu W, Yang J, Zeng N, Fan Y, Wen S, Xiang N, Jia F, Fang C. Real-time navigation for laparoscopic hepatectomy using image fusion of preoperative 3D surgical plan and intraoperative indocyanine green fluorescence imaging. Surg Endosc. 2020;34(8):3449–59.
32. Xu LX, He MH, Dai ZH, et al. Genomic and transcriptional heterogeneity of multifocal hepatocellular carcinoma. Ann Oncol. 2019;30:990–7.
33. Møller S, la Cour SE, Madsen JL, Bendtsen F. Indocyanine green retention test in cirrhosis and portal hypertension: accuracy and relation to severity of disease. J Gastroenterol Hepatol. 2019;34:1093–9.
34. Langella S, Ardito F, Russolillo N, Panettieri E, Perotti S, Mele C, Giuliante F, Ferrero A. Intraoperative ultrasound staging for colorectal liver metastases in the era of liver-specific magnetic resonance imaging: is it still worthwhile? J Oncol. 2019;2019:1369274.
35. Stigliano R, Marelli L, Yu D, Davies N, Patch D, Burroughs AK. Seeding following percutaneous diagnostic and therapeutic approaches for hepatocellular carcinoma. What is the risk and the outcome? Seeding risk for percutaneous approach of HCC. Cancer Treat Rev. 2007;33:437–47.
36. Aoki T, Murakami M, Koizumi T, Matsuda K, Fujimori A, Kusano T, Enami Y, Goto S, Watanabe M, Otsuka K. Determination of the surgical margin in laparoscopic liver resections using infrared indocyanine green fluorescence. Langenbecks Arch Surg. 2018;403(5):671–80.
37. Lu H, Gu J, Qian XF, Dai XZ. Indocyanine green fluorescence navigation in laparoscopic hepatectomy: a retrospective single-center study of 120 cases. Surg Today. 2021;51(5):695–702.
38. Lu H, Gu J, Qian XF, Dai XZ. Indocyanine green fluorescence navigation in laparoscopic hepatectomy: a retrospective single-center study of 120 cases. Surg Today. 2021;51(5):695–702. https://doi.org/10.1007/s00595-020-02163-8.
39. Handgraaf HJM, Boogerd LSF, Höppener DJ, Peloso A, Sibinga Mulder BG, Hoogstins CES, Hartgrink HH, van de Velde CJH, Mieog JSD, Swijnenburg RJ, Putter H, Maestri M, Braat AE, Frangioni JV, Vahrmeijer AL. Long-term follow-up after near-infrared fluorescence-guided resection of colorectal liver metastases: a retrospective multicenter analysis. Eur J Surg Oncol. 2017;43(8):1463–71.
40. Wada H, Eguchi H, Nagano H, et al. Perioperative allogenic blood transfusion is a poor prognostic factor after hepatocellular carcinoma surgery: a multi-center analysis. Surg Today. 2018;48:73–9.
41. Fang CH, Zhang P, Luo HL, et al. Application of augmented-reality surgical navigation technology combined with ICG molecular fluorescence imaging in laparoscopic hepatectomy. Zhonghua Wai Ke Za Zhi. 2019;57:578–84.

42. Aoki T, Yasuda D, Shimizu Y, Odaira M, Niiya T, Kusano T, Mitamura K, Hayashi K, Murai N, Koizumi T, Kato H, Enami Y, Miwa M, Kusano M. Image-guided liver mapping using fluorescence navigation system with indocyanine green for anatomical hepatic resection. World J Surg. 2008;32(8):1763–7.
43. Ishizawa T, Zuker NB, Kokudo N, Gayet B. Positive and negative staining of hepatic segments by use of fluorescent imaging techniques during laparoscopic hepatectomy. Arch Surg. 2012;147:393–4.
44. Makuuchi M, Hasegawa H, Yamazaki S. Ultrasonically guided subsegmentectomy. Surg Gynecol Obstet. 1985;161:346–50.
45. Takasaki K. Glissonean pedicle transection method for hepatic resection: a new concept of liver segmentation. J Hepatobiliary Pancreat Surg. 1998;5:286–91.
46. Aoki T, Koizumi T, Mansour DA, Fujimori A, Kusano T, Matsuda K, Tashiro Y, Watanabe M, Otsuka K, Murakami M. Ultrasound-guided preoperative positive percutaneous Indocyanine green fluorescence staining for laparoscopic anatomical liver resection. J Am Coll Surg. 2020;230:e7–e12.
47. Xu Y, Chen M, Meng X, Lu P, Wang X, Zhang W, Luo Y, Duan W, Lu S, Wang H. Laparoscopic anatomical liver resection guided by real-time indocyanine green fluorescence imaging: experience and lessons learned from the initial series in a single center. Surg Endosc. 2020;34(10):4683–91.
48. Chiow AKH, Rho SY, Wee IJY, Lee LS, Choi GH. Robotic ICG guided anatomical liver resection in a multi-Centre cohort: an evolution from "positive staining" into "negative staining" method. HPB (Oxford). 2021;23(3):475–82.
49. Wang X, Teh CSC, Ishizawa T, Aoki T, Cavallucci D, Lee SY, Panganiban KM, Perini MV, Shah SR, Wang H, Xu Y, Suh KS, Kokudo N. Consensus guidelines for the use of fluorescence imaging in hepatobiliary surgery. Ann Surg. 2021;274(1):97–106.
50. Nishino H, Seo S, Hatano E, Nitta T, Morino K, Toda R, Fukumitsu K, Ishii T, Taura K, Uemoto S. What is a precise anatomic resection of the liver? Proposal of a new evaluation method in the era of fluorescence navigation surgery. J Hepatobiliary Pancreat Sci. 2021;28(6):479–88. Epub 2020 Oct 4. https://doi.org/10.1002/jhbp.824.
51. Zhu K-S, Meng X-C, Huang M-S, Qian J-S, Guan S-H, Li Z-R, Jiang Z-B, Shan H, Yang Y, Chen G-H. The role of early hepatic artery ischemia on biliary complications after liver transplantation and hepatic arterial interventional therapy. Zhonghua Yi Xue Za Zhi. 2009;89:2195–8.
52. Hasegawa K, Kokudo N, Imamura H, et al. Prognostic impact of anatomic resection for hepatocellular carcinoma. Ann Surg. 2005;242:252–9.
53. Ray S, Mehta NN, Golhar A, Nundy S. Post hepatectomy liver failure - a comprehensive review of current concepts and controversies. Ann Med Surg (Lond). 2018;34:4–10.

54. Ishizawa T, Hasegawa K, Aoki T, Takahashi M, Inoue Y, Sano K, Imamura H, Sugawara Y, Kokudo N, Makuuchi M. Neither multiple tumors nor portal hypertension are surgical contraindications for hepatocellular carcinoma. Gastroenterology. 2008;134(7):1908–16.
55. Kuboki S, Furukawa K, Takayashiki T, Takano S, Miyazaki M, Ohtsuka M. Clinical implication of ICG test in major hepatectomy for biliary tract cancer. Minerva Surg. 2021;76:202–10.
56. Wang L, Xie L, Zhang N, Zhu W, Zhou J, Pan Q, Mao A, Lin Z, Wang L, Zhao Y. Predictive value of intraoperative Indocyanine green clearance measurement on postoperative liver function after anatomic major liver resection. J Gastrointest Surg. 2020;24:1342–51.
57. Kaneko J, Kokudo T, Inagaki Y, Hasegawa K. Innovative treatment for hepatocellular carcinoma (HCC). Transl Gastroenterol Hepatol. 2018;3:78.
58. Kaneko J, Inagaki Y, Ishizawa T, Gao J, Tang W, Aoki T, Sakamoto Y, Hasegawa K, Sugawara Y, Kokudo N. Photodynamic therapy for human hepatoma-cell-line tumors utilizing biliary excretion properties of indocyanine green. J Gastroenterol. 2014;49(1):110–6.
59. Miyata Y, Ishizawa T, Kamiya M, Yamashita S, Hasegawa K, Ushiku A, Shibahara J, Fukayama M, Urano Y, Kokudo N. Intraoperative imaging of hepatic cancers using γ-glutamyltranspeptidase-specific fluorophore enabling real-time identification and estimation of recurrence. Sci Rep. 2017;7(1):3542.
60. Meijer RPJ, de Valk KS, Deken MM, Boogerd LSF, Hoogstins CES, Bhairosingh SS, Swijnenburg RJ, Bonsing BA, Framery B, Fariña Sarasqueta A, Putter H, Hilling DE, Burggraaf J, Cailler F, Mieog JSD, Vahrmeijer AL. Intraoperative detection of colorectal and pancreatic liver metastases using SGM-101, a fluorescent antibody targeting CEA. Eur J Surg Oncol. 2021;47(3 Pt B):667–73.
61. Iimuro Y. ICG clearance test and 99mTc-GSA SPECT/CT fusion images. Visc Med. 2017;33:449–54.
62. Gon H, Komatsu S, Murakami S, Kido M, Tanaka M, Kuramitsu K, Tsugawa D, Awazu M, Toyama H, Fukumoto T. Real-time navigation during hepatectomy using fusion indocyanine green-fluorescence imaging: protocol for a prospective cohort study. BMJ Open. 2019;9:e030233.
63. Dip F, Boni L, Bouvet M, Carus T, Diana M, Falco J, Gurtner GC, Ishizawa T, Kokudo N, Lo Menzo E, Low PS, Masia J, Muehrcke D, Papay FA, Pulitano C, Schneider-Koraith S, Sherwinter D, Spinoglio G, Stassen L, Urano Y, Vahrmeijer A, Vibert E, Warram J, Wexner SD, White K, Rosenthal RJ. Consensus conference statement on the general use of near-infrared fluorescence imaging and Indocyanine green guided surgery: results of a modified Delphi study. Ann Surg. 2020;275:685. Epub ahead of print. PMID: 33214476. https://doi.org/10.1097/SLA.0000000000004412.

Use of Fluorescence Guidance in Endocrine Surgery

6

Jared Matson, Thinzar M. Lwin, and Michael Bouvet

Introduction

Surgeon interest in fluorescence-guided surgery (FGS) has existed since at least the 1950s. Some of the earliest applications were in ophthalmology and cataract surgery, although there was interest in applying the technology to gynecologic and hepatobiliary surgery as well [1–3]. While there were attempts at applying fluorescence in various surgical applications over the next five decades, including vascular surgery, thoracic surgery, otolaryngology, and more, the advent of high-quality commercially

J. Matson
Department of Surgery, UC San Diego, San Diego, CA, USA
e-mail: jsmatson@health.ucsd.edu

T. M. Lwin
Department of Surgery, UC San Diego, San Diego, CA, USA

Department of Surgical Oncology, Dana Farber Cancer Center, Boston, MA, USA
e-mail: thinzar_lwin@dfci.harvard.edu

M. Bouvet (✉)
Department of Surgery, UC San Diego, San Diego, CA, USA

VA San Diego Healthcare System, San Diego, CA, USA
e-mail: mbouvet@health.ucsd.edu

N. Szoka et al. (eds.), *The SAGES Manual of Fluorescence-Guided Surgery*, https://doi.org/10.1007/978-3-031-40685-0_6

available near-infrared (NIR) imaging systems in the 2000s allowed for rapid adoption and exploration of this technology in even more surgical fields, including breast surgery, colorectal surgery, plastic surgery, foregut surgery, and endocrine surgery [4–13]. This chapter will focus on the lattermost topic, and specifically on the use of indocyanine green (ICG) fluorescence guidance in adrenalectomy, parathyroidectomy, and thyroidectomy as well as the role of autofluorescence in parathyroid gland identification.

Background

Successful endocrine surgery relies on the identification and preservation of critical structures while removing pathologies that are often difficult to distinguish or separate from those normal structures. There has therefore been natural interest among endocrine surgeons in integrating NIR fluorescence imaging as the technology has become more widespread. In particular, several properties about ICG fluorescence guidance make it an intuitive choice in endocrine surgery.

It has been discovered that the thyroid and parathyroid glands possess inherent fluorescence when excited by NIR light. NIR light is chosen because of improved tissue penetration compared to other wavelengths as well as more selective autofluorescence [14, 15]. Paras et al. in 2011 described the use of custom software intraoperatively to assess this autofluorescence of the thyroid and parathyroid glands in real time and found that it could be used to distinguish thyroid and parathyroid tissue from surrounding structures as well as to differentiate the higher fluorescence parathyroid glands from the thyroid (this remained true whether the parathyroid glands were normal or hyperfunctioning) [16]. There now exist commercially available systems for detecting autofluorescence with either a probe (Fig. 6.1) or NIR imaging system (Fig. 6.2). Utilization of this natural property of parathyroid glands may be used

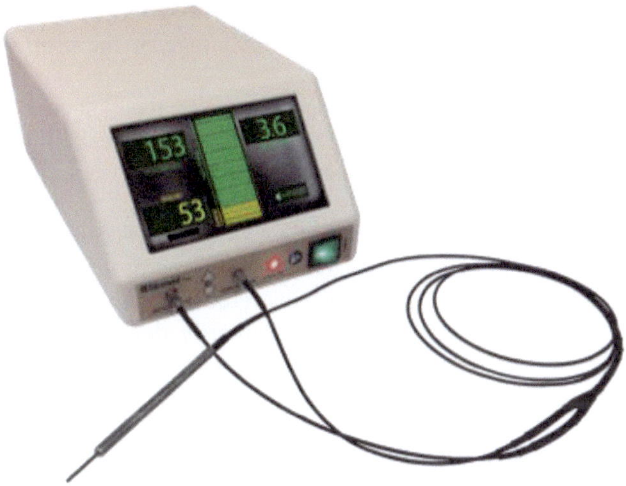

Fig. 6.1 PTeye™ (Medtronic, Minneapolis, MN, USA) near-infrared autofluorescence probe system. (Image from PTeye™ brochure https://www.medtronic.com/content/dam/medtronic-com/products/ear-nose-throat/pteye/documents/pteye-product-brochure.pdf)

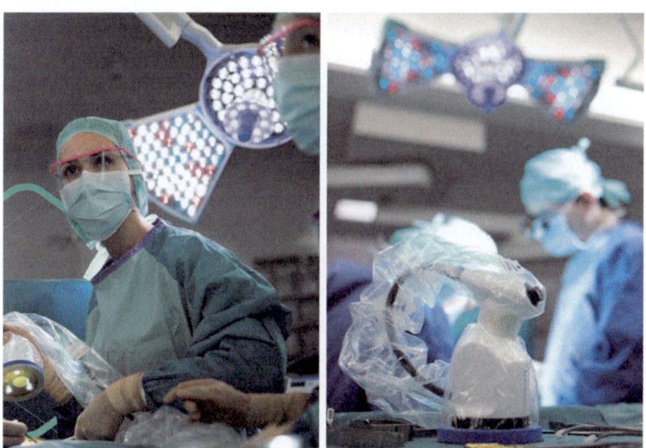

Fig. 6.2 Fluobeam® LX (Fluoptics, Grenoble, France) near-infrared autofluorescence imaging system; this system is also compatible with ICG for fluorescence angiography. (Image from Fluobeam® LX brochure https://fluoptics.us/wp-content/uploads/2019/10/Fluoptics-FluobeamLX-EN-web-2.pdf)

independently of or in combination with contrast-enhanced fluorescence angiography to take advantage of the properties unique to each system.

ICG is a water-soluble tricarbocyanine dye that has been used in humans since the 1950s [17]. It has an excellent safety profile with the primary concern potential cross-reactivity in patients with iodine allergies [18]. It fluoresces in the NIR spectrum (835 nm) when excited by NIR light (805 nm). When given intravenously, it binds avidly to plasma proteins and circulates intravascularly until it is excreted by the biliary system [19, 20]. Fluorescence therefore primarily depends on blood supply or the presence of biliary tissue. Endocrine organs require a rich blood supply and tend to be hypervascular compared to surrounding tissue. This property allows fluorescence imaging with ICG to differentiate endocrine organs from surrounding tissues, with theoretical increased distinction with hyperfunctioning and hypervascular glands. While other compounds, such as methylene blue, fluorescein green, and aminolevulinic acid, have been used as adjuncts for imaging of parathyroid glands, concerns over safety and usability have limited widespread adoption [21–24].

While initial studies required customized equipment and software to take advantage of these properties, the increased interest in and demand for NIR intraoperative imaging has resulted in standardized integration into newer models of laparoscopic and robotic imaging systems as well as the development of systems specific to open surgery (Fig. 6.3). As there is no longer a need to utilize unwieldy and complex systems, the barriers to using this technology continue to decrease. Fluorescence imaging may now be seamlessly integrated into parathyroid, thyroid, and adrenal operations with the ability to transition instantaneously between fluorescent overlays, grayscale images, and traditional white light to allow the surgeon to customize their operation for the safest and most effective operation possible.

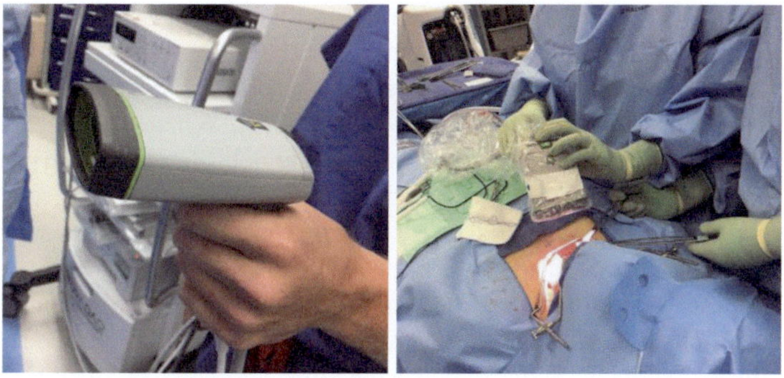

Fig. 6.3 The SPY Portable Handheld Imaging (SPY-PHI) System by Stryker (Kalamazoo, MI). The image on the left shows the handheld imaging device in the foreground with the associated imaging tower in the background. The image on the right shows the SPY-PHI System in use intraoperatively. (Figure and caption reproduced from Matson et al. [45])

Thyroid Surgery

Thyroidectomy, or removal of the thyroid gland, may be performed for several benign or malignant conditions, including Graves' disease, goiter, or thyroid cancer. The parathyroid glands are four pea-sized endocrine glands primarily responsible for calcium balance in the body. Failure to identify and protect the parathyroid glands are some of the factors associated with postoperative hypocalcemia [25]. The most common complication following thyroid surgery is postoperative hypocalcemia, occurring transiently in approximately 10–30% of patients, with permanent deficiency in about 1–10% [25, 26]. When hypocalcemia is mild, it is typically asymptomatic. However, when hypocalcemia is symptomatic, it can have a significant impact on patients' quality of life as well as duration of hospitalization and healthcare costs. Typical symptoms are related to the key role of calcium in muscle contraction and neurotransmitter release and include paresthesias, perioral numbness and tingling, and muscle spasms/tetany (such as the classic Chvostek sign, contraction of the ipsilateral facial muscles when tapping the facial nerve, and Trousseau sign, a carpopedal spasm with inflation of a blood pressure cuff over the upper arm) [27–29]. Life-threatening symptoms include seizures, laryngospasm, cardiac arrhythmias, and cardiomyopathy [27]. When permanent, even asymptomatic hypocalcemia can be debilitating, requiring lifelong supplementation with calcium and vitamin D and routine follow-up, particularly for patients with comorbidities or women of childbearing age.

Parathyroid glands can be difficult to identify even for experienced surgeons in ideal circumstances; they can be highly variable in their location (particularly the inferior glands); preoperative imaging often lacks sensitivity and/or specificity (especially for normal glands); they can be difficult to distinguish from thyroid tissue, lymph nodes, or fat tissue; and they can vary in number. This task may be even more challenging in the case of a large goiter or invasive thyroid cancer. Even when identified, preserving the delicate blood supply of parathyroid glands and ensuring adequate postoperative function presents another challenge. If devascularized, the need to autotransplant one or more parathyroid glands can also be unclear. The use of NIR imaging to visualize the presence and function of the parathyroid glands during thyroid surgery offers surgeons an intraoperative adjunct.

Autofluorescence

In 2016, Falco et al. published a feasibility study demonstrating that the parathyroid glands could be reliably identified using autofluorescence with NIR imaging in various pathologies of the thyroid and parathyroid glands and that the parathyroid glands could be distinguished from the thyroid glands using fluorescence intensity (Fig. 6.4) [30]. This led to increased interest in the practical implications of using this technology, and a randomized controlled trial by Dip et al. in 2019 included 170 patients and demonstrated that the use of NIR autofluorescence (NIRAF) imaging of the parathyroid glands increased the number of parathyroid glands identified prior to initiating the thyroid gland dissection over white light from 2.6 to 3.5 ($p < 0.001$), including at least one

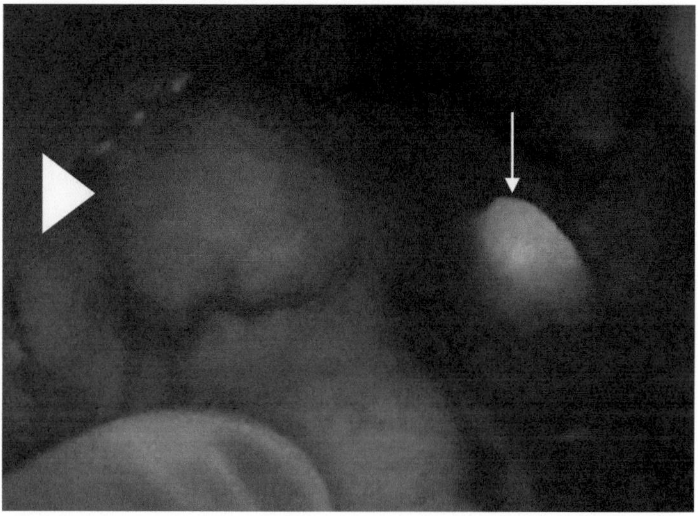

Fig. 6.4 Near-infrared autofluorescence viewed using Fluobeam® LX (Fluoptics, Grenoble, France) of a normal parathyroid gland (long arrow) demonstrating clear differentiation from the thyroid gland (arrowhead)

previously missed gland in 2/3 of patients [31]. More importantly, it reduced the rate of hypocalcemia (defined as calcium level ≤7.5 mg/dL) by 90% compared to the control group undergoing dissection under white light alone ($p = 0.005$). They did not find a significant difference between the total number of parathyroid glands identified after thyroid gland dissection under white light and pre-dissection with NIR light (3.6 vs. 3.5, respectively).

These findings were supported by the PARAFLUO multicenter randomized trial comparing rates of hypocalcemia on postoperative day (POD) 1 or 2 (corrected calcium <8.0 mg/dL). In that study, Benmiloud et al. randomized 241 patients to conventional thyroidectomy versus NIRAF-assisted thyroidectomy and found that the rates of temporary hypocalcemia were 9.1% for the NIRAF group and 21.7% for the controls ($p = 0.007$), though they did not detect a significant difference in permanent hypocalcemia (0% vs. 1.6%, respectively) [32]. These findings persisted on multivariate analysis, with an odds ratio of 0.35 for hypocalcemia in the NIRAF group. Secondary outcomes further demonstrated that the rates of autotransplantation (3.3% vs. 13.3%, $p = 0.009$) and inadvertently resected glands (2.5% vs. 11.7%, $p = 0.006$) were also lower for the NIRAF-assisted compared to traditional thyroidectomy.

While other studies have had conflicting results regarding the ability of NIRAF imaging to reduce hypocalcemia, these two large randomized trials provide level II evidence that NIRAF can improve the identification and preservation of parathyroid glands during thyroid surgery [31–35]. This may increase surgeon confidence in identification of glands and allow them to proceed more freely with thyroid gland dissection, or it could reduce the need for frozen section analysis or intraoperative parathyroid hormone (PTH) measurement and therefore save time in the operating room, as well as potentially reducing the rates of transient postoperative hypocalcemia and incidental parathyroidectomy. While NIRAF can assist in identification of parathyroid glands, it does not provide information regarding adequate parathyroid gland perfusion, which is essential for proper function in the perioperative period.

Fluorescent Dyes

One of the advantages of incorporating the use of fluorescent dyes is that they can give real-time information about the blood flow to various tissues. Early studies on the use of ICG FA during thyroid surgery suggested that having well-vascularized parathyroid glands on NIR imaging was associated with normal PTH levels following thyroid surgery [36–38]. Case series summarized by Spartalis et al. further supported the idea that adequate perfusion of parathyroid glands on ICG FA correlated with postoperative PTH levels and even that poor perfusion was associated with increased risk of hypocalcemia [39]. However, there was significant heterogeneity in the doses of ICG and protocols summarized in this review.

A randomized controlled trial by Vidal Fortuny et al. compared the need for calcium and PTH as well as vitamin D and calcium supplementation if patients had at least one well-perfused parathyroid gland by ICG FA [40]. Patients were randomized to either standard measurement of calcium and PTH on POD 1 with vitamin D and calcium supplementation or neither blood tests nor supplementation. Rates of hypocalcemia on POD 10–15 were compared. One hundred forty-six of the196 patients undergoing ICG FA had at least one well-perfused gland and were randomized; of the 50 patients who did not have a well-perfused parathyroid gland, 11 had hypoparathyroidism on POD 1 with six having persistent hypoparathyroidism on POD 10–15, while none of the randomized patients developed hypoparathyroidism ($p = 0.007$). The intervention group (no supplementation or measurement of PTH or calcium levels) was therefore found to be noninferior, suggesting that patients with at least one well-vascularized parathyroid gland by ICG FA during thyroidectomy do not need routine supplementation or lab draws. However, there are no randomized trials comparing the use of ICG FA during thyroidectomy to traditional surgery. The most impactful results would be a demonstration of reduced complications such as hypocalcemia and hypoparathyroidism with NIR imaging; while transient hypocalcemia and hypoparathyroidism are relatively common and may be observed with a single-institution study, the infrequent nature of permanent hypocalcemia will likely require a large, multicenter trial to reach adequate statistical power.

It has also been theorized that the use of ICG FA may guide more appropriate autotransplantation, preventing unnecessary autotransplantation or encouraging autotransplantation of compromised glands, but the literature in this field is limited. While Rudin et al. found that the autotransplantation rate was 36% with ICG FA compared to 12% in the control group ($p = 0.0001$), Razavi et al. concluded that low-flow patterns with ICG FA were not associated with postoperative hypoparathyroidism or hypocalcemia and may result in unnecessary autotransplantation [41, 42].

Other dye alternatives to ICG have been examined. Enny et al. evaluated the use of fluorescein green (FG) dye as a low-cost alternative to ICG [23]. FG has long been used for ophthalmologic purposes but had not previously been applied to the identification of parathyroid glands. It absorbs light in the blue spectrum (465–490 nm) and fluoresces in the green spectrum (520–530 nm). Enny et al. administered 500 mg (2 mL of 25% FG) of dye after resection of the thyroid gland followed by visualization of the parathyroid glands under white light vs. fluorescence light [23]. They found that FG fluorescence did appear to be correlated with function postoperatively, as patients who had three to four fluorescent glands did not experience hypocalcemia, whereas visualization of three or four glands with the naked eye still resulted in rates of hypocalcemia of 23% and 28%, respectively. They also found that postoperative PTH and calcium levels correlated with the number of fluorescent parathyroid glands seen with FG. While additional studies are required, this may be a viable option in low-resource areas to predict the need for postoperative supplementation and laboratory monitoring in patients undergoing thyroid surgery. As newer base models of laparoscopic and robotic imaging systems incorporate NIR capabilities, this is likely irrelevant for first-world countries. However, it may allow for application of similar principles without the required investment in expensive imaging systems in resource-limited situations.

Potential Pitfalls

While both NIRAF and dye-enhanced NIR fluorescence imaging appear to offer some advantages over traditional thyroid surgery, there are important limitations of the technologies of which surgeons must be aware while using the technology (Table 6.1).

For NIRAF, the fluorescence signal can only be detected through two to three millimeters of soft tissue. This poor tissue penetration can result in missed glands if the overlying tissues have not been sufficiently dissected. However, it can also result in devascularization if care is not taken to protect the blood supply during exposure. Intrathyroidal glands pose a particular challenge in this regard. There is also significant variability in relative fluorescence of parathyroid and thyroid glands, so it may be of limited utility in certain patients. There have been reports of false positives with brown fat, colloidal thyroid nodules, and even metastatic lymph nodes [43]. The lattermost situation is particularly concerning since the consequences of mistaking a metastatic lymph node for an inadequately perfused parathyroid gland and autotransplanting it could be catastrophic. Another limitation is that NIRAF does not offer any information on the perfusion status of the parathyroid glands. While this limits the utility in predicting postoperative function, it does allow for more ready identification

Table 6.1 Utility and limitations of fluorescence guidance during thyroid surgery

system	Benefits/utility	Limitations
Autofluorescence	Does not require any exogenous contrast agent	Occasionally, contrast between thyroid and parathyroid glands is not significant
	Distinguishes between thyroid and parathyroid glands	Does not provide information on perfusion/ viability
	Distinguishes between thyroid/parathyroid glands and surrounding tissues	Limited tissue penetration
	Improves identification of parathyroid glands before dissection	Potential false positives with metastatic lymph nodes, brown fat, colloidal thyroid nodules
	Reduces rate of inadvertently resected parathyroid glands	Requires purchase of imaging system
	Reduces rate of autotransplantation	Unclear effect on operative duration
	Helps identify inadvertently removed parathyroid glands in resection specimen for autotransplantation	
	Reduces rates of short- and medium-term hypocalcemia	

(continued)

Table 6.1 (continued)

system	Benefits/utility	Limitations
Contrast-enhanced	Provides real-time information on parathyroid gland perfusion	Limited ability to distinguish between thyroid and parathyroid glands
	May help identify and preserve parathyroid gland blood supply	Limited tissue penetration
	Can guide decision-making regarding need for autotransplantation	Subjective interpretation of degree of fluorescence/perfusion
	Helps determine which patients are at risk for postoperative hypocalcemia	ICG contraindicated in patients with iodine allergy
	Can help determine need for postoperative labs and calcium and vitamin D supplementation	Requires purchase of imaging system and dye
	Rapid cycling between fluorescence imaging, white light, and fluorescence overlay	Unclear effect on operative duration

of inadvertently removed glands in the resection specimen that could then be autotransplanted. Finally, there is an upfront cost to acquire the imaging system. There is conflicting data on the effect on operative duration and the ability to prevent hypocalcemia, and no cost-effectiveness studies have been published, so it is unclear what the overall financial impact of incorporating this technology into a thyroid surgery practice would be.

ICG FA has several similar limitations. The penetration is also limited to only several millimeters, so overlying soft tissue can obscure the parathyroid glands. There is also rapid enhancement of the thyroid gland by ICG as it is also a hypervascular organ. Therefore, ICG FA should not be used to distinguish between the thyroid and parathyroid glands. Furthermore, current systems depend on subjective interpretation of fluorescence, which limits standardization and the ability to determine cutoffs associated with postoperative hypocalcemia and hypoparathyroidism. Quantitative fluorescence is not currently integrated into imaging systems and requires customization of equipment for real-time visualization or later analysis of videos with appropriate software, which does not provide immediate feedback to the surgeon. While the capability for NIR fluorescence imaging is being integrated into newer laparoscopic and robotic imaging systems, purchasing these newer models requires significant investment. Additionally, the greatest utility in thyroid surgery is likely using systems specifically designed for open surgery that do not require using the unwieldy laparoscopic or robotic cameras to visualize the neck (and which also do not require sterilization of the camera between cases). ICG dye also presents an added cost, though it is insignificant compared to the overall operative costs. It is also contraindicated in patients with allergies to iodine. Finally, like NIRAF, there is conflicting data on the effect of the technology on duration of the operation. There is undeniably a requirement to wait for fluorescence after administration of the dye, but most studies have shown this to range from less than a minute to no more than 3 min [44, 45]. This may also result in time-savings if it allows surgeons to proceed with the operation and wound closure without waiting for intraoperative PTH levels or frozen section analysis or avoid unnecessary autotransplantation.

Summary and Vision for Application

Based on early results, there has been a good deal of excitement and numerous publications about the use of fluorescence image guidance in thyroid surgery. While the vast majority of studies are retrospective, single-institution case series or cohort studies, there are several large, randomized trials that seem to show superiority of NIRAF visualization of the parathyroid glands compared to traditional surgery [31, 32]. ICG FA may provide additional insight into the perfusion status of identified glands to help guide autotransplantation and the need for postoperative monitoring and supplementation. The systematic review by Demarchi et al. summarized 25 studies utilizing either NIRAF or dye-enhanced NIR imaging in thyroid surgery; they concluded that the use of the technology was feasible and safe and several benefits including improved identification and preservation of the parathyroid glands as well as early identification of mistakenly resected glands that might allow autotransplantation [44]. Together, this may result in reduced postoperative hypoparathyroidism and hypocalcemia. This is supported by the findings of Barbieri et al.; the authors performed a meta-analysis of 13 studies looking at fluorescence imaging in total thyroidectomy and included 1484 operations [46]. They found that fluorescence-guided surgery resulted in improvements in both short- and medium-term hypocalcemia rates compared to traditional surgery (8% vs. 15% and 1% vs. 5%, respectively).

Taking this information into consideration, we believe that these techniques can be used in complementary fashion for optimal results. In any case, a pre-incision PTH level should be drawn. The utility of NIRAF seems to primarily be in the early identification and preservation of parathyroid glands and in examining the resection specimen for missed glands. Therefore, once adequate exposure of the thyroid gland has been achieved through incision of the skin, soft tissue, and platysma and retraction of the strap muscles, the surgical field should be examined with the use of a device designed for detection of parathyroid gland autofluorescence. The location of identified parathyroid glands should be noted, and they should be protected while the dissection carefully continues, periodically reexamining the field if candidate structures are found. Once the thyroid specimen has been removed, it may also be examined briefly for any missed glands, noting the limitations of penetration in identifying deeper intrathyroidal glands.

The previously identified glands should be confirmed, and then 2.5 mg of ICG (1 mL of reconstituted solution, 25 mg vial with 10 mL of sterile water) should be administered through a peripheral IV immediately followed by a 10 cc flush of normal saline or lactated ringers by the anesthesia provider while the surgical field is visualized with an NIR imaging device. The parathyroid glands should fluoresce within 30–90 s if they remain well-vascularized, and the peak intensity of their fluorescence as well as the rate of increase in fluorescence intensity may provide evidence for the adequacy of their perfusion. Glands that appear to be devascularized (minimal or no fluorescence) can be incised with a scalpel and if there is no bleeding can be considered for autotransplantation. If there are at least two well-vascularized glands, autotransplantation of any remaining glands is likely unnecessary. Similarly, in the case of at least two well-vascularized glands, providers may choose to forego postoperative PTH/calcium monitoring or prophylactic vitamin D and calcium supplementation.

If there is concern that a candidate gland may be a metastatic lymph node, this structure should be sampled and sent for frozen section analysis before autotransplantation. Otherwise, frozen section analysis and rapid PTH assays are not necessary and should be used at surgeon discretion on a case-by-case basis.

Parathyroid Surgery

The utility of fluorescence-guided surgery in identifying parathyroid glands and determining their perfusion status may also be applied to parathyroid surgery. Parathyroid surgery is primarily performed to prevent complications or alleviate symptoms related to hypercalcemia secondary to elevated PTH levels (i.e., kidney stones, fatigue, depression, osteoporosis, and other symptoms). The most common indication for parathyroidectomy is primary hyperparathyroidism, or abnormally elevated PTH and calcium levels, which is usually due to a single hyperfunctional parathyroid adenoma. Less common causes of primary hyperparathyroidism are multiple adenomas, diffuse hyperplasia, and parathyroid carcinoma. In patients with single or multiple adenomas, their disease process can typically be cured and calcium/PTH normalized by removal of the pathologic gland(s). Patients with diffuse hyperplasia as well as those with secondary (caused by constant stimulation from low calcium and elevated phosphate levels in renal disease) or tertiary (hyperparathyroidism from renal disease that persists after kidney transplant) hyperparathyroidism require subtotal parathyroidectomy, or removal of most parathyroid glands and leaving about 1/2 gland in situ or autotransplanted to a more easily accessible area such as the forearm or sternocleidomastoid. Failure to remove diseased glands may result in persistent hyperparathyroidism, while leaving or autotransplanting inadequately perfused glands during subtotal parathyroidectomy could result in hypoparathyroidism and hypocalcemia. Preoperative imaging is most effective at localizing single adenomas but has far less sensitivity and specificity for multiple adenomas or diffuse hyperplasia; even in the case of a single adenoma, however, intraoperative localization may present a challenge [47–50]. Using near-infrared imaging either to elicit autofluorescence of the parathyroid gland or in combination with fluorescent dye such as ICG may facilitate localization of the abnormal glands, and the latter may be used to help determine which gland is most appropriate for preservation/autotransplantation.

Autofluorescence

Parathyroid gland autofluorescence has been found to be helpful in identifying parathyroid glands during parathyroid surgery for various indications as well as during thyroid surgery. Parras et al. found a significant difference in autofluorescence intensity between parathyroid and thyroid glands ($p = 0.00000235$) [16]. McWade et al. corroborated this (parathyroid gland autofluorescence is between 1.2 and 29 times higher than thyroid autofluorescence) and found a sensitivity for intraoperative parathyroid gland detection of 97% [51]. The clinical significance of autofluorescence in parathyroidectomy is to help identify parathyroid glands in order to prevent persistent hyperparathyroidism due to a missed adenoma or insufficient resection in diffuse hyperplasia. Given current high cure rates at specialist centers (up to 97%), superiority over traditional surgery is difficult to demonstrate [52]. In their 2019 review of NIRAF in thyroid and parathyroid surgery, DiMarco and Palazzo determined that 902 patients would need to be included to demonstrate an improvement in persistent hyperparathyroidism from 2% to 0.1% [34]. Thus far, no studies have been performed looking at that outcome. However, Demarchi et al. recently described a characteristic autofluorescent pattern for parathyroid adenomas (heterogenous fluorescence with a more highly fluorescent cap that correlated with normal parathyroid tissue in 74% of specimens); all patients in their study demonstrated cure of their primary hyperparathyroidism [53]. If this finding is confirmed in larger studies, the characteristic pattern may permit the use of NIRAF in further distinguishing normal from abnormal gland(s) and obviating the need to wait for confirmation with a 50% reduction in PTH levels post-resection, as is the current standard.

Fluorescent Dyes

The use of dye-based techniques to help identify the parathyroid glands has existed for half a century [21]. The combination of dye administration with NIR fluorescence imaging has seen a significant uptick in interest and use in the last decade. While various compounds have been explored for his purpose, including methylene blue and aminolevulinic acid, the dye that has been the most studied is ICG [12, 22, 24, 39].

It has been proposed that ICG FA may be particularly helpful in identifying abnormal parathyroid glands because of their potential increased blood flow. The initial case study by Chakedis et al. demonstrated that ICG FA could effectively assist with localization of a recurrent parathyroid adenoma in redo parathyroidectomy [54]. Several case series confirmed its utility in reoperative parathyroidectomy as well as in initial parathyroid surgery [55–59]. These studies showed superior sensitivity of ICG FA compared to traditional techniques such as ultrasound or sestamibi, and even compared to newer imaging modalities such as 4D CT.

When compared to NIRAF, ICG FA can also give insight into the perfusion status of the parathyroid glands (Fig. 6.5). This is important in subtotal parathyroidectomy to ensure that an adequately perfused remnant is selected for either preservation or autotransplantation. Studies have demonstrated that ICG FA may be useful in this regard, as none of the patients in these reported case series developed hypoparathyroidism [39, 58, 60]. This was one of

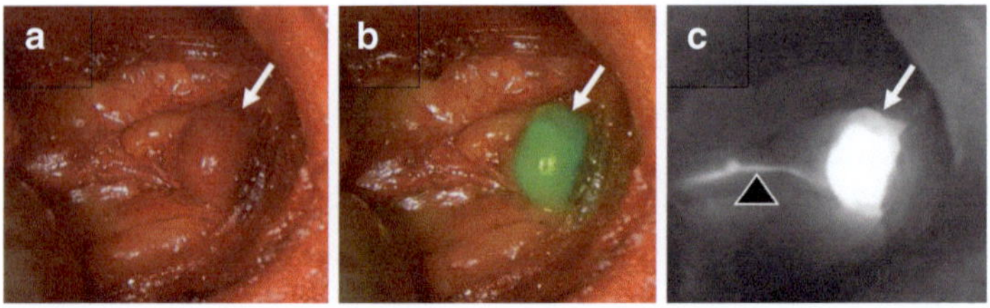

Fig. 6.5 A representative image of parathyroid adenoma fluorescence following injection of ICG and excitement with NIR light. All are from the same patient and injection of ICG. (**a**) Parathyroid adenoma (white arrow) under white light prior to injection of ICG. (**b**) The adenoma (white arrow) with computer-generated green overlay after peak fluorescence was achieved. (**c**) Fluorescence of the adenoma (white arrow) and its feeding vessel (black triangle) seen in grayscale viewing mode. (Figure and caption reproduced from Matson et al. [45])

the proposed uses for contrast-enhanced NIR fluorescence imaging in parathyroidectomy described by Solórzano et al. in their recent review of NIR fluorescence in endocrine surgery of the neck [12].

Doses of ICG administered for the detection of parathyroid glands during parathyroidectomy were variable [39]. As little as 2.5 mg can be used effectively, and repeat administration of ICG can still provide adequate fluorescence visualization, such as for bilateral neck exploration, with ICG FA first performed on one side of the neck before repeating the procedure on the contralateral side [39, 45]. The parathyroid glands will typically reach peak fluorescence in less than a minute; the authors' recently published study found an average time to initial fluorescence of 26.7 s and average time to peak fluorescence of 38.0 s, with a significant association between time to fluorescence and how quickly the anesthesia provider flushed the IV following injection of the dye [39, 45].

Potential Pitfalls

Like thyroid surgery, both NIRAF and dye-enhanced fluorescence imaging have a potential role in parathyroid surgery. This role is variable depending on the exact indication for surgery, and the limitations vary accordingly (Table 6.2).

Table 6.2 Utility and limitations of fluorescence guidance during parathyroid surgery

system	Benefits/utility	Limitations
Autofluorescence	Does not require any exogenous contrast agent	Occasionally, contrast between thyroid and parathyroid glands is not significant
	Distinguishes between thyroid and parathyroid glands	Does not provide information on perfusion/viability
	Distinguishes between thyroid/parathyroid glands and surrounding tissues	Limited tissue penetration
	May improve intraoperative identification of parathyroid glands over traditional surgery	Potential false positives with metastatic lymph nodes, brown fat, colloidal thyroid nodules
	Potential to identify parathyroid adenomas based on characteristic fluorescence pattern in some cases	Requires purchase of imaging system
	Potential to reduce rates of persistent hyperparathyroidism	Unclear effect on operative duration
Contrast-enhanced	Provides real-time information on parathyroid gland perfusion	Limited ability to distinguish between thyroid and parathyroid glands
	May help guide selection of remnant gland for subtotal parathyroidectomy	Limited tissue penetration
	May reduce hypoparathyroidism/hypocalcemia after subtotal parathyroidectomy	Subjective interpretation of degree of fluorescence/perfusion
	May improve localization of parathyroid adenomas over traditional preoperative imaging techniques	ICG contraindicated in patients with iodine allergy
	Dosing may be safely repeated for bilateral neck exploration	Requires purchase of imaging system and dye
	Uptake of ICG is rapid in both normal and pathologic glands	Unclear effect on operative duration
	Rapid cycling between fluorescence imaging, white light, and fluorescence overlay	

The primary role of NIRAF in parathyroid surgery is in identification of the parathyroid glands, similar to its role in thyroid surgery. Therefore, some of the potential issues with its use are the same: the limited depth of penetration (just a couple millimeters) could result in missed glands, potentially causing persistent hyperparathyroidism and requiring reoperation, or could result in devascularization of glands that should be preserved, potentially resulting in hypoparathyroidism and hypocalcemia; the lack of information about perfusion status could result in selection for preservation or autotransplantation of a suboptimally perfused gland and hypocalcemia. In parathyroid surgery, it is also important to be aware of the variable autofluorescence of pathologic parathyroid glands (often less brightly fluorescent than normal glands or heterogenous in enhancement, and sometimes even hypofluorescent compared to surrounding tissues), which is particularly true for secondary hyperparathyroidism and multiple endocrine neoplasia type (MEN1).

Dye-enhanced NIR fluorescence imaging may be used for either the identification of normal or abnormal parathyroid glands during parathyroidectomy or for the assessment of perfusion status of the remnant gland in subtotal parathyroidectomy. The limitations are essentially the same as for thyroid surgery: limited tissue penetration and ability to detect intrathyroidal or other "buried" glands, inability to differentiate thyroid and parathyroid tissue, and potentially increased costs and OR time associated with its use. However, in parathyroid surgery, there may be better delineation between thyroid and parathyroid tissue since the parathyroid gland being localized is usually hyperplastic and therefore should theoretically have increased uptake of ICG and greater relative fluorescence.

Summary and Vision for Application

Overall, the data supporting the use of both NIRAF and ICG FA in parathyroid surgery is limited, with no randomized trials or meta-analyses supporting its use. There are several case series that seem to demonstrate superior sensitivity compared to traditional methods of preoperative localization and multiple systematic reviews that highlight the potential uses of these technologies. There remains a need for large cohort studies and randomized controlled trials to better support widespread adoption of these techniques.

Because the data is more limited, the optimal use of either or both NIRAF and ICG FA in parathyroid surgery is unclear. For a surgeon who already uses one or both technologies in their thyroid operations, they may prefer to continue integrating that technology into their parathyroid operations. However, the authors believe that ICG FA offers more advantages in parathyroid surgery over autofluorescence. First, pathologic parathyroid glands have variable autofluorescence, which may include heterogenous enhancement or global hypoenhancement [34]. This is particularly true in the diffuse hyperplasia of secondary hyperparathyroidism and multiple endocrine neoplasia type 1 (MEN1). Second, the use of ICG can provide information on the perfusion status of the parathyroid glands and guide autotransplantation or subtotal parathyroidectomy to reduce the risk of postoperative hypoparathyroidism. The following represents our technique.

The beginning of the operation is no different than for thyroid surgery, beginning with the anesthesia provider drawing a pre-incision PTH level followed by the surgeon making a transverse cervical neck incision and carrying the dissection down through the platysma and retracting the strap muscles. Once the thyroid gland is identified, it is retracted toward the midline from the presumed site of pathology (based on preoperative imaging) or from the surgeon's preferred initial side if addressing 4-gland disease. Gentle dissection is then performed to attempt to identify the parathyroid glands on that side without disrupting their blood supply. Particular attention is given to attempting to find the enlarged gland in the case of an assumed single adenoma. After identifying the candidate gland(s), the surgical field is visualized through the fluorescence imaging system to ensure appropriate image quality. This may require adjustment of the OR lights away from the surgical field or dimming of the room lights. 2.5 mg of ICG (1 mL of reconstituted solution) is then injected by the anesthesia provider through a peripheral IV followed immediately by a flush of at least 10 cc of normal saline or lactated ringers solution. The parathyroid glands fluoresce within 30–90 s if they remain well-vascularized, and the time to reach peak intensity of their fluorescence as well as the degree of peak fluorescence intensity may provide qualitative information for the adequacy of their perfusion. If a likely single adenoma is confirmed, the blood supply to that gland may be ligated and the specimen removed; the surgeon may proceed with wound closure if they have sufficient confidence in removal of the pathologic gland. If there is uncertainty, the gland may be sent for frozen section, an intraoperative PTH level may be sent (with a 50% drop in PTH at 10 min after resection confirming cure), and/or the contralateral side may be explored. In the case of diffuse hyperplasia, the perfusion status of the glands on ICG FA should be noted and attention turned to the contralateral side. Once the presumed parathyroid glands on that side have been identified, the procedure with visualization of the field using the fluorescence imaging system and injection of ICG should be repeated. A gland that exhibits adequate enhancement with ICG should be selected to reduce the risk of postoperative hypoparathyroidism. Successive clipping of the gland chosen for partial preservation should then be performed until an appropriate remnant has been created, with a final assessment of perfusion with the fluorescence imaging system. If this process results in damage to the gland such that it appears inadequate, the gland should be excised, and the procedure repeated with one of the remaining glands. Once an appropriate remnant is created, the blood supply to the remaining glands may be ligated and the specimens removed.

We routinely draw a PTH level and calcium level in the recovery area. For patients with one or multiple adenomas, if there has been an appropriate drop in the PTH level and the patient is otherwise meeting criteria for discharge and without risk factors for complications, they may be allowed to discharge. If the PTH level does not experience an adequate drop, it is at the surgeon's discretion and OR availability to return to the OR later the same day or the next for removal of a possible missed adenoma versus continued observation and trending of PTH levels. For patients who have undergone subtotal parathyroidectomy, we admit them for serial calcium checks and monitoring for symptoms until their calcium levels have stabilized and their degree of supplementation has been determined.

Adrenal Surgery

The adrenal glands are small, bilateral retroperitoneal endocrine organs positioned just cephalad to the kidneys whose normal function is the production of several essential hormones, including cortisol, sex hormones, aldosterone, and catecholamines. Tumors that develop in the adrenal glands may be either benign or malignant and may additionally produce one or more of those substances. When these tumors are functional, the excess hormones may lead to symptoms such as tachycardia and hypertension (catecholamines) or various syndromes such as Cushing's syndrome (hypercortisolism), Conn syndrome (hyperaldosteronism), virilization, and/or feminization.

Adrenalectomy is recommended for functional tumors, malignant tumors, and tumors at risk for malignancy (typically benign-appearing lesions that are greater than 4–6 cm, though some are so characteristic on imaging that even larger lesions do not require resection unless symptomatic, such as myelolipomas or simple cysts), with minimally invasive adrenalectomy being the standard of care for benign lesions. Adrenalectomy poses several challenges for surgeons. It may be difficult to distinguish the adrenal gland from the surrounding retroperitoneal fat or between the tumor and normal adrenal tissue (as may be required in partial adrenalectomy for bilateral benign tumors or in patients with genetic diseases putting them at increased risk of recurrence), particularly in minimally invasive surgery where surgeons lack the tactile feedback of open operations. It is also essential to identify critical vascular structures early in the operation, including the inferior vena cava (IVC), renal vessels, and adrenal vein. For example, expeditious identification of the adrenal vein is essential during resection of a pheochromocytoma; the vein must be ligated before manipulating the tumor to prevent catecholamine surge and hemodynamic instability. The right adrenal vein is short and connects directly to the IVC, whereas the left connects to the renal vein. Technical errors during surgery can result in significant hemorrhage, potentially leading to blood transfusions or even death [61, 62]. NIR fluorescence imaging offers a natural opportunity for safer and more efficient surgery, particularly for minimally invasive approaches.

Fluorescence Guidance During Adrenalectomy

The earliest studies of contrast enhancement for adrenalectomy are less than two decades old. In 2003, Obermeyer et al. demonstrated reduced operative times using methylene blue in a preclinical study of laparoscopic adrenalectomy in pigs [63]. However, the doses required for adequate color change in the glands were several times higher than typical doses used clinically, and it has known potential toxic side effects [22]. Additionally, the duration of the visualization enhancement was less than 15 min, and the high doses required would not allow for repeated injections, further decreasing its utility. In 2013, Manny et al. published the first clinical use of ICG for fluorescence-guided adrenal surgery [64]. Their feasibility study on three patients undergoing robotic partial adrenalectomy demonstrated the safety and the potential of the technique, as the masses were all hypofluorescent compared to normal adrenal tissue. While other fluorophores have been studied, ICG remains the most used and studied compound for fluorescence imaging guidance during adrenal surgery [13, 65, 66].

Following the study by Manny et al. exploring the use of ICG in robotic partial adrenalectomy, DeLong, et al. published the first description of ICG FA-aided laparoscopic adrenalectomy in a four-patient case series in 2015 [64, 67]. They highlighted the value of the technique in defining the vascular anatomy and guiding an efficient and hemostatic dissection (Fig. 6.6). Colvin et al. then compared ICG fluorescence imaging to conventional view in 40 consecutive patients undergoing robotic adrenalectomy; they found that contrast-enhanced imaging was superior to conventional view in 46.5% of cases and equivalent in another

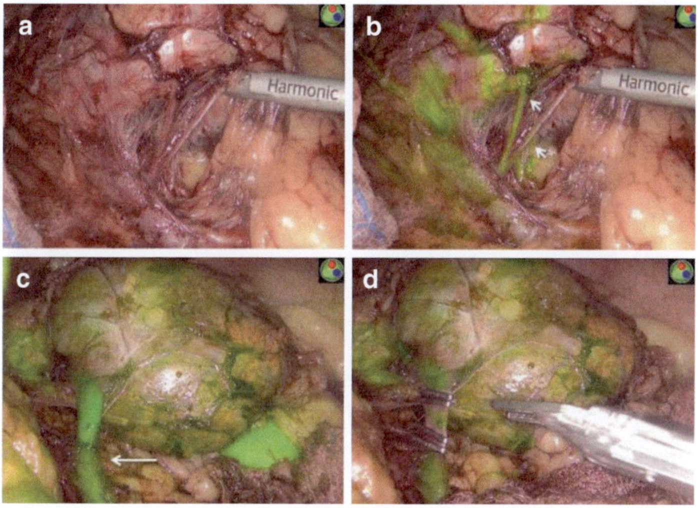

Fig. 6.6 View of the abnormal adrenal gland in Case 2 (left adrenalectomy) prior to administration of ICG (**a**); view of the adrenal gland after early administration of ICG, enhancing the arterial vasculature (short arrows), facilitating meticulous hemostatic dissection with the harmonic scalpel (**b**); the ICG subsequently illuminates the adrenal parenchyma and strongly enhances the adrenal vein (long arrow) (**c**); surgical navigation is not disrupted in the fluorescent mode; the adrenal vein is clipped under fluorescence guidance (**d**). *ICG* indocyanine green. (Figure and caption reproduced from DeLong et al. [55])

25.6% [68]. The only parameter that was predictive of fluorescence imaging superiority over conventional was tumor type. Since these early studies, several other studies have been performed in robotic and laparoscopic total or partial adrenalectomy, demonstrating several important features:

1. The technique is rapid, with fluorescence of critical structures beginning within 30–90 s of injection of ICG and waning within 20 min of injection [68–71].
2. The technique is safe, with no complications reported due to the ICG and multiple injections well-tolerated without nearing maximum safe doses [68–71].

3. Different fluorescent patterns may be expected depending on tumor type, with adrenocortical tumors characteristically showing hyperfluorescence compared to surrounding adrenal tissue, while other tumor types, such as pheochromocytoma, may be hypofluorescent [68, 70]. This may help with distinction between normal and pathologic tissue and improve the likelihood of complete resection of the tumor while leaving adequate functional remnant during partial adrenalectomy.

The quality of evidence supporting the use of ICG FA in adrenalectomy remains low, however, with no cohort studies or randomized controlled trials.

Potential Pitfalls

While ICG FA shows promise in enhancing laparoscopic and robotic adrenalectomy, there are several potential limitations (Table 6.3). For instance, ICG is excreted through the biliary system and is taken up by hepatocytes shortly after administration. The fluorescence of biliary tissue lingers much longer than does that of other tissues or the vasculature, however, and thus may limit the utility of ICG FA, particularly for posterior approach to right adrenalectomy. Therefore, if bilateral lesions are present, the surgeon should consider beginning on the right so that the repeat administration for the second side is less significantly impacted by this property of ICG and if there is an isolated right-sided lesion, a lateral or anterior approach should be considered. Additionally, the current technology doesn't have the capability for quantitative assessment of fluorescence intraoperatively, so relative fluorescence depends on subjective surgeon assessment. This limits the generalizability of results from prior studies. As with other uses of ICG FA, there is also a significant upfront cost required for acquisition of the NIR imaging system. However, this capability is being integrated into newer laparoscopic and robotic platforms, which would then not require purchase of a separate NIR-capable device. There is then a nominal cost for the ICG required for each case. It is also unclear what the effect is of

Table 6.3 Utility and limitations of fluorescence guidance during adrenal surgery

system	Benefits/utility	Limitations
Contrast-enhanced	May help in identification of critical vascular structures, thereby decreasing bleeding complications	Use in R adrenalectomy limited by hepatic contrast uptake and prolonged fluorescence
	Distinguishes between adrenal gland and retroperitoneal adipose tissue	ICG contraindicated in patients with iodine allergy
	May distinguish between normal adrenal tissue and tumor (especially pheochromocytoma) for partial adrenalectomy	Limited tissue penetration
	Allows for real-time assessment of perfusion of remnant adrenal tissue	Subjective interpretation of degree of fluorescence/perfusion
	Uptake of ICG is rapid	Requires purchase of imaging system
	Dosing may be safely repeated	Unclear effect on operative duration
	Rapid cycling between fluorescence imaging, white light, and fluorescence overlay	

implementing ICG FA on operative duration; while in theory it could improve operative efficiency by allowing for more rapid identification of critical structures such as the adrenal vein and for easier delineation of tissue planes, there is time required after the administration of ICG before peak fluorescence is achieved.

Summary and Vision for Application

ICG FA has been studied in several applications for minimally invasive adrenal surgery. It has been shown to have superiority over conventional imaging for the majority of cases during robotic adrenalectomy, especially with adrenocortical tumors [68]. It is also effective during partial adrenalectomy at ensuring complete resection of the lesion while sparing uninvolved tissue and assessing the vascularization of that tissue [64, 71]. Other studies have shown that it is helpful during laparoscopic adrenalectomy at distinguishing between tissues of interest and identifying critical vascular structures [67, 69]. Support for more widespread use will require large, multicenter studies with clear definitions of outcomes of interest (e.g., recurrence rates, sufficient remnant adrenal tissue, operative duration, complication rates).

We believe that ICG FA may be effectively used in either laparoscopic or robotic total or partial adrenalectomy and offers similar advantages regardless of the surgical approach. At our institution, we most commonly utilize a transperitoneal approach for laparoscopic adrenalectomy. Patient positioning is then dependent on the laterality of the pathology, with the patient in lateral decubitus position with the side of interest up. For a right-sided lesion, entry into the abdomen is typically gained under direct visualization through a 5 mm port. The abdomen is then insufflated through this port and three additional trocars are placed in the right upper quadrant. The liver is retracted cephalad and dissected from the retroperitoneum with an energy device to preserve hemostasis. Once the IVC and right adrenal gland are visualized, 5 mg of ICG (2.5 mg/mL) may then be administered via a peripheral vein by the anesthesia provider followed by a 10 mL flush with normal saline or lactated ringers solution. The adrenal vein is then identified, clipped, and divided before proceeding with completion of the dissection of the adrenal gland and tumor. Once dissected free, the gland and tumor are then placed intact into a laparoscopic bag and removed through a 10 mm port.

Left adrenalectomy is performed in similar fashion with the exception that after insufflating through the 5 mm port, only two additional ports are placed in the left upper quadrant. In this case, the splenic flexure is initially mobilized with an energy device to expose the left kidney and adrenal gland. The spleen and pancreas are mobilized anteriorly to improve visualization of the tumor. ICG is then administered to identify the left adrenal vein which is then clipped and divided, and fluorescence guidance is used to complete dissection of the adrenal gland and tumor. The gland and tumor are then removed intact via a laparoscopic bag through a 10 or 12 mm port.

Discussion

Safe and successful endocrine surgery requires a detailed understanding of the relevant anatomy. However, even experienced endocrine surgeons sometimes have trouble identifying and preserving essential structures while removing the pathology. Fluorescence-guided surgery provides an adjunct that can aid surgeons in identifying relevant structures and minimizing complications.

In thyroid and parathyroid surgery, autofluorescence has been shown to reliably improve identification of the thyroid glands and differentiate between the parathyroid glands and surrounding tissues, including the thyroid gland, with randomized controlled trials demonstrating decreased rates of hypocalcemia following thyroidectomy [31, 32]. Meanwhile, ICG FA may provide surgeons with information on the perfusion status of the parathyroid glands in addition to helping to identify them during parathyroidectomy. A randomized controlled trial has shown that prophylactic vitamin D and calcium supplementation may be safely foregone in patients with at least one well-perfused parathyroid gland by ICG FA post-thyroidectomy [40]. Other applications include selecting an appropriate gland for preservation during subtotal parathyroidectomy to minimize the risk of postoperative hypothyroidism and hypocalcemia.

During adrenal surgery, ICG FA has been shown to aid in identification of critical vascular structures and distinguishing tissue planes during robotic and laparoscopic adrenalectomy [67–70]. It also offers the potential to ensure complete removal of pathologic tissue while preserving an adequate functional remnant during bilateral partial adrenalectomy [64, 71].

Conclusion

Overall, the use of various fluorescence imaging techniques in endocrine surgery shows promise but requires further investigation. It has been shown to be safe and helpful in several applications but optimal procedures and uses are only beginning to be defined.

Large, well-designed randomized trials with long-term follow-up are needed to determine the utility in preventing permanent hypocalcemia in thyroid surgery and subtotal parathyroidectomy. Randomized trials and larger cohort studies are needed comparing traditional techniques with ICG FA during adrenal surgery to define its effect on critical outcomes such as complete resection, recurrence, and preservation of a sufficient functional remnant during partial adrenalectomy. Quality data regarding operative duration using fluorescence guidance compared to traditional surgery in all fields will also help to define its optimal use and cost-effectiveness. Additionally, investigation into tissue-targeted fluorophores, such as for identification of peripheral nerves in head and neck surgery, is in its infancy but has the potential to radically alter the landscape of FGS [72]. As FGS becomes more accessible and integrated into imaging platforms, perhaps the barriers to adopting the technology will fall and fluorescence imaging will become even more broadly adopted by endocrine surgeons around the world.

References

1. Hague EB. Fluorescing illumination in cataract surgery. Am J Ophthalmol. 1959;47(5 Pt 1):663–6. https://doi.org/10.1016/s0002-9394(14)78191-7.
2. Peck GC, Mack HP, Holbrook WA, Figge FH. Use of hematoporphyrin fluorescence in biliary and cancer surgery. Am Surg. 1955;21(3):181–8.
3. Sussman W. Detection of gynecologic cancer by fluorescence microscopy. Obstet Gynecol. 1959;13(3):273–7.
4. Homasson JP, Bonniot JP, Angebault M, Renault P, Carnot F, Santelli G. Fluorescence as a guide to bronchial biopsy. Thorax. 1985;40(1):38–40. https://doi.org/10.1136/thx.40.1.38.
5. Leon MB, Almagor Y, Bartorelli AL, Prevosti LG, Teirstein PS, Chang R, et al. Fluorescence-guided laser-assisted balloon angioplasty in patients with femoropopliteal occlusions. Circulation. 1990;81(1):143–55. https://doi.org/10.1161/01.cir.81.1.143.
6. Mehlmann M, Betz CS, Stepp H, Arbogast S, Baumgartner R, Grevers G, et al. Fluorescence staining of laryngeal neoplasms after topical application of 5-aminolevulinic acid: preliminary results. Lasers Surg Med. 1999;25(5):414–20. https://doi.org/10.1002/(sici)1096-9101(1999)25:5<414::aid-lsm8>3.0.co;2-e.

7. Silverman DG, Roberts A, Reilly CA, Brousseau DA, Norton KJ, Bartley E, et al. Fluorometric quantification of low-dose fluorescein delivery to predict amputation site healing. Surgery. 1987;101(3):335–41.
8. Girard N, Delomenie M, Malhaire C, Sebbag D, Roulot A, Sabaila A, et al. Innovative DIEP flap perfusion evaluation tool: qualitative and quantitative analysis of indocyanine green-based fluorescence angiography with the SPY-Q proprietary software. PloS One. 2019;14(6):e0217698. https://doi.org/10.1371/journal.pone.0217698.
9. Reinhart MB, Huntington CR, Blair LJ, Heniford BT, Augenstein VA. Indocyanine green: historical context, current applications, and future considerations. Surg Innov. 2016;23(2):166–75. https://doi.org/10.1177/1553350615604053.
10. Jafari MD, Lee KH, Halabi WJ, Mills SD, Carmichael JC, Stamos MJ, et al. The use of indocyanine green fluorescence to assess anastomotic perfusion during robotic assisted laparoscopic rectal surgery. Surg Endosc. 2013;27(8):3003–8. https://doi.org/10.1007/s00464-013-2832-8.
11. Griffiths M, Chae MP, Rozen WM. Indocyanine green-based fluorescent angiography in breast reconstruction. Gland Surg. 2016;5(2):133–49. https://doi.org/10.3978/j.issn.2227-684X.2016.02.01.
12. Solórzano CC, Thomas G, Berber E, Wang TS, Randolph GW, Duh QY, et al. Current state of intraoperative use of near infrared fluorescence for parathyroid identification and preservation. Surgery. 2021;169(4):868–78. https://doi.org/10.1016/j.surg.2020.09.014.
13. Agcaoglu O, Kulle CB, Berber E. Indocyanine green fluorescence imaging for robotic adrenalectomy. Gland Surg. 2020;9(3):849–52. https://doi.org/10.21037/gs-2019-ra-06.
14. Solórzano CC, Thomas G, Baregamian N, Mahadevan-Jansen A. Detecting the near infrared autofluorescence of the human parathyroid: hype or opportunity? Ann Surg. 2020;272(6):973–85. https://doi.org/10.1097/sla.0000000000003700.
15. van Manen L, Handgraaf HJM, Diana M, Dijkstra J, Ishizawa T, Vahrmeijer AL, et al. A practical guide for the use of indocyanine green and methylene blue in fluorescence-guided abdominal surgery. J Surg Oncol. 2018;118(2):283–300. https://doi.org/10.1002/jso.25105.
16. Paras C, Keller M, White L, Phay J, Mahadevan-Jansen A. Near-infrared autofluorescence for the detection of parathyroid glands. J Biomed Opt. 2011;16(6):067012. https://doi.org/10.1117/1.3583571.
17. Winkler K, Tygstrup N. Determination of hepatic blood flow in man by cardio green. Scand J Clin Lab Invest. 1960;12:353–6. https://doi.org/10.3109/00365516009062449.
18. Hope-Ross M, Yannuzzi LA, Gragoudas ES, Guyer DR, Slakter JS, Sorenson JA, et al. Adverse reactions due to indocyanine green. Ophthalmology. 1994;101(3):529–33. https://doi.org/10.1016/s0161-6420(94)31303-0.

19. Alander JT, Kaartinen I, Laakso A, Pätilä T, Spillmann T, Tuchin VV, et al. A review of indocyanine green fluorescent imaging in surgery. Int J Biomed Imaging. 2012;2012:940585. https://doi.org/10.1155/2012/940585.
20. Desmettre T, Devoisselle JM, Mordon S. Fluorescence properties and metabolic features of indocyanine green (ICG) as related to angiography. Surv Ophthalmol. 2000;45(1):15–27. https://doi.org/10.1016/s0039-6257(00)00123-5.
21. Dudley NE. Methylene blue for rapid identification of the parathyroids. Br Med J. 1971;3(5776):680–1. https://doi.org/10.1136/bmj.3.5776.680.
22. Khan MA, North AP, Chadwick DR. Prolonged postoperative altered mental status after methylene blue infusion during parathyroidectomy: a case report and review of the literature. Ann R Coll Surg Engl. 2007;89(2):W9–11. https://doi.org/10.1308/147870807x160434.
23. Enny L, Ramakant P, Singh KR, Rana C, Garg S, Mishra AK. Efficacy of fluorescein green dye in assessing intra-operative parathyroid gland vascularity and predicting Post-thyroidectomy hypocalcaemia- a novel prospective cohort study. Indian J Endocrinol Metab. 2020;24(5):446–51. https://doi.org/10.4103/ijem.IJEM_499_20.
24. Prosst RL, Weiss J, Hupp L, Willeke F, Post S. Fluorescence-guided minimally invasive parathyroidectomy: clinical experience with a novel intraoperative detection technique for parathyroid glands. World J Surg. 2010;34(9):2217–22. https://doi.org/10.1007/s00268-010-0621-2.
25. Edafe O, Antakia R, Laskar N, Uttley L, Balasubramanian SP. Systematic review and meta-analysis of predictors of post-thyroidectomy hypocalcaemia. Br J Surg. 2014;101(4):307–20. https://doi.org/10.1002/bjs.9384.
26. Rosato L, Avenia N, Bernante P, De Palma M, Gulino G, Nasi PG, et al. Complications of thyroid surgery: analysis of a multicentric study on 14,934 patients operated on in Italy over 5 years. World J Surg. 2004;28(3):271–6. https://doi.org/10.1007/s00268-003-6903-1.
27. Pepe J, Colangelo L, Biamonte F, Sonato C, Danese VC, Cecchetti V, et al. Diagnosis and management of hypocalcemia. Endocrine. 2020;69(3):485–95. https://doi.org/10.1007/s12020-020-02324-2.
28. Bove-Fenderson E, Mannstadt M. Hypocalcemic disorders. Best Pract Res Clin Endocrinol Metab. 2018;32(5):639–56. https://doi.org/10.1016/j.beem.2018.05.006.
29. Hujoel IA. The association between serum calcium levels and Chvostek sign: a population-based study. Neurol Clin Pract. 2016;6(4):321–8. https://doi.org/10.1212/cpj.0000000000000270.
30. Falco J, Dip F, Quadri P, de la Fuente M, Rosenthal R. Cutting edge in thyroid surgery: autofluorescence of parathyroid glands. J Am Coll Surg. 2016;223(2):374–80. https://doi.org/10.1016/j.jamcollsurg.2016.04.049.
31. Dip F, Falco J, Verna S, Prunello M, Loccisano M, Quadri P, et al. Randomized controlled trial comparing White light with near-infrared autofluorescence for parathyroid gland identification during Total thy-

roidectomy. J Am Coll Surg. 2019;228(5):744–51. https://doi.org/10.1016/j.jamcollsurg.2018.12.044.
32. Benmiloud F, Godiris-Petit G, Gras R, Gillot JC, Turrin N, Penaranda G, et al. Association of Autofluorescence-Based Detection of the parathyroid glands during Total thyroidectomy with postoperative hypocalcemia risk: results of the PARAFLUO multicenter randomized clinical trial. JAMA Surg. 2020;155(2):106–12. https://doi.org/10.1001/jamasurg.2019.4613.
33. Kim YS, Erten O, Kahramangil B, Aydin H, Donmez M, Berber E. The impact of near infrared fluorescence imaging on parathyroid function after total thyroidectomy. J Surg Oncol. 2020;122(5):973–9. https://doi.org/10.1002/jso.26098.
34. Di Marco AN, Palazzo FF. Near-infrared autofluorescence in thyroid and parathyroid surgery. Gland Surg. 2020;9(Suppl 2):S136–s46. https://doi.org/10.21037/gs.2020.01.04.
35. DiMarco A, Chotalia R, Bloxham R, McIntyre C, Tolley N, Palazzo FF. Does fluoroscopy prevent inadvertent parathyroidectomy in thyroid surgery? Ann R Coll Surg Engl. 2019;101(7):508–13. https://doi.org/10.1308/rcsann.2019.0065.
36. Vidal Fortuny J, Belfontali V, Sadowski SM, Karenovics W, Guigard S, Triponez F. Parathyroid gland angiography with indocyanine green fluorescence to predict parathyroid function after thyroid surgery. Br J Surg. 2016;103(5):537–43. https://doi.org/10.1002/bjs.10101.
37. Jin H, Dong Q, He Z, Fan J, Liao K, Cui M. Application of a fluorescence imaging system with Indocyanine green to protect the parathyroid gland intraoperatively and to predict postoperative Parathyroidism. Adv Ther. 2018;35(12):2167–75. https://doi.org/10.1007/s12325-018-0834-6.
38. Zaidi N, Bucak E, Yazici P, Soundararajan S, Okoh A, Yigitbas H, et al. The feasibility of indocyanine green fluorescence imaging for identifying and assessing the perfusion of parathyroid glands during total thyroidectomy. J Surg Oncol. 2016;113(7):775–8. https://doi.org/10.1002/jso.24237.
39. Spartalis E, Ntokos G, Georgiou K, Zografos G, Tsourouflis G, Dimitroulis D, et al. Intraoperative Indocyanine green (ICG) angiography for the identification of the parathyroid glands: current evidence and future perspectives. In Vivo. 2020;34(1):23–32. https://doi.org/10.21873/invivo.11741.
40. Vidal Fortuny J, Sadowski SM, Belfontali V, Guigard S, Poncet A, Ris F, et al. Randomized clinical trial of intraoperative parathyroid gland angiography with indocyanine green fluorescence predicting parathyroid function after thyroid surgery. Br J Surg. 2018;105(4):350–7. https://doi.org/10.1002/bjs.10783.
41. Rudin AV, McKenzie TJ, Thompson GB, Farley DR, Lyden ML. Evaluation of parathyroid glands with Indocyanine green fluorescence angiography after thyroidectomy. World J Surg. 2019;43(6):1538–43. https://doi.org/10.1007/s00268-019-04909-z.

42. Razavi AC, Ibraheem K, Haddad A, Saparova L, Shalaby H, Abdelgawad M, et al. Efficacy of indocyanine green fluorescence in predicting parathyroid vascularization during thyroid surgery. Head Neck. 2019;41(9):3276–81. https://doi.org/10.1002/hed.25837.
43. Hartl DOR, Guerlain J, Breuskin I, Abbaci M, Laplace-Builhé C. Intraoperative parathyroid gland identification using autofluorescence: pearls and pitfalls. World J Surg Surg Res. 2019;2(1):1166.
44. Demarchi MS, Seeliger B, Lifante JC, Alesina PF, Triponez F. Fluorescence image-guided surgery for thyroid cancer: utility for preventing hypoparathyroidism. Cancers (Basel). 2021;13(15):3792. https://doi.org/10.3390/cancers13153792.
45. Matson J, Lwin TM, Bouvet M. Rapid intraoperative perfusion assessment of parathyroid adenomas with ICG using a wide-field portable hand-held fluorescence imaging system. Am J Surg. 2021;223:686. https://doi.org/10.1016/j.amjsurg.2021.07.027.
46. Barbieri D, Indelicato P, Vinciguerra A, Di Marco F, Formenti AM, Trimarchi M, et al. Autofluorescence and Indocyanine green in thyroid surgery: a systematic review and meta-analysis. Laryngoscope. 2021;131(7):1683–92. https://doi.org/10.1002/lary.29297.
47. Bunch PM, Kelly HR. Preoperative imaging techniques in primary hyperparathyroidism: a review. JAMA Otolaryngol Head Neck Surg. 2018;144(10):929–37. https://doi.org/10.1001/jamaoto.2018.1671.
48. Feo MLD, Colagrande S, Biagini C, Tonarelli A, Bisi G, Vaggelli L, et al. Parathyroid glands: combination of 99mTc MIBI scintigraphy and US for demonstration of parathyroid glands and nodules. Radiology. 2000;214(2):393–402. https://doi.org/10.1148/radiology.214.2.r00fe04393.
49. Haber RS, Kim CK, Inabnet WB. Ultrasonography for preoperative localization of enlarged parathyroid glands in primary hyperparathyroidism: comparison with (99m)technetium sestamibi scintigraphy. Clin Endocrinol (Oxf). 2002;57(2):241–9. https://doi.org/10.1046/j.1365-2265.2002.01583.x.
50. Hamidi M, Sullivan M, Hunter G, Hamberg L, Cho NL, Gawande AA, et al. 4D-CT is superior to ultrasound and Sestamibi for localizing recurrent parathyroid disease. Ann Surg Oncol. 2018;25(5):1403–9. https://doi.org/10.1245/s10434-018-6367-z.
51. McWade MA, Sanders ME, Broome JT, Solórzano CC, Mahadevan-Jansen A. Establishing the clinical utility of autofluorescence spectroscopy for parathyroid detection. Surgery. 2016;159(1):193–202. https://doi.org/10.1016/j.surg.2015.06.047.
52. Norlén O, Wang KC, Tay YK, Johnson WR, Grodski S, Yeung M, et al. No need to abandon focused parathyroidectomy: a multicenter study of long-term outcome after surgery for primary hyperparathyroidism. Ann Surg. 2015;261(5):991–6. https://doi.org/10.1097/sla.0000000000000715.

53. Demarchi MS, Karenovics W, Bédat B, De Vito C, Triponez F. Autofluorescence pattern of parathyroid adenomas. BJS Open. 2021;5(1):zraa047. https://doi.org/10.1093/bjsopen/zraa047.
54. Chakedis JM, Maser C, Brumund KT, Bouvet M. Indocyanine green fluorescence-guided redo parathyroidectomy. BMJ Case Rep. 2015;2015:bcr2015211778. https://doi.org/10.1136/bcr-2015-211778.
55. DeLong JC, Ward EP, Lwin TM, Brumund KT, Kelly KJ, Horgan S, et al. Indocyanine green fluorescence-guided parathyroidectomy for primary hyperparathyroidism. Surgery. 2018;163(2):388–92. https://doi.org/10.1016/j.surg.2017.08.018.
56. Di Meo G, Karampinis I, Gerken A, Lammert A, Pellicani S, Nowak K. Indocyanine green fluorescence angiography can guide intraoperative localization during parathyroid surgery. Scand J Surg. 2019;110:1457496919877581. https://doi.org/10.1177/1457496919877581.
57. Sound S, Okoh A, Yigitbas H, Yazici P, Berber E. Utility of Indocyanine green fluorescence imaging for intraoperative localization in reoperative parathyroid surgery. Surg Innov. 2019;26(6):774–9. https://doi.org/10.1177/1553350615613450.
58. Zaidi N, Bucak E, Okoh A, Yazici P, Yigitbas H, Berber E. The utility of indocyanine green near infrared fluorescent imaging in the identification of parathyroid glands during surgery for primary hyperparathyroidism. J Surg Oncol. 2016;113(7):771–4. https://doi.org/10.1002/jso.24240.
59. Cui L, Gao Y, Yu H, Li M, Wang B, Zhou T, et al. Intraoperative parathyroid localization with near-infrared fluorescence imaging using Indocyanine green during total parathyroidectomy for secondary hyperparathyroidism. Sci Rep. 2017;7(1):8193. https://doi.org/10.1038/s41598-017-08347-6.
60. Vidal Fortuny J, Guigard S, Diaper J, Karenovics W, Triponez F. Subtotal parathyroidectomy under Indocyanine green angiography. VideoEndocrinology. 2016;3(1):ve.2015.0056. https://doi.org/10.1089/ve.2015.0056.
61. Coste T, Caiazzo R, Torres F, Vantyghem MC, Carnaille B, Pattou F, et al. Laparoscopic adrenalectomy by transabdominal lateral approach: 20 years of experience. Surg Endosc. 2017;31(7):2743–51. https://doi.org/10.1007/s00464-016-4830-0.
62. Sommerey S, Foroghi Y, Chiapponi C, Baumbach SF, Hallfeldt KK, Ladurner R, et al. Laparoscopic adrenalectomy—10-year experience at a teaching hospital. Langenbecks Arch Surg. 2015;400(3):341–7. https://doi.org/10.1007/s00423-015-1287-x.
63. Obermeyer RJ, Knauer EM, Millie MP, Ojeda H, Peters MB Jr, Sweeney JF. Intravenous methylene blue as an aid to intraoperative localization and removal of the adrenal glands during laparoscopic adrenalectomy. Am J Surg. 2003;186(5):531–4. https://doi.org/10.1016/j.amjsurg.2003.07.011.

64. Manny TB, Pompeo AS, Hemal AK. Robotic partial adrenalectomy using indocyanine green dye with near-infrared imaging: the initial clinical experience. Urology. 2013;82(3):738–42. https://doi.org/10.1016/j.urology.2013.03.074.
65. Ashitate Y, Levitz A, Park MH, Hyun H, Venugopal V, Park G, et al. Endocrine-specific NIR fluorophores for adrenal gland targeting. Chem Commun (Camb). 2016;52(67):10305–8. https://doi.org/10.1039/c6cc03845j.
66. Moore EC, Berber E. Fluorescence techniques in adrenal surgery. Gland Surg. 2019;8(Suppl 1):S22–s7. https://doi.org/10.21037/gs.2019.03.01.
67. DeLong JC, Chakedis JM, Hosseini A, Kelly KJ, Horgan S, Bouvet M. Indocyanine green (ICG) fluorescence-guided laparoscopic adrenalectomy. J Surg Oncol. 2015;112(6):650–3. https://doi.org/10.1002/jso.24057.
68. Colvin J, Zaidi N, Berber E. The utility of indocyanine green fluorescence imaging during robotic adrenalectomy. J Surg Oncol. 2016;114(2):153–6. https://doi.org/10.1002/jso.24296.
69. Arora E, Bhandarwar A, Wagh A, Gandhi S, Patel C, Gupta S, et al. Role of indo-cyanine green (ICG) fluorescence in laparoscopic adrenalectomy: a retrospective review of 55 cases. Surg Endosc. 2018;32(11):4649–57. https://doi.org/10.1007/s00464-018-6309-7.
70. Kahramangil B, Kose E, Berber E. Characterization of fluorescence patterns exhibited by different adrenal tumors: determining the indications for indocyanine green use in adrenalectomy. Surgery. 2018;164(5):972–7. https://doi.org/10.1016/j.surg.2018.06.012.
71. Lerchenberger M, Gündogar U, Al Arabi N, Gallwas JKS, Stepp H, Hallfeldt KKJ, et al. Indocyanine green fluorescence imaging during partial adrenalectomy. Surg Endosc. 2020;34(5):2050–5. https://doi.org/10.1007/s00464-019-06985-7.
72. Crawford KL, Pacheco FV, Lee YJ, Hom M, Rosenthal EL, Nguyen QT, et al. A scoping review of ongoing fluorescence-guided surgery clinical trials in otolaryngology. Laryngoscope. 2021;132:36. https://doi.org/10.1002/lary.29891.

7 Use of Fluorescence Guidance in Bariatric Surgery

Edmund B. Chen, Mark A. Burroughs, Andrea Trinh, Sachin Kukreja, and Keri A. Seymour

Introduction

Bariatric surgery is a durable treatment for morbid obesity with long-term resolution of obesity-related diseases. In the United States, the recommendations for bariatric surgery are based on the National Institutes of Health guidelines from 1991. The indication for surgery is a body mass index (BMI) greater or equal to 35 kg/m^2 with an associated obesity-related comorbidity, or a BMI of greater or equal to 40 kg/m^2 [1]. The Roux-en-Y gastric bypass

Supplementary Information The online version contains supplementary material available at https://doi.org/10.1007/978-3-031-40685-0_7.

E. B. Chen · K. A. Seymour (✉)
Department of Surgery, School of Medicine, Duke University, Durham, NC, USA
e-mail: keri.seymour@duke.edu

M. A. Burroughs · A. Trinh
Department of Surgery, Methodist Dallas Medical Center, Dallas, TX, USA

S. Kukreja
Department of Surgery, Methodist Dallas Medical Center, Dallas, TX, USA

Dallas-Fort Worth Bariatrics and General Surgery, Dallas, TX, USA

N. Szoka et al. (eds.), *The SAGES Manual of Fluorescence-Guided Surgery*, https://doi.org/10.1007/978-3-031-40685-0_7

(RYGB) and vertical banded gastroplasty were the two approved bariatric procedures when these guidelines were first implemented. According to the American Society for Metabolic and Bariatric Surgery (ASMBS), an estimated 256,000 bariatric procedures were performed in 2019. Of these procedures, sleeve gastrectomy (SG) comprised 60% of all bariatric surgeries performed, RYGB was 18%, biliopancreatic diversion with duodenal switch (BPD/DS) was 1%, and revisional bariatric surgery constituted 17% of all procedures [2]. This chapter will review the indications and technique of both primary and revisional bariatric surgery and describe how intraoperative ICG is utilized during these surgeries.

Primary Bariatric Surgery

Sleeve Gastrectomy (SG)

The SG was initially performed in 1999 as the first stage of a BPD/DS operation for patients with super morbid obesity [3]. The intestinal bypass was reportedly easier and safer to perform at the second stage, after patients lost weight. Ultimately, some patients were able to achieve substantial weight loss with the SG alone. The SG became a separate procedure and acquired a unique common procedural terminology code in 2011 [4]. The benefits of SG include an average of 55% excess weight loss (%EWL) [5]. Percent EWL is defined as:

$$\%EWL = (\text{Weight loss}/\text{Excess weight}) \times 100$$
$$\text{Excess weight} = \text{Baseline weight} - \text{Ideal weight.}$$

The definition of ideal weight can differ, yet a BMI of 2 kg/m^2 is commonly applied [6].

The SG may be preferable to other primary bariatric surgeries for specific patients. The International Sleeve Gastrectomy Expert Panel Consensus Statement recommends SG for transplant candidates, patients with inflammatory bowel disease, and elderly patients. In addition, SG is commonly performed for adolescent patients undergoing bariatric surgery [7, 8]. The SG results in fewer vitamin and mineral deficiencies and is technically easier to perform since there is no anastomosis. There is no risk of marginal ulcers or internal hernias associated with SG like the risk associated with the RYGB and BPD/DS [9].

A notable disadvantage for SG is the possibility of worsening gastroesophageal reflux disease (GERD), or the incidence of de novo reflux occurring in 5–21% of post-SG patients [10, 11]. Therefore, the International Sleeve Gastrectomy Expert Panel views the preoperative presence of Barrett's esophagus as a contraindication to performing SG [7]. In addition, SG may result in less robust weight loss and weight recidivism, when compared to other primary bariatric procedures [12, 13].

Technique of Sleeve Gastrectomy

After gaining intraperitoneal access, the SG procedure starts with mobilization of the greater omentum via hemostatic division of both the gastrocolic and gastrosplenic ligaments. The fundus is fully mobilized, and the left crus is cleared of peritoneal attachments to expose the angle of His. If encountered, a hiatal hernia is reduced, and the hiatus is repaired to prevent migration of the sleeve stomach into the mediastinum. A gastric calibration tube (typically 34 to 40 French) is then passed into the lumen of the stomach to prevent narrowing at the incisura and establish symmetry of the SG. Serial staple fires create a long staple line starting approximately 3 cm to 5 cm proximal from the pylorus and ending lateral to the angle of His. A leak test is performed based on surgeon preference and may utilize air insufflation, methylene blue, or indocyanine green (ICG) [8].

Incidence and Management of Leaks After Sleeve Gastrectomy

The leak rate after SG is low at 2.4% according to a meta-analysis of 29 publications, including 4888 patients [14]. Leak after SG is associated with a varied range of presentations and subsequent clinical sequala. According to the International Sleeve Gastrectomy Expert Panel Consensus Statement, leaks after SG are classified as acute, early, late, and chronic [7]. Acute leaks are recognized within 7 days of the SG procedure. Early leaks are defined as those that occur between 1 week and 6 weeks after SG. Late leaks are observed 6 weeks after the SG and a chronic leak persists after 12 weeks [7]. A gastrointestinal leak that is not well-contained, with dissemination into the abdominal or pleural (typically left) cavity, and with major systemic clinical manifestations will require immediate intervention [7].

Leaks after SG are generally related to mechanical causes or from tissue ischemia. Mechanical causes for a leak are often linked to incomplete staple formation. Some surgeons use the same staple height for the entire sleeve gastrectomy while other surgeons vary the staple height based on location and tissue characteristics [15]. The International Sleeve Gastrectomy Expert Panel Consensus Statement stated it is not appropriate to use a staple height of less than 1.5 mm for any portion of the SG [7]. Operative technique is especially important when understanding the mechanical causes of sleeve leak. A smaller bougie size and use of buttressing materials are associated with increased rates of leak after SG [16, 17]. Narrowing the sleeve at the incisura will also create high intraluminal pressures and lead to disruption of the staple line. As esophageal tissue lacks serosa, inclusion of this weaker tissue into the staple line is another potential source of leak after SG. Depending on the mechanism, leaks that are the result of mechanical issues may manifest as early postoperative day 1 or 2 [18].

In contrast, leaks due to tissue ischemia typically occur later, around the fifth to seventh day after surgery [18]. Poor tissue perfusion and resultant ischemia can occur from overly aggressive dissection and devascularization of the resultant stomach. In addition, inadvertent thermal injury to the stomach during mobilization may also result in tissue ischemia and an eventual leak.

Gastrointestinal leak after SG is an uncommon and challenging complication to manage. Treatment options are individualized to the patient and based on location, timing of presentation, and systemic signs of illness. Patients may present with signs of fulminant sepsis, diffuse intra-abdominal fluid, well-contained abscesses, an associated fistula, or minimal clinical signs [19]. Conversative methods for controlling SG leak include antimicrobial therapy, percutaneous drainage of intra-abdominal collections, and nutritional support often in the form of parenteral nutrition. Management of SG leaks via a conservative approach was successful in 82% of patients [19]. If supportive measures fail, the next step includes endoscopic therapies that use covered stents, clips, endoluminal vacuum therapy, or internal drainage [19]. In the appropriate patient, these endoscopic therapies can be highly effective. In a meta-analysis, endoscopic stent placement had an initial success rate of 62% [19]. Endoscopic internal drainage was successful for 85% of patients [20].

Surgical intervention is the recommended initial management for toxic and symptomatic patients and necessary if the above conservative and endoscopic methods fail. Surgery can be performed both via either laparoscopic or open techniques. Peritoneal washout with drain placement is the procedure most often performed during the management of the acute SG leak [19]. In the appropriate patients, surgery was successful as the initial management of acute SG leak in 76% cases. Unfortunately, surgical management was associated with a 9.7% mortality rate [19]. In the chronic setting for unresolved leak with a chronic fistula, surgery often entails resection of the fistula tissue and conversion to RYGB or esophagojejunostomy.

Intraoperative Application of ICG During Sleeve Gastrectomy

Prevention of a leak after SG is of intense interest to bariatric surgeons, and fluorescence imaging using ICG has emerged as a promising imaging modality. Given the numerous operative techniques that contribute to staple line disruption and leak after SG, the ability to perform an intraoperative assessment is of high value to surgeons. ICG is a water-soluble anionic probe, with excitation and emission wavelengths of around 778 nm and 830 nm, respectively. When administered intravenously, the molecule binds to plasma lipoproteins. ICG is then metabolized by the liver and excreted into the bile. Tests incorporating ICG have elevated sensitivity, as extremely small concentrations of ICG are visible. In addition, ICG uniquely offers extraordinary contrast versus other imaging modalities. The target is illuminated, while the background remains dark because separate wavelengths are employed for excitation and reading [21]. When intravenous ICG is used for a leak test, it is quickly detected in the extraluminal space. Operative repair can be performed immediately and before leaving the operative theater.

The use of ICG during a SG is extremely safe, since ICG is an inert molecule with a very favorable safety profile. The contraindication to ICG is an allergy to iodine or iodinated imaging agents, as the molecule is manufactured with a small amount of sodium iodine. The incidence of adverse reactions to ICG is exceedingly rare, roughly 0.003%, and occurs when doses exceed 0.5 mg/kg [22].

Given its application, numerous studies have evaluated the use of ICG angiography and ICG as a leak test after SG (Table 7.1).

Steps to Use ICG Angiography to Test Perfusion During SG

Intravenous injection of ICG allows for assessment of tissue perfusion and evaluation of hemostasis. First, the 2.5 mg/mL solution of ICG is mixed. A 25 mg vial of ICG is reconstituted with 10 mL of water and then shaken until dissolved. For perfusion assessment, a 3 mL of the 2.5 mg/mL ICG solution is injected and followed with a 10 mL saline bolus. This can be repeated to a maximum dose of 2 mg/kg. Near-infrared light will highlight the perfusing blood vessels within 5 s and visibility will persist for up to 30 s. Organs perfused from numerous blood vessels (e.g., stomach, liver, and small bowel) are visible within 1 min to 2 min with visibility lasting for 20 min to 120 min. When given intravenously, ICG can also be utilized to assess the perfusion of the stomach prior to stapling. This allows the surgeon to identify and protect accessory blood vessels at the proximal stomach. ICG angiography can also be injected after creation of the gastric conduit to verify adequate perfusion to the SG (Video 7.1). Active bleeding will be revealed as an intraperitoneal, continuous fluorescent stream. Thus, ICG has an additional benefit of assessing hemostasis at the end of the procedure.

Table 7.1 Review of studies using intraoperative indocyanine green (ICG) during primary and revisional bariatric surgery

Author (year published)	Type of study (level of evidence)	Application of ICG	Type of procedure	Study cohort (*n*)	Major findings
ICG angiography					
Olmi et al. (2019) [23]	Case study (Level V)	Vascular perfusion of sleeve stomach	SG	1	Staple line was well perfused after transection
Frattini et al. (2015) [24]	Case series (Level IV)	Vascular perfusion of sleeve stomach	SG	15	Perfusion of the gastric conduit was consistent and uniform No perfusion observed in the excised stomach
Ortega et al. (2018) [25]	Case series (Level IV)	Vascular perfusion of stomach identified both prior and after stapling	SG	86	Vascular patterns were identified at the gastroesophageal junction
Di Furla et al. (2019) [26]	Case series (Level IV)	Vascular perfusion of sleeve stomach	SG	43	One SG leak occurred despite adequate perfusion
Billy et al. (2019) [27]	Case series (Level IV)	Vascular perfusion	Primary or revisional SG, RYGB, or BPD/DS	50 (Procedure numbers were not provided)	The duodenal stump showed delayed but effective perfusion

(continued)

Table 7.1 (continued)

Author (year published)	Type of study (level of evidence)	Application of ICG	Type of procedure	Study cohort (n)	Major findings
Intraluminal ICG					
Hagen et al. (2019) [28]	Case series (Level IV)	Leak test of GJ anastomosis	Robotic RYGB	95	No leaks were detected via the air insufflation or methylene blue tests. These anastomoses were reexamined with ICG and 4 had a positive test. ICG may be a more sensitive test
Kalmar et al. (2020) [29]	Retrospective cohort study (Level III)	Air sufflation leak test vs. ICG leak test	SG and RYGB	Air insufflation ($n = 196$) vs. ICG ($n = 59$)	Negative predictive value of air insufflation was 98.47% vs. ICG negative predictive value was 100% Sensitivity of ICG was 100%

ICG indocyanine green, *SG* sleeve gastrectomy, *RYGB* Roux-en-Y gastric bypass, *BPD/DS* biliopancreatic diversion with duodenal switch, *GJ* gastrojejunal

Outcomes of ICG Angiography to Determine Perfusion During SG

Fluorescence imaging using ICG has emerged as a promising imaging modality for intraoperative assessment of leak and tissue perfusion. Studies that report the indications for ICG and application for bariatric surgery procedures are summarized in Table 7.1. Given the early application of ICG in bariatric surgery, a number of these studies are retrospective with a small sample size.

The use of ICG angiography to augment the intraoperative tests for tissue perfusion after SG was first introduced by Frattini et al. in 2014 [24]. ICG was administered intraoperatively to 15 patients during routine SG. Consistent and homogenous perfusion was observed along the entirety of gastric conduit and compared to the devascularized specimens. Strong fluorescence patterns were visualized in the SG and no clinical leak was reported. Another study by Di Furia et al. added a timepoint to declare adequate tissue perfusion. This study injected ICG intravenously and then compared fluorescence presence in the gastric tube to the gastric specimen between 150 s and 180 s. Even though all patients had adequate intraoperative perfusion, one patient developed a gastric leak on the fifth day after SG [26].

The above studies utilized ICG angiography after the SG was fashioned, to assess whether there was still adequate perfusion after stapling and transection. ICG angiography also helps determine the individualized blood supply to the stomach prior to stapling. This allows the surgeon to fashion the sleeve in a manner that ensures the maximum perfusion to the gastric tube. Vascular mapping was utilized in 86 patients during SG in a study by Ortega et al. Intravenous injection of 1 mL ICG was followed by fluorescence visualization to identify several patterns of blood supply to the gastroesophageal junction. Intraoperative ICG angiography allowed for visualization and preservation of vessels in proximity to the crus and gastroesophageal area [25]. Applications for intraoperative ICG continue to evolve beyond angiography to include intraluminal use, with the common goal of preventing SG leak.

Steps to Use Intraluminal ICG for a Leak Test After SG

An intraluminal ICG leak test is performed after completion of the SG. A larger volume of ICG is required with 12.5 mg of ICG dissolved in 100 mL of sterile 0.9% normal saline. Next, the entire 100 mL of the 1.25 mg/mL ICG solution is introduced through an orogastric tube. The staple line is inspected for the next 30 s to 1 min, paying particular attention to the angle of His. A positive leak test occurs when a line of bright neon green fluorescence is appreciated on the extraluminal side of the staple line and pools in the peritoneal cavity (Video 7.2). This is not to be confused with the dull green hue detected through the gastric wall [29]. A positive intraluminal ICG leak test can be confirmed with a second intraluminal leak test. This confirmatory test can be a repeated ICG intraluminal leak test with an additional bolus of intraluminal ICG or another leak test modality such as endoscopy with air insufflation. Once confirmed, options for repair of a gastric leak include suture repair at the injury, buttressing with omentum, applying tissue sealants, resection of the involved segment, or a combination of these methods. The ICG leak test should be repeated after repair of the damaged tissue to confirm the integrity of the repair. Revision to RYGB is reserved as definitive repair of a non-salvageable sleeve leak. A surgical drain may be placed if additional procedures are performed, and upper gastrointestinal imaging series should be considered during the postoperative period.

Outcomes of Intraluminal ICG to Determine Leak After SG

Intraluminal ICG offers advantages over an air sufflation test. In a retrospective study, 196 patients (SG $n = 77$, RYGB $n = 119$) underwent an intraoperative leak test via air sufflation with an endoscope. Of those undergoing an air leak test, there were 3 false-negative and 193 true-negative results. Another 59 patients (SG $n = 29$, RYGB $n = 30$) underwent an ICG intraluminal leak test. This resulted in 1 true-positive, 1 false-positive, and 57 true-negative tests. There were no false-negative results with the use of ICG as a leak test. Therefore, the negative predictive value of intraluminal ICG for a leak was 100% compared to the negative predictive value of 98.5% with an air insufflation test after SG and RYGB [29].

Considerations for ICG During Sleeve Gastrectomy

The utility of a routine intraoperative leak test after SG is controversial. In a retrospective study of 1550 patients, a routine intraoperative leak test was performed in 86% of cases versus 14% of cases that did not use a leak test. Despite a negative intraoperative leak test, 15 patients (1%) developed a gastric leak in the postoperative period. There was no significant difference in postoperative leak rates between the patients who underwent an intraoperative leak test and the patients who did not have a leak test performed [30]. Another study evaluated 7 years of SG, without a single positive intraoperative leak test. Despite the negative intraoperative leak test, 2.4% of patients developed a leak [31]. Therefore, it is important to always be vigilant for a postoperative leak after a SG, even after a reassuring intraoperative leak test.

The use of intraluminal ICG for a leak test still has advantages to colored dye and air insufflation. Colored dye penetrates the surrounding tissue and can obscure the area of injury, making a definitive repair more challenging. ICG is visible when combined with the near-infrared camera and not visible with white light. This allows a surgeon to oscillate between ICG fluorescence and visible light to precisely identify the injured tissue. The ICG leak test is technically easier to perform and does not require the same level of trained assistance that is necessary with use of air insufflation. During an air insufflation test, the endoscope is placed by an experienced surgeon and the stomach is distended while a trained surgical assistant irrigates and inspects the staple line. Identifying the precise location of the leak requires a coordinated effort between two skilled individuals. In contrast, ICG is administered by the anesthesia team which allows the surgeon to remain at the bedside. The surgeon is then able to identify and manage the SG leak in real time.

Roux-en-Y Gastric Bypass (RYGB)

The Roux-en-Y gastric bypass (RYGB) is the gold standard for bariatric procedures and results in durable and consistent weight loss. When compared to SG in a randomized control trial, the mean postoperative weight loss after RYGB was 75% EWL versus SG with 65% EWL at 5 years [32].

RYGB also offers significant rates of resolution or improvement of obesity-related diseases. Diabetes resolution occurred in 84% of patients, hypertension in 68%, and hyperlipidemia in 97% of patients after RYGB when a meta-analysis analyzed a large of cohort of patients involved in retrospective studies [33]. The RYGB is more effective at glucose control when compared to the SG, as reported in the Surgical Treatment and Medications Potentially Eradicate Diabetes Efficiently (STAMPEDE) trial. After RYGB, significantly more patients no longer required glucose-lowering medications compared to patients after SG (44.9% vs. 25.5%, $p < 0.05$) [34]. Furthermore, remission of diabetes continued to occur more frequently after RYGB (49%) versus SG (28%) at 7 years ($p < 0.001$) [35]. An evidence-based calculator assists both patients and providers when selecting between RYGB and SG to treat type 2 diabetes [35].

RYGB is also a preferred procedure for patients with severe or refractory GERD. The choice of SG versus RYGB depends on the presence of GERD symptoms, acid exposure, esophageal motility, and presence of hiatal hernias. GERD is extremely common, as up to 50% of patients with obesity report GERD symptoms. Short-term resolution of GERD was better after RYGB patients (56.6%) compared to SG (41%) in an analysis of the Bariatric Outcomes Longitudinal Database [36]. Similarly, resolution of GERD was significantly more common after RYGB (60% of patients) than after SG (25% of patients) in the Swiss Multicenter Bypass or Sleeve Study (SM-BOSS) randomized study. Of note, GERD worsened after SG in 31% of patients compared to RYGB 6% of patients in the SM-BOSS study [37].

Relative contraindications to RYGB include a behavior associated with marginal ulcers, including the use of nonsteroidal anti-inflammatory drugs and steroids and exposure to cigarette smoke. If these risk factors are not modifiable, the patient may be better suited for a SG. RYGB may also be technically challenging in patients with large abdominal wall hernias or patients with numerous intra-abdominal surgeries and dense interloop and intra-abdominal adhesions.

Technique of RYGB

RYGB is commonly performed with a 50 cm to 100 cm biliopancreatic limb, a 100 to 150 cm alimentary limb, and creation of a 15 mL to 30 mL gastric pouch. The RYGB is performed using a laparoscopic, robotic, or open surgical approach. The two anastomoses, the gastrojejunostomy (GJ) and jejunojejunostomy, are created with a stapled or handsewn technique. The rate of marginal ulcer and anastomotic leak between the circular-stapled, linear-stapled, and handsewn techniques has conflicting results [38, 39].

The jejunojejunostomy is the first anastomosis performed in our practice. After establishing laparoscopic access, the duodenojejunal junction is identified and the jejunum is measured 50 cm to 100 cm distally. The area of transection is then lifted to the stomach to confirm tension-free contact with the stomach. If necessary, the jejunum is mobilized another 10 cm to 20 cm until there is a lack of tension. The jejunum is transected, and the associated mesentery is divided with adequate hemostasis. The alimentary limb is measured for additional 100 cm to 150 cm of jejunum. The jejunojejunostomy is created at this location and the mesenteric defect is closed with permanent suture. The gastric pouch is then created with identification and protection of the left gastric artery. The stomach is stapled and transected near the second transverse vessels. A 15 mL to 30 mL gastric pouch is then fashioned from the lesser curvature of the stomach. The alimentary limb is mobilized in an antecolic, ante-gastric fashion unless tautness or hostility requires a retrocolic or retrogastric approach. The GJ is created, and then permanent suture collapses the mesenteric defect at the transverse mesocolon (Peterson's defect). A leak test of the GJ anastomosis is routinely performed in our practice.

Incidence and Management of Leaks After RYGB

Leaks after RYGB are also associated with noteworthy morbidity and mortality. Even though the overall incidence of anastomotic leak was 1% in a study of RYGB performed at ASMBS Bariatric Surgery Centers of Excellence [40], the diagnosis and management was individualized to the patient. A gastrointestinal leak after RYGB involves four areas with varied reported incidence. The majority of leaks occurred at the GJ (68%) followed by the gastric pouch (10%), then the jejunojejunal anastomosis (5%), and also the excluded stomach (4%) in an assessment of 1200 RYGB patients [41].

Management of leak after RYGB follows the surgical pillars of source control with wide drainage, broad-spectrum antibiotic therapy, and proper nutrition (including parenteral and/or enteral nutrition) [42, 43]. Septic patients require immediate surgery. The defect is treated with a patched tongue of omentum, with or without suture repair. If the anastomosis is not salvageable, then resection may be necessary [44]. Endoluminal stenting or placement of endoluminal vacuum dressings is an innovative option to control the drainage from the injured tissue [45]. Overall, the majority of patients (93%) recovered after the above options were explored [40].

Technical considerations include tension, tissue quality, and type of anastomosis. The method of GJ creation (linear-stapled, circular-stapled, or handsewn) was compared in relation to leak rates. The GJ leak rate was highest after the handsewn technique (1.7%) compared to the circular-stapled (0.7%) and the linear-stapled GJ (0.4%, $p = 0.02$) [40]. Remarkably, another study did not show a significant difference in rates of leak rate, marginal ulcer, or stricture among the three techniques for GJ formation [36]. Prophylactic use of synthetic materials at the anastomosis, oversewing the staple line, buttressing materials, and intraoperative leak tests have not shown to effectively reduce the incidence of anastomotic leak after RYGB with high-quality evidence [44].

An intraoperative leak test can diagnose a technique failure at the time of GJ creation that allows the surgeon to promptly repair the defect. During a leak test, the gastric pouch is distended with air or contrast dye (e.g., methylene blue). If a leak is identified intraoperatively, the anastomosis should be repaired and retested until a negative leak test is obtained. Tissue quality will not be sufficiently assessed during an intraoperative leak test and thus leaks may still occur in the postoperative period. A closed suction drain may be placed near the anastomosis if there are any concerns. Additional imaging with upper gastrointestinal series or testing the level of drain amylase is an additional option to investigate for postoperative GJ leak. The use of selective, rather than routine, upper gastrointestinal series was more appropriate to diagnose an anastomotic leak during the postoperative period [46, 47]. The use of ICG, predominantly as an intraoperative anastomotic leak test, offers potential benefits to the bariatric surgeon performing a RYGB, as detailed below.

Steps to Use Intraluminal ICG for a Leak Test After RYGB

An intraluminal ICG leak test can then be performed during RYGB (Video 7.3). As discussed with SG, 12.5 mg of ICG is dissolved in 100 mL of sterile 0.9% normal saline. The proximal alimentary limb is occluded with a bowel clamp and the GJ anastomosis is distended. The entire 100 mL of the ICG solution is then instilled via the orogastric tube. The white light is exchanged for the near-infrared lens and the ICG fluorescence is visible. The entire anastomosis is scrutinized, with attention to the medial and lateral corners of the anastomosis, as well as the anterior and posterior surfaces. Any extravasation of fluorescence is a positive leak test (Video 7.4). A positive test can be quickly repaired, and then a second leak test with another 100 mL of ICG solution or air insufflation will confirm patency of the GJ anastomosis. A persistent leak will require additional procedures including possible resection. An esophagojejunal anastomosis may be performed if additional gastric resection would lead to an inadequate perfusion or limited stomach tissue for a GJ.

Outcomes of Intraluminal ICG to Determine Leak After RYGB

There are even fewer studies reporting on the intraoperative use of ICG in RYGB than studies reporting ICG use during SG (Table 7.1). Kalmar et al. studied 196 patients who underwent either a SG or RYGB [29]. An intraluminal ICG leak test was compared to the air insufflation test to assess GJ continuity. The use of intraluminal ICG as a leak test had negative predictive value of 100% compared to the negative predictive value for air insufflation of 98.5%. This was not limited to the RYGB since the authors did not stratify the results of ICG based on operation type [29].

Hagen et al. exclusively evaluated the use of intraluminal ICG to perform a leak test after robotic-assisted RYGB [31]. In this study, patients underwent a series of GJ anastomotic leak tests. Patients first underwent an air insufflation test, followed by a methylene blue leak test, and then an ICG leak test. No leaks were detected using air insufflation or methylene blue; however, there were four positive ICG leak tests. The leak was repaired intraoperatively and without complications. The authors concluded the intraluminal ICG was a more sensitive leak test than air insufflation or colored dye [31]. Utilization of intraluminal ICG as a leak test after RYGB appears promising and warrants further investigation.

ICG Angiography in RYGB

Currently, there are no published reports on the use of ICG for assessment of tissue perfusion during RYGB. ICG angiography may be beneficial to surgeons when tissue perfusion is a concern. Future research is necessary to understand the benefits of ICG angiography as it applies to RYGB.

Biliopancreatic Diversion with Duodenal Switch (BPD/DS)

The BPD/DS was first described by Hess and Hess in 1988 [48]. Of all the primary bariatric operations, the BPD/DS results in the greatest amount of weight loss from 65%EWL to 80%EWL [49, 50]. The BPD/DS is of particular benefit to patients with super obesity (BMI greater than and equal to 50 kg/m^2). In a randomized trial comparing patients with a BMI of 50 kg/m^2 to 60 kg/m^2, the mean reduction in BMI after a BPD/DS was 22.1 kg/m^2 compared to RYGB with a loss of 13.6 kg/m^2 at 5 years ($p < 0.001$) [49].

The BPD/DS offers the substantial improvements in metabolic profile of patients compared to other bariatric procedures. Specifically, the BPD/DS leads to superior and steady glycemic control when directly compared to RYGB. Patients with a BMI of 35 kg/m^2 and higher were randomized to conventional medication therapy or undergo RYGB or biliopancreatic diversion (BPD)

[51]. Of note, the authors compared patients undergoing a BPD as described by Scopinaro et al., which includes a distal gastrectomy, 200 cm alimentary limb, 50 cm common channel, and the small bowel anastomosed to the transected stomach [52]. The primary end point was remission of diabetes, defined as a fasting glucose of less than 100 mg/dL and a hemoglobin A1c of less than 6.5% in the absence of pharmacologic therapy. After 2 years of follow-up, 95% of patients who received a BPD achieved remission of diabetes, compared to 75% in the RYGB group, and 0% in the conventional medical therapy group ($p < 0.001$) [51]. The distal delivery of food instigates a complex interaction of incretins, bile acids, and the microbiome that contribute to the remarkable metabolic impact of the BPD/DS compared to other bariatric surgeries [53–55].

Despite the advantages of BPD/DS, the operation accounts for roughly 1% of total bariatric procedures performed every year [2]. This is likely due to the combination of technical challenges, the lack of a unique current procedural technology code for the laparoscopic BPD/DS, and intense metabolic impact that requires appropriate patient selection. Of note, the single anastomosis duodenoileostomy with sleeve gastrectomy (SADI-S) and stomach-intestinal pyloric sparing (SIPS) have recently emerged as modifications of the BPD/DS. These procedures are a simplification of the BPD/DS, as they do not include the Roux-en-Y ileoileal anastomosis. Instead, the SADIS/SIPS has a loop configuration at the duodenoileostomy with an associated longer common channel, typically 250 cm to 300 cm [56]. Recent studies show comparable weight loss and similar nutritional profiles when the SADIS/SIPS is compared to RYGB or BPD/DS [57–59]. The ASMBS now formally recognizes the SADIS/SIPS as a modification of the BPD/DS, and the SADIS/SIPS is "endorsed by the ASMBS as an appropriate metabolic bariatric surgical procedure" [60].

Technique of BPD/DS

The BPD/DS is a technically challenging procedure that has been performed using the laparoscopic and robotic approach since 2000 [61, 62]. The BPD/DS consists of several procedures: SG, cholecystectomy, creation of an alimentary limb with duodenoileostomy, and construction of an ileoileostomy to connect the biliopancreatic limb and common channel. The first step includes measuring the small bowel. Starting from the terminal ileum, the bowel is marked at the site of the ileoileostomy (100 cm to 150 cm) and then again at the site of the future duodenoileostomy (200 cm to 300 cm). The next step is to perform the SG as previously described. Some surgeons opt to create a larger gastric reservoir over a bigger calibration tube, for example, a 50 French bougie. After performing a cholecystectomy, the peri-duodenal dissection is begun 3 cm to 5 cm distal to the pylorus. The gastroduodenal artery is identified, and a retro-duodenal tunnel is created above the artery. The duodenum is transected near the junction of the first and second portions of the duodenum. The duodenoileostomy is fashioned between the proximal duodenal stump and the previously marked ileum. The duodenoileostomy can be created via a handsewn or stapled technique. Next, the ileum is transected proximal to the duodenoileostomy, and a leak test is performed. The ileoileostomy is created between the previously marked distal ileum and the newly created biliopancreatic limb. Both unidirectional and bidirectional techniques have been described. The mesenteric defects at the ileoileostomy and transverse colon are closed with permanent suture. The results are a 100 cm to 150 cm alimentary limb and a 100 cm to 150 cm common channel for a combined 200 cm to 300 cm total limb length and an extremely long biliopancreatic limb. To perform the SADIS/SIPS, a loop duodenoileostomy is constructed around 300 cm from the terminal ileum.

Incidence and Management of Leaks After BPD/DS

BPD/DS leaks occur in the area of the gastric staple line, duodenoileal anastomosis, and ileoileal anastomosis. Leak rates at these sites are 1.5%, 1.5%, and 0.1%, respectively [63]. In a more recent study of 566 patients over 4 years, there was a 0.7% (n = 4 patients) leak rate at the duodenoileal anastomosis and a 0.2% (n = 1 patient) leak rate from the gastric staple line [50]. Notably, when BPD/DS is compared to RYGB, there is a small increase in rate of leak [64].

Ischemia of the duodenal stump, excessive tension on the anastomosis, and aggressive dissection are similarly a concern for leak after BPD/DS. With an extended medial mobilization of the greater curvature past the pylorus, the branches from the right gastroepiploic are cauterized. Care must be taken to preserve as much of the remaining blood supply of the duodenal stump as possible. Aside from the right gastroepiploic artery, the duodenal stump is also supplied by branches from the supraduodenal artery, the superior pancreaticoduodenal arteries, the gastroduodenal artery, and the right gastric artery. Cottam et al. described a safe method for dissecting and transecting the duodenum, with step-by-step description to protect the blood supply for the future duodenoileal anastomosis [65].

Leaks after BPD/DS are managed using many of the same tools previously described. Gastric body leaks are treated in similar manner to SG leak, with consideration for endoscopic stenting and injury to the duodenoileostomy. Leaks at the duodenoileal anastomosis can be especially difficult to control given associated high volume of output. Duodenal perforation or disruption of the anastomosis is similarly treated with placement of an omental patch and wide drainage. Endoscopic vacuum therapy is also a newer and promising method of treating duodenoileostomy leaks. Prognosis depends on the location of the leak as well as the patient's clinical status and presentation [45, 66, 67].

Steps to Use ICG Angiography to Test Perfusion During BPD/DS

ICG can be incorporated into a BPS/DS in three methods. First, ICG angiography will confirm perfusion of the duodenal stump after transection. Second, intraluminal ICG is placed in an orogastric tube to assess the integrity and patency of the duodenoileal anastomosis. Finally, ICG cholangiogram will evaluate the biliary tree during a concomitant cholecystectomy. The three techniques are reviewed below.

ICG angiography is performed in a similar manner as previously described in the SG section. ICG is reconstituted for intravenous administration according to manufacturer instructions; a

25 mg vial of ICG is reconstituted with 10 mL of sterile water to create a 2.5 mg/mL solution. Three mL of the reconstituted 2.5 mg/mL ICG solution (2.5 mg of ICG) is then given intravenously after transection of the duodenum, followed by a 10 mL saline flush. The transected duodenum is evaluated under near-infrared light to evaluate perfusion. A bright or dull fluorescence hue is interrupted as sufficient perfusion to continue with the next steps in the BPD/DS procedure. The absence of fluorescence is considered restricted perfusion. An extended time to reevaluate the perfusion or resection of the duodenum is performed based on surgeon judgment.

Outcomes of ICG Angiography to Determine Perfusion During BPD/DS

The BPD/DS is not a commonly performed procedure, and there are limited studies involving intraoperative ICG use during BPD/DS or SADIS/SIPS. Currently, only one abstract mentions the use of ICG during a BPD/DS [27]. This study includes a combination of the procedures already mentioned: SG, RYGB, and BPD/DS. Intravenous ICG was injected to assess perfusion of the tissue and anastomoses. Perfusion of the duodenum was evaluated in an unspecified number of BPD/DS procedures and deemed to be adequate, although decreased, in the transected duodenal stump. The authors do not mention any operative interventions as a result of the ICG angiography of the duodenal stump.

Pearls and Pitfalls

There are a few pitfalls to consider when incorporating ICG angiography into the BPD/DS or SADIS/SIPS procedures. At times, due to the extended dissection, the duodenal stump may appear dusky and the ICG angiogram will show diminished perfusion. The options are to the resect this portion of the duodenum or create an anastomosis to the dusky tissue. Resection is complicated by the location of the pylorus and possibility of needing to convert to a gastroileal anastomosis or RYGB. In our experience, despite an ICG perfusion test with diminished blood flow, continuing with the duodenoileal anastomosis is a reasonable option. The duodenum has a concentrated submucosal vasculature that leads to adequate mucosal perfusion even when the serosa appears ischemic. This allows for a viable duodenoileal anastomosis. The decision to resect or persist is often part of the learning curve of this procedure.

Steps to Use Intraluminal ICG for a Leak Test After BPD/DS

Although it is not reported, intraluminal ICG has been used to evaluate for a leak at the duodenoileostomy in our practice. Like previously mentioned, a solution is created with 12.5 mg of ICG dissolved in 100 mL of sterile 0.9% normal saline. The premixed solution is then instilled through the orogastric tube by the anesthesiology team. The duodenoileal anastomosis is inspected with the near-infrared laser of the camera enabled. Patency of the anastomosis is confirmed when the ICG is observed shining through the wall of the duodenal bulb and across the anastomosis into the lumen of small bowel (Video 7.5). The anterior and posterior sides of the anastomosis are evaluated for intraperitoneal leakage of fluorescence. The sharp contrast of ICG and the background tissue is especially obvious under the near-infrared light. A positive leak occurs when bright green fluorescence is located outside of the lumen within the peritoneal cavity. The area of concern is oversewn, and a second leak test is performed. If the second leak test is positive, the surgeon must decide on another attempt at repair versus resecting and recreating the anastomosis.

Outcomes of Intraluminal ICG to Determine Leak After BPD/DS

The benefits of using ICG as a leak test relate to the invisibility of ICG in white light. This allows the surgeon to toggle back and forth between near-infrared light and white light to isolate and repair a leak under direct visualization. If the leak test is negative, the next steps of the BPD/DS are performed while the SADI/SIPS procedure is complete. If a leak is positive, the tissue is repaired, and a second test is performed. The falciform ligament may be mobilized and wrapped around the anastomosis as a patch. External drainage is also an option after a positive leak test.

If there is a delay of contrast moving past the anastomosis and into the small bowel, additional time is warranted. For the BPD/DS, the ileoileostomy is created and the mesenteric defect is closed. The duodenoileal anastomosis is reevaluated under near-infrared light. At this point, the intraluminal ICG should be present in the small bowel to confirm a patent anastomosis without intraperitoneal leakage of ICG. Given the paucity of data, bariatric surgery would benefit from further research about the use of intraluminal ICG during BPD/DS and SADI/SIPS.

Cholecystectomy Performed During BPD/DS

The inclusion of concomitant cholecystectomy during BPD/DS and SADI/SIPS is controversial. The rate of biliary symptoms after BPD/DS is higher than after RYGB or for other primary bariatric surgeries. This is attributed to the more drastic weight loss and aggressive malabsorption associated with a BPD/DS. Up to 23% of patients develop biliary symptoms if the gallbladder is not removed at the time of BPD/DS. This risk continues for the first 3 years after BPD/DS and peaks during the second year [68]. If laparoscopic cholecystectomy is performed after BPD/DS, the dissection of the gallbladder and cystic duct may be complicated by the proximity to the duodenal stump and duodenoileostomy. Another concern of chronic and intense inflammation includes damage to the duodenal stump or DI anastomosis during cholecystectomy. Furthermore, if choledocholithiasis occurs after BPD/DS or SADIS/SIPS, endoscopic retrograde cholangiopancreatography requires surgical assistance via laparoscopic jejunal access. Another option at clearing the common bile duct is laparoscopic or open common bile duct exploration. At last, the mesenteric defects should be evaluated to ensure closure at the time of laparoscopic cholecystectomy.

ICG Cholangiogram

If prophylactic cholecystectomy is included in the BPD/DS, then ICG cholangiography can delineate the biliary system. ICG cholangiography during a standalone cholecystectomy is discussed in a previous chapter. We will review the benefits and challenges of ICG cholangiography as it relates to BPD/DS.

Steps to Use ICG Cholangiogram During BPD/DS

The benefits of ICG cholangiography compared to contrast cholangiogram include cheaper cost, ease of use, a shorter learning curve, and lack of radiation exposure to patients and staff [69]. For ICG cholangiogram, 25 mg of ICG is mixed with 10 mL of sterile water. Then 3 mL of the 2.5 mg/mL solution (5 mg ICG) is injected followed by 10 mL of sterile saline, approximately 45 min before the ICG cholangiogram is performed. The ICG is metabolized by the liver and secreted into the bile. During the dissection of the hepatocystic triangle, the near-infrared light will delineate biliary system, to allow differentiation between the cystic duct and the common bile duct. The ICG fluorescence also can delineate the borders of the gallbladder and liver as the gallbladder is dissected from the cystic plate. This technique is especially helpful when intrahepatic gallbladders, chronic inflammation, or dense layers of pericholecystic adipose tissue are encountered. More detail about performing an isolated ICG cholangiogram is included in a previous chapter.

Pearls and Pitfalls for ICG Cholangiogram During BPD/DS

Using ICG cholangiography during BPD/DS is complicated for two reasons. First, care must be taken to prevent bile spillage during the cholecystectomy. If bile is spilled, irrigation should be limited to allow for the ICG leak test to be performed in the same area. Second, bile is often released during creation of the duodenoileostomy. Bile staining during any portion of the procedure will obscure and confuse further intraluminal leak tests. For these reasons, some surgeons do not use ICG for cholangiogram if there is interest in performing an intraluminal leak test with ICG.

Revisional Bariatric Surgery

The number of primary bariatric procedures continues to grow as does the number of revisional bariatric procedures [70]. Revisional bariatric surgery is associated with increased morbidity and mortality compared to primary bariatric surgery, with an overall complication rate as high as 10% to 50% [71]. The rate of anastomotic leak is also significantly higher in revisional cases [70, 71]. In a 13-year study at a tertiary care referral center, the incidence of anastomotic leak after revisional surgery was 13% [71].

Indications for revisional bariatric surgery include intolerable adverse effects, severe nutritional deficiencies, and/or inadequate weight loss, [71]. The type of revisional procedure performed depends on the index operation and the indication for the revision. The range of revisional bariatric surgeries is extremely broad, but typical examples involve creation of a GJ. Three revisional procedures will be discussed along with the potential use for intraoperative ICG. The more common revisional procedures that create a GJ are (1) removal of laparoscopic adjustable gastric band (LAGB) with conversion to RYGB, (2) conversion of SG to RYGB, and (3) revision of GJ anastomosis in a RYGB.

Laparoscopic Adjustable Gastric Band (LAGB) to RYGB

The removal of LAGB and conversion to RYGB is a revisional bariatric surgery that is frequently performed. This revisional surgery is often due to intolerance of the adjustable gastric band with refractory GERD, esophageal dysmotility, or failure of weight loss. Long-term studies show that LAGB has a notable failure rate of 20% to 56%. Associated complications from LAGB include band slippage, band erosion, esophageal and pouch dilation, and gastric necrosis, in addition to failure to achieve adequate weight loss [72]. Removal of the LAGB and conversion to RYGB can be performed in a single operation or as a staged procedure. The LAGB and port are removed at the initial procedure, and if adhesions, bleeding, or manipulation of the stomach is excessive, then the RYGB is completed after a period of time. As a revisional procedure, the complication risk of a LAGB to RYGB is higher than that for a primary RYGB (8.6% vs. 5.5%, respectively) [73]. ICG may again help reduce the complication profile.

ICG may be of particular use during a removal of LAGB and conversion to RYGB as an intraluminal leak test. First, ICG will determine if there is any gastric leak after the removal of the band or after the takedown of the anterior fundoplication. This is especially important if there was any concern for band erosion preoperatively. If a gastric leak is seen, the leak can be repaired primarily with oversewing or with an omental patch. In this case, strong consideration should be given to performing the operation as a staged procedure and converting to a RYGB at a later point. Intraluminal ICG may be employed in the same manner previously described during the conversion to a RYGB to assess the integrity of the GJ anastomosis.

Sleeve Gastrectomy (SG) to Roux-en-Y Gastric Bypass (RYGB)

Conversion of SG to RYGB is another revisional bariatric surgery that creates a GJ and use of ICG may be beneficial. Indications for conversion of SG include insufficient weight loss, stricture of the sleeve stomach, and/or refractory GERD [13]. Early revisions of SG to RYGB may be performed to correct perioperative complications, including SG staple line leaks. SG revision to RYGB performed after a year or more is often due to medically refractory GERD, fistula, or obstruction, including stenosis and helical twist of the stomach [13].

Complications after SG to RYGB include GJ anastomotic dehiscence, remnant staple line leaks, and surgical site infections (including organ space, deep, and superficial). Notably, in a single-institution study of SG to RYGB cases, the incidence of anastomotic leak at the GJ was 3.4% [13]. ICG may help reduce the complication rate during a conversion of SG to RYGB. For example, ICG is administered intravenously to help identify the blood supply of the sleeve stomach, particularly the left gastric artery. The left gastric artery is an important landmark to identify during the creation of a gastric pouch from a sleeve stomach, as it is the main blood supply to the future gastric pouch. Once identified, the gastric pouch is created by cutting across the sleeve below the level of the left gastric artery. Indocyanine green can also be injected to highlight the biliary system and edge of the liver during revisional bariatric surgery (Video 7.6). In the situation where the sleeve is dilated or a large redundant fundus is identified, the sleeve may require tailoring vertically to the angle of His to make an appropriate gastric pouch. This situation leaves an island of stomach tissue that was previously stripped of its blood supply from the left gastroepiploic artery and now loses more blood flow generated from the left gastric artery. As such, it is at risk of ischemia, and an evaluation with ICG may also be useful in this situation in determining the need for resection (Video 7.7). Following the gastric pouch formation, assuming no ischemia concerns exist, a GJ and jejunojejunal anastomosis is then created. After the new GJ anastomosis is constructed, ICG is placed inside the stomach lumen to verify the integrity of the GJ anastomosis. The leak test is performed in the same method as it was previously explained during primary RYGB operations.

Revision of GJ Anastomosis

Marginal ulcers are a known complication after RYGB. The rate of marginal ulcers ranges from 0.6% to 25% [74]. Though most marginal ulcers resolve with medical and endoscopic therapies, surgery is required for refractory marginal ulcers. Rates of reoperation for marginal ulcers are as high as 32% [75]. Refractory marginal ulcers are typically surgically corrected with a resection of the GJ anastomosis and jejunum with recreation of the GJ anastomosis or formation of an esophagojejunostomy. Given the reoperative nature in a hostile, inflammatory area, the rate of complications from this type of surgery is considerable compared to primary bariatric surgery. In a small study by Chau et al., 25% of patients who required revisional surgery for marginal ulcers had a postoperative complication that required a reoperation [76]. Patel et al. indicated a 5% chance of anastomotic leak [75]. In these high-risk anastomoses, ICG may again be beneficial when given intraluminally to ensure the integrity of the new GJ anastomosis and potentially reduce the incidence of complications. Intraluminal ICG would be delivered in the same solution and manner as described previously in this chapter. Intravenous ICG can also be used to assess perfusion of the GJ (Video 7.8) and gastric pouch during revisional surgery (Video 7.9).

Novel Fluorescence-Guided Gastric Calibration Tube

The Endolumik Fluorescence-Guided Gastric Calibration Tube (Figs. 7.1 and 7.2) is a novel single-use, fluorescence-guided calibration tube indicated for use in bariatric, gastric, and esophageal

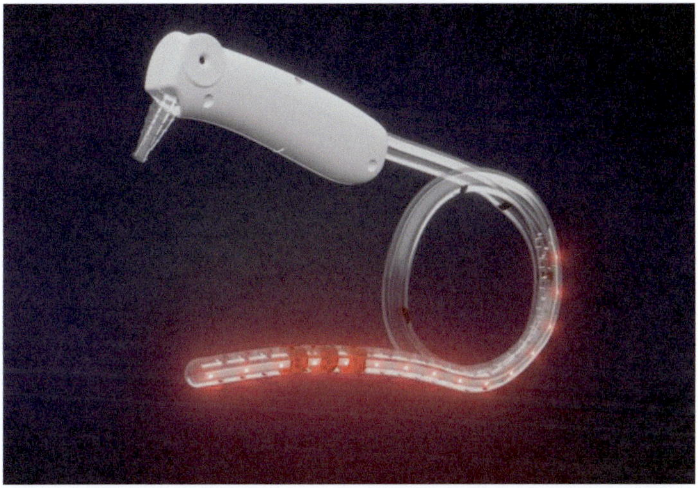

Fig. 7.1 The Endolumik Fluorescence-Guided Gastric Calibration Tube after turning on NIR lighting system, white light view

surgery to improve visualization of tube position and to serve as a sizing and measurement guide, for the application of suction, gastric decompression/drainage of gastric fluids, and irrigation and leak testing [77]. This device combines the functionality of a nasogastric or orogastric tube, a calibration tube, and a leak testing system. The device was designed to improve intraoperative visualization and provide surgeons with additional visual cues to identify anatomic structures and delineate tissue planes with the goal of improving the precision of surgical dissection.

The Endolumik Gastric Calibration Tube is lit using NIR spectrum LEDs which enable transillumination through esophagogastric tissues. The tube is 80 cm long and is available in two different diameters: 36 and 40 French. It has a rounded tip and small side holes at the distal end to enable gastric decompression and/or irrigation. The proximal end includes a handle with an integral suction regulator. An additional squeeze bulb with pressure gauge may be attached to the end of the regulator to perform leak testing. Pilot studies have been completed using the device to improve visualization during laparoscopic sleeve gastrectomy and laparoscopic gastric bypass (Figs. 7.3, 7.4 and 7.5). The three black

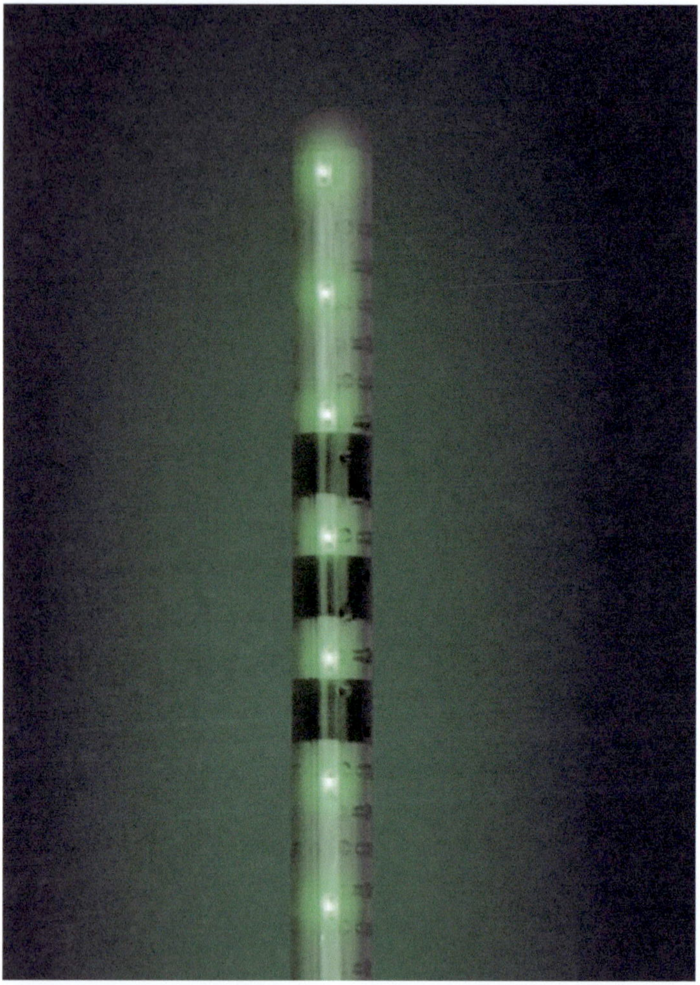

Fig. 7.2 The Endolumik Fluorescence-Guided Gastric Calibration Tube after turning on NIR lighting system, NIR light view

stripes at the distal end of the device enable fluorescence-guided measurement of up to 10 cm of length (Fig. 7.6). The device was FDA approved on March 3, 2023, via the 510 K pathway. It is the

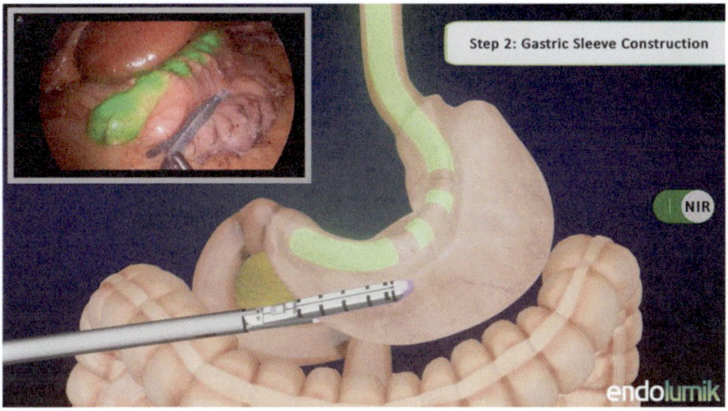

Fig. 7.3 Use of the Endolumik Fluorescence-Guided Gastric Calibration Tube during gastric sleeve construction

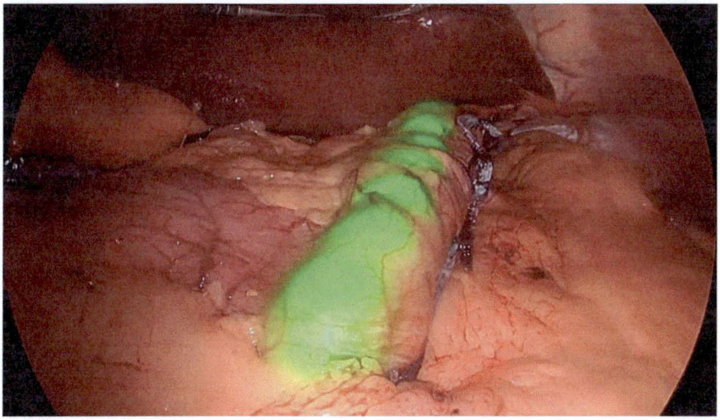

Fig. 7.4 Fluorescence-guided gastric sleeve construction during sleeve gastrectomy operation using the Endolumik calibration tube

first device to be approved through the Safer Technologies Program (STeP) [78], a voluntary program for medical devices that are reasonably expected to significantly improve the safety of currently available treatments.

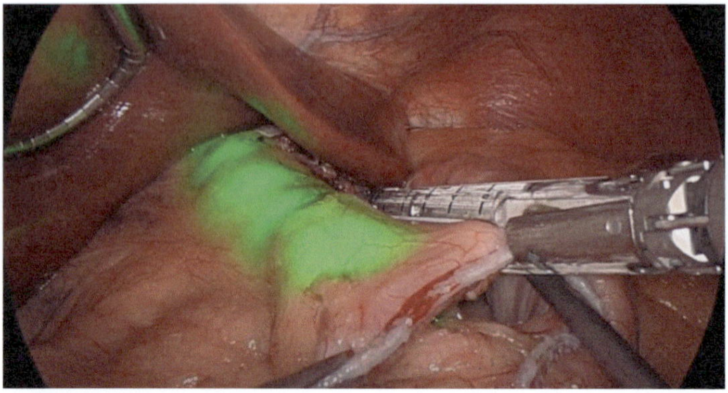

Fig. 7.5 Fluorescence-guided gastric pouch construction during gastric bypass operation using the Endolumik calibration tube

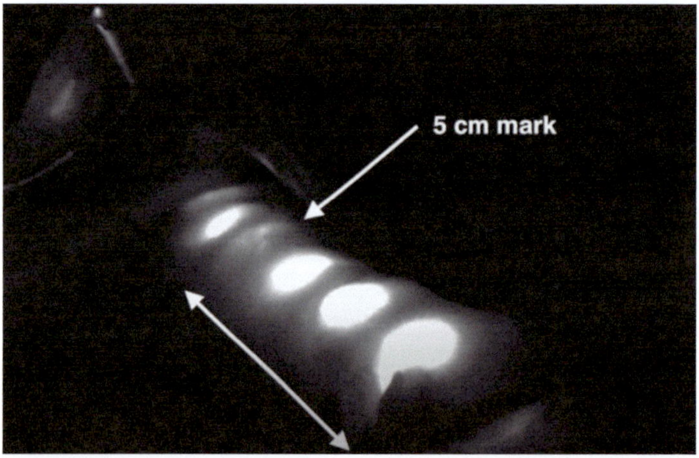

Fig. 7.6 Use of the Endolumik Fluorescence-Guided Gastric Calibration Tube to make fluorescence-guided measurements of gastric pouch length during gastric bypass

Pearls and Pitfalls

- Transillumination device which provides enhanced intraoperative visualization to enable more precise surgical dissection.
- Combines functionality of orogastric tube, calibration tube, and leak testing system.
- Compatible with all NIR surgical camera systems.
- LED-powered NIR device obviates the need for ICG dye injection.

Conclusion

Bariatric surgery is a powerful tool for treating obesity and its associated comorbidities. Sleeve gastrectomy (SG), Roux-en-Y gastric bypass (RYGB), and biliopancreatic diversion with duodenal switch (BPD/DS) are the main primary operations. The number of revisional bariatric surgeries continues to grow and often involves creation of a gastrojejunostomy. ICG has emerged as a useful tool in assessing perfusion and the integrity of the tissue perfusion and anastomoses in these surgeries. Further investigation into the application of intraoperative fluorescence guidance will make the primary and revisional bariatric surgeries a safer and more effective option for patients.

Conflicts of Interest None.

References

1. The National Institutes of Health (NIH) Consensus Development Program: Gastrointestinal Surgery for Severe Obesity. https://consensus.nih.gov/1991/1991gisurgeryobesity084html.htm. Accessed 11 Sep 2021.
2. Estimate of Bariatric Surgery Numbers, 2011–2019 | American Society for Metabolic and Bariatric Surgery. https://asmbs.org/resources/estimate-of-bariatric-surgery-numbers. Accessed 5 Sep 2021.

3. Ren CJ, Patterson E, Gagner M. Early results of laparoscopic biliopancreatic diversion with duodenal switch: a case series of 40 consecutive patients. Obes Surg. 2000;10:514–23.
4. Brethauer SA. Sleeve gastrectomy. Surg Clin N Am. 2011;91:1265–79.
5. Brethauer SA, Hammel JP, Schauer PR. Systematic review of sleeve gastrectomy as staging and primary bariatric procedure. Surg Obes Relat Dis. 2009;5:469–75.
6. Dixon JB, McPhail T, O'Brien PE. Minimal reporting requirements for weight loss: current methods not ideal. Obes Surg. 2005;15:1034–9.
7. Rosenthal RJ. International sleeve gastrectomy expert panel consensus statement: best practice guidelines based on experience of >12,000 cases. Surg Obes Relat Dis. 2012;8:8–19.
8. Gagner M, Hutchinson C, Rosenthal R. Fifth International Consensus Conference: current status of sleeve gastrectomy. Surg Obes Relat Dis. 2016;12:750–6. https://doi.org/10.1016/j.soard.2016.01.022.
9. Zellmer JD, Mathiason MA, Kallies KJ, Kothari SN. Is laparoscopic sleeve gastrectomy a lower risk bariatric procedure compared with laparoscopic roux-en-Y gastric bypass? A meta-analysis. Am J Surg. 2014;208:903–10.
10. Rebecchi F, Allaix ME, Giaccone C, Ugliono E, Scozzari G, Morino M. Gastroesophageal reflux disease and laparoscopic sleeve gastrectomy : a physiopathologic evaluation. Ann Surg. 2014;260:909–15.
11. Himpens J, Dobbeleir J, Peeters G. Long-term results of laparoscopic sleeve gastrectomy for obesity. Ann Surg. 2010;252:319–24.
12. Lauti M, Kularatna M, Hill AG, Maccormick AD. Weight regain following sleeve gastrectomy—a systematic review. Obes Surg. 2016;26:1326–34.
13. Landreneau JP, Strong AT, Rodriguez JH, Aleassa EM, Aminian A, Brethauer S, Schauer PR, Kroh MD. Conversion of sleeve gastrectomy to Roux-en-Y gastric bypass. Obes Surg. 2018;28:3843–50.
14. Aurora A, Khaitan L, Saber A. Sleeve gastrectomy and the risk of leak: a systematic analysis of 4,888 patients. Surg Endosc. 2012;26:1509–15.
15. Silecchia G, Iossa A. Complications of staple line and anastomoses following laparoscopic bariatric surgery. Ann Gastroenterol. 2018;31:56.
16. Berger ER, Clements RH, Morton JM, Huffman KM, Wolfe BM, Nguyen NT, Ko CY, Hutter MM. The impact of different surgical techniques on outcomes in laparoscopic sleeve gastrectomies: the first report from the metabolic and bariatric surgery accreditation and quality improvement program (MBSAQIP). Ann Surg. 2016;264:464–71.
17. Gagner M, Buchwald JN. Comparison of laparoscopic sleeve gastrectomy leak rates in four staple-line reinforcement options: a systematic review. Surg Obes Relat Dis. 2014;10:713–23.
18. Baker RS, Foote J, Kemmeter P, Brady R, Vroegop T, Serveld M. The science of stapling and leaks. Obes Surg. 2004;14:1290–8.

19. Hughes D, Hughes I, Khanna A. Management of staple line leaks following sleeve gastrectomy—a systematic review. Obes Surg. 2019;29:2759–72.
20. Giuliani A, Romano L, Marchese M, Necozione S, Cianca G, Schietroma M, Carlei F. Gastric leak after laparoscopic sleeve gastrectomy: management with endoscopic double pigtail drainage. A systematic review. Surg Obes Relat Dis. 2019;15:1414–9.
21. Alander JT, Kaartinen I, Laakso A, Pätilä T, Spillmann T, Tuchin VV, Venermo M, Välisuo P. A review of Indocyanine green fluorescent imaging in surgery. Int J Biomed Imaging. 2012;2012:1. https://doi.org/10.1155/2012/940585.
22. Benya R, Quintana J, Brundage B. Adverse reactions to indocyanine green: a case report and a review of the literature. Cathet Cardiovasc Diagn. 1989;17:231–3.
23. Olmi S, David G, Cesana G, Ciccarese F, Giorgi R, de Carli S, Uccelli M. Modified sleeve gastrectomy combined with laparoscopic Rossetti fundoplication and vascularization assessment with Indocyanine green. Obes Surg. 2049;29:3086–8.
24. Frattini F, Lavazza M, Mangano A, Amico F, Rausei S, Rovera F, Boni L, Dionigi G. Indocyanine green-enhanced fluorescence in laparoscopic sleeve gastrectomy. Obes Surg. 2015;25:949–50.
25. Ortega CB, Guerron AD, Yoo JS. The use of fluorescence angiography during laparoscopic sleeve gastrectomy. JSLS. 2018;22:e2018.00005. https://doi.org/10.4293/JSLS.2018.00005.
26. di Furia M, Romano L, Salvatorelli A, Brandolin D, Lomanto D, Cianca G, Schietroma M, Carlei F, Giuliani A. Indocyanine green fluorescent angiography during laparoscopic sleeve gastrectomy: preliminary results. Obes Surg. 2019;29:2786–90.
27. Billy H, Jones G. Indocyanine green mesenteric angiography as an intraoperative assessment of bowel perfusion in revisional and primary bariatric operations. Assessment of 50 cases, operative findings, and surgical interventions taken. Surg Obes Relat Dis. 2019;15:S228.
28. Hagen ME, Diaper J, Douissard J, Jung MK, Buehler L, Aldenkortt F, Barcelos GK, Morel P. Early experience with intraoperative leak test using a blend of methylene blue and Indocyanine green during robotic gastric bypass surgery. Obes Surg. 2019;29:949–52.
29. Kalmar CL, Reed CM, Peery CL, Salzberg AD. Intraluminal indocyanine green for intraoperative staple line leak testing in bariatric surgery. Surg Endosc. 2020;34:4194–9.
30. Sethi M, Zagzag J, Patel K, et al. Intraoperative leak testing has no correlation with leak after laparoscopic sleeve gastrectomy. Surg Endosc. 2016;30:883–91.
31. Bingham J, Lallemand M, Barron M, Kuckelman J, Carter P, Blair K, Martin M. North Pacific surgical association routine intraoperative leak

testing for sleeve gastrectomy: is the leak test full of hot air? Am J Surg. 2016;211:943–7.
32. Ignat M, Vix M, Imad I, D'Urso A, Perretta S, Marescaux J, Mutter D. Randomized trial of Roux-en-Y gastric bypass versus sleeve gastrectomy in achieving excess weight loss. Br J Surg. 2017;104:248–56.
33. Buchwald H, Avidor Y, Braunwald E, Jensen MD, Pories W, Fahrbach K, Schoelles K. Bariatric surgery: a systematic review and meta-analysis. JAMA. 2004;292:1724–37.
34. Schauer PR, Bhatt DL, Kirwan JP, et al. Bariatric surgery versus intensive medical therapy for diabetes—5-year outcomes. N Engl J Med. 2017;376:641–51.
35. Aminian A, Brethauer SA, Andalib A, et al. Individualized metabolic surgery score: procedure selection based on diabetes severity. Ann Surg. 2017;266:650–7.
36. Pallati PK, Shaligram A, Shostrom VK, Oleynikov D, Mcbride CL, Goede MR. Improvement in gastroesophageal reflux disease symptoms after various bariatric procedures: review of the bariatric outcomes longitudinal database. Surg Obes Relat Dis. 2014;10:502–7.
37. Peterli R, Wolnerhanssen BK, Peters T, et al. Effect of laparoscopic sleeve gastrectomy vs laparoscopic Roux-en-Y gastric bypass on weight loss in patients with morbid obesity: the SM-BOSS randomized clinical trial. JAMA. 2018;319:255–65.
38. Bendewald FP, Choi JN, Blythe LS, Selzer DJ, Ditslear JH, Mattar SG. Comparison of hand-sewn, linear-stapled, and circular-stapled gastrojejunostomy in laparoscopic Roux-en-y gastric bypass. Obes Surg. 2004;21:1671. https://doi.org/10.1007/s11695-011-0470-6.
39. Sundaresan N, Sullivan M, Hiticas BA, et al. Impacts of gastrojejunal anastomotic technique on rates of marginal ulcer formation and anastomotic bleeding following Roux-en-Y gastric bypass. Obes Surg. 2021;31:2921–6.
40. Smith MD, Adeniji A, Wahed AS, et al. Technical factors associated with anastomotic leak after Roux–en–Y gastric bypass. Surg Obes Relat Dis. 2015;11:313–20.
41. Ballesta C, Berindoague R, Cabrera M, Palau M, Gonzales M. Management of anastomotic leaks after laparoscopic Roux-en-Y gastric bypass. Obes Surg. 2008;18:623–30.
42. Griffith PS, Birch DW, Sharma AM, Karmali S. Managing complications associated with laparoscopic Roux-en-Y gastric bypass for morbid obesity. Can J Surg. 2012;55:329.
43. Gonzalez R, Sarr MG, Smith D, Baghai M, Kendrick M, Szomstein S, Rosenthal R, Murr MM. Diagnosis and contemporary management of anastomotic leaks after gastric bypass for obesity. J Am Coll Surg. 2007;204:47–55.
44. Kim J, Azagury D, Eisenberg D, DeMaria E, Campos GM. ASMBS position statement on prevention, detection, and treatment of gastrointestinal

leak after gastric bypass and sleeve gastrectomy, including the roles of imaging, surgical exploration, and nonoperative management. Surg Obes Relat Dis. 2015;11:739–48.
45. de Moura DTH, de Moura BFBH, Manfredi MA, Hathorn KE, Bazarbashi AN, Ribeiro IB, de Moura EGH, Thompson CC. Role of endoscopic vacuum therapy in the management of gastrointestinal transmural defects. World J Gastrointest Endosc. 2019;11:329–44.
46. Carter JT, Tafreshian S, Campos GM, Tiwari U, Herbella F, Cello JP, Patti MG, Rogers SJ, Posselt AM. Routine upper GI series after gastric bypass does not reliably identify anastomotic leaks or predict stricture formation. Surg Endosc Other Interv Tech. 2007;21:2172–7.
47. Lee SD, Khouzam MN, Kellum JM, DeMaria EJ, Meador JG, Wolfe LG, Maher JW. Selective, versus routine, upper gastrointestinal series leads to equal morbidity and reduced hospital stay in laparoscopic gastric bypass patients. Surg Obes Relat Dis. 2007;3:413–6.
48. Hess DS, Hess DW. Biliopancreatic diversion with a duodenal switch. Obes Surg. 1998;8:267–82.
49. Sethi M, Chau E, Youn A, Jiang Y, Fielding G, Ren-Fielding C. Surgery for long-term outcomes after biliopancreatic diversion with and without duodenal switch: 2-, 5-, and 10-year data. Surg Obes Relat Dis. 2016;12:1697–705.
50. Biertho L, Simon-Hould F, Marceau S, Lebel S, Lescelleur O, Biron S. Current outcomes of laparoscopic duodenal switch. Ann Surg Innov Res. 2016;10:1.
51. Mingrone G, Panunzi S, de Gaetano A, et al. Bariatric surgery versus conventional medical therapy for type 2 diabetes. N Engl J Med. 2012;366:1577–85.
52. Scopinaro N, Adami GF, Marinari GM, Gianetta E, Traverso E, Friedman D, Camerini G, Baschieri G, Simonelli A. Biliopancreatic diversion. World J Surg. 1998;22:936–46.
53. Albaugh VL, Banan B, Antoun J, Xiong Y, Guo Y, Ping J, Alikhan M, Clements BA, Abumrad NN, Flynn CR. Role of bile acids and GLP-1 in mediating the metabolic improvements of bariatric surgery. Gastroenterology. 2019;156:1041–1051.e4.
54. Raghow R. Ménage-à-trois of bariatric surgery, bile acids and the gut microbiome. World J Diabetes. 2015;6:367.
55. Albaugh VL, Banan B, Ajouz H, Abumrad NN, Flynn CR. Bile acids and bariatric surgery. Mol Aspects Med. 2017;56:75–89.
56. Sánchez-Pernaute A, Rubio Herrera MA, Pérez-Aguirre E, García Pérez JC, Cabrerizo L, Díez Valladares L, Fernández C, Talavera P, Torres A. Proximal duodenal-ileal end-to-side bypass with sleeve gastrectomy: proposed technique. Obes Surg. 2007;17:1614–8.
57. Yashkov Y, Bordan N, Torres A, Malykhina A, Bekuzarov D. SADI-S 250 vs roux-en-Y duodenal switch (RY-DS): results of 5-year observational study. Obes Surg. 2021;31:570–9.

58. Surve A, Cottam D, Richards C, Medlin W, Belnap L. A matched cohort comparison of long-term outcomes of roux-en-Y gastric bypass (RYGB) versus single-anastomosis Duodeno-ileostomy with sleeve gastrectomy (SADI-S). Obes Surg. 2021;31:1438–48.
59. Brown WA, Ooi G, Higa K, Himpens J, Torres A. Single anastomosis duodenal-Ileal bypass with sleeve gastrectomy/one anastomosis duodenal switch (SADI-S/OADS) IFSO position statement. Obes Surg. 2018;28:1207–16.
60. Kallies K, Rogers AM. ASMBS guidelines/statements American Society for Metabolic and Bariatric Surgery updated statement on single-anastomosis duodenal switch. Surg Obes Relat Dis. 2020;16:825–30.
61. Sudan R, Puri V, Sudan D. Robotically assisted biliary pancreatic diversion with a duodenal switch: a new technique. Surg Endosc. 2007;21:729–33.
62. Biertho L, Lebel S, Marceau S, Hould F-S, Julien F, Biron S. Biliopancreatic diversion with duodenal switch surgical technique and perioperative care. Surg Clin North Am. 2016;96:815–26.
63. Biertho L, Lebel S, Marceau S, Hould FS, Lescelleur O, Moustarah F, Simard S, Biron S, Marceau P. Perioperative complications in a consecutive series of 1000 duodenal switches. Surg Obes Relat Dis. 2013;9:63–8.
64. Dorman RB, Rasmus NF, Al-Haddad BJS, Serrot FJ, Slusarek BM, Sampson BK, Buchwald H, Leslie DB, Ikramuddin S. Benefits and complications of the duodenal switch/biliopancreatic diversion compared to the Roux-en-Y gastric bypass. Surgery. 2012;152:758–67.
65. Surve A, Zaveri H, Cottam D. Video case report a safer and simpler technique of duodenal dissection and transection of the duodenal bulb for duodenal switch-NC-ND license. Surg Obes Relat Dis. 2016;12:923–4. http://creativecommons.org/licenses/by-nc-nd/4.0/.
66. Yoo T, Hou LA, Reicher S, Chen KT, Eysselein VE. Successful repair of duodenal perforation with endoscopic vacuum therapy. Gastrointest Endosc. 2018;87:1363–4.
67. Loske G, Liedke M, Schlöricke E, Herrmann T, Rucktaeschel F. Endoscopic negative-pressure therapy for duodenal leakage using new open-pore film and polyurethane foam drains with the pull-through technique. Endoscopy. 2017;49:E300–2.
68. Sucandy I, Abulfaraj M, Naglak M, Antanavicius G. Risk of biliary events after selective cholecystectomy during biliopancreatic diversion with duodenal switch. Obes Surg. 2016;26:531–7.
69. Buddingh KT, Nieuwenhuijs VB, van Buuren L, Hulscher JBF, de Jong JS, van Dam GM. Intraoperative assessment of biliary anatomy for prevention of bile duct injury: a review of current and future patient safety interventions. Surg Endosc. 2011;25:2449.
70. Shimizu H, Annaberdyev S, Motamarry I, Kroh M, Schauer PR, Brethauer SA. Revisional bariatric surgery for unsuccessful weight loss and complications. Obes Surg. 2013;23:1766–73.

71. Spyropoulos C, Kehagias I, Panagiotopoulos S, Mead N, Kalfarentzos F. Revisional bariatric surgery: 13-year experience from a tertiary institution. Arch Surg. 2010;145:173–7.
72. Ramly EP, Safadi BY, Dakour Aridi H, Kantar R, Mailhac A, Alami RS. Concomitant removal of gastric band and gastric bypass: analysis of outcomes and complications from the ACS-NSQIP database. Obes Surg. 2017;27:462–8.
73. Topart P, Becouarn G, Ritz P. One-year weight loss after primary or revisional Roux-en-Y gastric bypass for failed adjustable gastric banding. SOARD. 2009;5:459–62.
74. Coblijn UK, Goucham AB, Lagarde SM, Kuiken SD, van Wagensveld BA. Development of ulcer disease after Roux-en-Y gastric bypass, incidence, risk factors, and patient presentation: a systematic review. Obes Surg. 2014;24:299–309.
75. Patel RA, Brolin RE, Gandhi A. Revisional operations for marginal ulcer after Roux-en-Y gastric bypass. SOARD. 2009;5:317–22.
76. Chau E, Youn H, Ren-Fielding CJ, Fielding GA, Schwack BF, Kurian MS. Surgical management and outcomes of patients with marginal ulcer after Roux-en-Y gastric bypass. Surg Obes Relat Dis. 2015;11:1071–5.
77. https://endolumik.com/wp-content/uploads/2023/03/Endolumik-Gastric-Calibration-Tube-IFU-V3.pdf.
78. https://www.accessdata.fda.gov/cdrh_docs/pdf22/K222880.pdf.

Use of Fluorescence Guidance in Breast Reconstruction

8

Acara Turner, Luis Quiroga,
Sebastian Brooke, and Kerri Woodberry

Introduction

The assessment of tissue perfusion is a critical step in the planning and success of every plastic surgery procedure. Plastic surgeons rely on the clinical evaluation of tissue perfusion, including tissue color, capillary refill, and bleeding at the edge of a flap. Recently, several objective assessment adjuncts have been developed in order to reduce complication rates of fat necrosis, mastectomy skin flap necrosis, and partial flap loss [1, 2]. These objective adjuncts utilize various surrogate markers via tissue oximetry measurements, ultrasound-based tools, dye-based and

Supplementary Information The online version contains supplementary material available at https://doi.org/10.1007/978-3-031-40685-0_8.

A. Turner · L. Quiroga · S. Brooke · K. Woodberry (✉)
Department of Surgery, Division of Plastic, Reconstructive, and Hand Surgery, West Virginia University School of Medicine,
Morgantown, WV, USA
e-mail: acara.turner@hsc.wvu.edu; luis.quiroga@hsc.wvu.edu; sebastian.brooke@hsc.wvu.edu; kerri.woodberry@hsc.wvu.edu

N. Szoka et al. (eds.), *The SAGES Manual of Fluorescence-Guided Surgery*, https://doi.org/10.1007/978-3-031-40685-0_8

non-dye-based angiography, or temperature as a relative measurement of well-perfused tissue. While these methods are more sophisticated than clinical evaluation, some are superior to others. For example, thermography has been found to be less reliable than others due to multiple factors that interfere with the accuracy of its reading [1]. On the other hand, fluorescent angiography has proved to be a reliable and more accurate form of intraoperative perfusion assessment. Since the mid-1950s, indocyanine green (ICG) angiography has become a popular method to assess tissue perfusion with applications in multiple specialties [3]. ICG was first used in plastic surgery in 1999 by Still et al. who used the technology as a tool to assess flap perfusion in burn reconstruction. Since then, it has had multiple applications throughout the field including management of diabetic ulcers, assessment of flap perfusion, lymph flow reconstruction, and breast reconstruction, with experimental use in face transplant preoperative planning. This chapter focuses on the application of ICG in breast reconstruction and treatment of associated lymphedema. We will discuss its use in implant-based reconstruction, autologous reconstruction, and postmastectomy surgical correction of lymphedema. More importantly, we will discuss the implications of its use in intraoperative decision-making, postoperative complications, patient costs, and overall patient satisfaction. Overall, the use of ICG has been found to reduce rates of fat necrosis and partial flap necrosis, facilitate early detection of lymphedema in breast cancer reconstruction, reduce patient costs associated with management of complications, and improve patient satisfaction [2, 4, 5]. ICG angiography is not only a cost-effective adjunct to breast reconstruction but also an effective tool to assess tissue perfusion in breast reconstruction.

History

Indocyanine green was initially developed by Kodak during World War II and used as a forming layer of Technicolor films. In the mid-1950s, an executive of Kodak offered to help Dr. Irwin Fox search for a biocompatible dye that could be detected in the blood.

Kodak sent several dyes, including ICG, for testing. ICG showed a distinguished absorption of near-infrared light at 805 nm (the same wavelength at which the optical densities of oxygenated and reduced hemoglobin in blood are approximately equal). In 1955, ICG dye was developed for near-infrared (NIR) photography by the Kodak research laboratories. It was then approved for clinical use in 1959 by the FDA. Hynson, Westcott & Dunning, a small pharmaceutical company in Baltimore, developed the stable lyophilized form in use today. ICG had its first medical application in 1956 in the field of cardiology. By measuring the time-variant dilution of ICG in whole blood, cardiac output could be measured, and valvular septal defects could be determined. It was then discovered that the dye was excreted exclusively by the liver, leading to his application for measuring hepatic function. In 1969, Kogure and co-workers attempted the first ICG angiography when they demonstrated infrared absorption of the canine brain vasculature following intra-arterial ICG injection. Since its initial use in burn patients, ICG angiography has become an important tool for assessing tissue perfusion and lymphatics. Today, the SPY Elite system is the most common and accessible indocyanine green angiography system in the USA. It was first used in cardiac surgery to assess vascular flow and transplant surgery. In 2009, Newman and Samsom introduced the SPY Elite system as a tool to assess free flap perfusion. Jones and Pestana then described its ability to assess both mastectomy skin flap perfusion and microvascular anastomoses in autologous tissue transfer. These were the first of many studies that have proven its efficacy in improving intraoperative decision-making and reducing postoperative complications.

Mechanism of Action

Indocyanine green is an anionic, hydrophobic tricarbocyanine molecule. Immediately following IV injection, ICG rapidly binds to plasma proteins, especially lipoproteins with no known metabolites. ICG has a short half-life of only 2.5 to 3 min as it is extracted rapidly by the liver without modifications and excreted into the bile approximately 8 min after injection. When injected interstitially, ICG binds to protein and is then found in lymphatic channels. It can be found in the nearest draining lymph nodes within 15 min and reaches regional lymph nodes within 1–2 h. ICG absorbs light in the near-infrared region at 800 to 810 nm in blood plasma and emits fluorescent light at a slightly longer wavelength, with peak emission at a wavelength of 830 nm. The fluorescence imaging devices provide external energy as near-infrared light for the indocyanine green to absorb. This causes excitation of the indocyanine greens and emits a fluorescent light which is transferred from the field to an image on the monitor. At this wavelength, ICG allows visualization of blood vessels at 2 cm depth without significant absorption by water, tissue, or hemoglobin. The dye is eventually taken up by the liver cells and secreted in the bile. The plasma fractional disappearance rate is 0.5 mg/kg and is slightly higher in women than in men. The pharmacokinetic properties of ICG have two main benefits. First, it allows a practical application of ICG in bile system assessment during surgery. Second and more importantly, the short half-life of ICG enables repeated examinations via multiple injections without reaching toxic levels, which is vital to plastic surgery applications. This property separates ICG from fluorescein, which can only be used once as it remains within the tissues.

Indications in Plastic Surgery

The use of indocyanine green angiography in breast reconstruction has increased in the past 20 years as a useful tool to assess mastectomy skin and autologous tissue viability with real-time imaging. Complication rates associated with assessment of flap perfusion via clinical assessment alone highlighted the need for an improved means of skin flap and autologous tissue evaluation [1, 6]. Indocyanine green angiography in implant-based and autologous breast reconstruction is a useful tool that has been associated with decreased rates of mastectomy skin necrosis, partial flap loss, and fat necrosis by guiding intraoperative decision-making [6]. Its use allows surgeons to excise poorly perfused tissue, place implants in the proper plane, and determine the appropriate timeline for breast reconstruction. ICG angiography provides surgeons with visual evidence of poor perfusion that may not manifest clinically until several days postoperatively, thereby allowing surgeons to excise specific areas of poor tissue perfusion (Video 8.1). In implant-based reconstruction, ICG angiography provides an objective assessment of mastectomy skin flap perfusion that helps determine which plane is most appropriate for implant placement. This is especially important in high-risk patients, such as those who are smokers, those with a BMI greater than 30, or those who have undergone radiotherapy. In autologous reconstruction, ICG angiography centers around the assessment of autologous tissue perfusion and patency of microvascular anastomoses, which has led to decreased rates of fat necrosis and partial flap loss, as poorly perfused tissue can be primarily excised. For patients who have undergone axillary lymph node surgery with resultant lymphedema, ICG angiography has been found to outperform lymphoscintigraphy, which is currently the main lymphatic imaging modality [4, 7]. Lymphoscintigraphy does not provide the detailed characteristics or real-time dynamic flow needed to perform lymphatic surgery. ICG angiography evaluates lymphatic channels in order to determine the adequate timing of surgical intervention and guide preoperative planning and intraoperative performance of lymphedema surgery. Overall, indocyanine green angiography has become a useful tool in breast reconstruction that has decreased overall complication rates.

Implant-Based Reconstruction

Immediate Reconstruction

Immediate breast reconstruction with a direct-to-implant (DTI) reconstruction has the clear advantage of a single operation, which is offset by higher complication rates especially in the early postoperative period. Early complications include mastectomy skin necrosis, infection, delayed wound healing, and implant exposure—the majority of which are due to inadequate tissue perfusion. Having a tool for objective assessment of tissue perfusion to complement clinical evaluation allows surgeons to make intraoperative decisions based on ICG angiography findings. The use of ICG angiography guides two main surgical decisions:

1. The quantity and location of mastectomy skin flap excision based on surface area of tissue perfusion.
2. The feasibility of direct-to-implant reconstruction versus tissue expander placement based on skin flap vascular integrity.

In immediate breast reconstruction with direct-to-implant reconstruction, implants may be placed in the prepectoral plane or in the submuscular plane with total coverage or partial coverage by the pectoralis major muscle, the serratus muscle, or an acellular dermal matrix. While submuscular placement has historically been the predominant location of implants, prepectoral placement has increased in popularity as patients experience less postoperative pain and have lower rates of animation distortion seen in submuscular placement. The use of SPY angiography allows patients to undergo DTI reconstruction in the prepectoral plane with lower rates of postoperative complications [6]. Using this tool permits surgeons to assess the vascular integrity of mastectomy skin flaps, thereby guiding intraoperative decision-making. When mastectomy skin flaps display an adequate percentage of skin perfusion, surgeons may move forward with prepectoral implant placement. However, when mastectomy skin flaps display a lack of vascular integrity proven by SPY fluorescent imaging, prepectoral placement is no longer the best option and necessitates conversion to submuscular implant or expander. Following movement of the implant, a repeated vascular assessment according to the SPY ELITE or SPY Portable Handheld Imager protocol can then be used to confirm the absence of implant-induced vascular compromise. In both planes of implant placement, the use of acellular dermal matrix is important. Its use in the prepectoral plane provides superior pole fullness and provides adequate coverage that is comparable to the pectoralis major muscle coverage. In the submuscular plane, the acellular dermal matrix provides lower pole coverage, often needed during the tissue expansion process which muscular coverage is inadequate [6].

There are special considerations that the plastic surgeon should address when following this decision-making algorithm. They are based on the angiography assessment as well as patient factors. Cutoffs for skin perfusion values that necessitate conversion to submuscular range from 25% to 45% relative perfusion. Skin with 25% or less relative tissue perfusion is nonviable in most patients, and skin with 45% relative tissue perfusion will survive in most patients. Therefore, a gray area exists between these values. Moyer et al. studied this "gray area" and found that the use of a 33% cutoff is associated with a positive predictive value of removing nonviable skin of 88% with a negative predictive value of removing healthy skin of 16% [8]. These values, however, should be determined on an individual basis after evaluating the patient's risk factors for increased mastectomy skin flap necrosis. The main risk factors that affect skin flap necrosis and therefore contribute to angiography success in predicting skin flap necrosis are smoking status, BMI, and mastectomy weight [9]. In patients who are smokers, have a BMI greater than 30, and have a mastectomy weight greater than 800 g, rates of mastectomy skin flap necrosis are higher compared to nonsmokers, patients with a BMI less than 30, or patients with lower mastectomy weights [9]. After accounting for values of tissue perfusion and patient risk factors, the plastic surgeon can then determine an adequate amount of tissue that can be excised without compromising the skin envelope. SPY angiography provides both qualitative and quantitative assessments that allow plastic surgeons to make informed decisions regarding patient eligibility for DTI reconstruction. In doing so, it guides excision of poorly perfused areas and determination of the best plane of implant placement. When factoring in patient factors, these two surgical decisions lead to reduced rates of mastectomy skin flap necrosis and reduce the need for subsequent surgical revision.

Tissue Expander Reconstruction

In patients who undergo immediate or delayed breast reconstruction with tissue expanders, SPY angiography serves to maximize tissue expansion and allows surgeons to assess the amount of initial fill of the tissue expander. In immediate breast reconstruction, the tissue expander can be filled to a significant volume—particularly with the use of ADM—which speeds the overall timing of expansion. The use of acellular dermal matrix and skin sparing mastectomies has allowed greater intraoperative filling of expanders. Delayed breast reconstruction occurs for multiple reasons, including patient preference, need for radiotherapy, or inadequate tissue perfusion in the immediate setting. In patients who undergo tissue expander placement after mastectomy, the initial fill of the tissue expander is vital to skin flap perfusion throughout expansion. Following intraoperative tissue expander fill, SPY angiography may be used to assess skin flap perfusion [2] (Video 8.2). If the tissue is shown to have inadequate perfusion, saline should be removed, and the skin flap should be reassessed. This should be repeated until tissue perfusion is adequate, after which closure can take place. While not a requirement, SPY angiography may be used in the intraoperative setting to determine safe rates of tissue expander fill [9].

Autologous Reconstruction

For patients who choose to undergo breast reconstruction but do not want to undergo implant-based reconstruction, autologous reconstruction is an alternative option. Autologous reconstruction, though associated with longer operative times and length of hospital stay, touts the benefits of a breast mound with a more natural shape and feel without the use of a foreign body. Complications of fat necrosis associated with autologous reconstruction can include either partial or complete fat necrosis. Fat necrosis after autologous breast reconstruction not only is a source of patient discomfort and anxiety but also leads to contour abnormalities that may construe the breast exam. Fat necrosis, in addition to partial and total flap loss, has many implications ranging from the need for biopsy to surgical excision.

SPY angiography in autologous breast reconstruction can be used to assess flap perfusion based on perforators present [5, 10]. When used to assess flap perfusion, the plastic surgeon should use

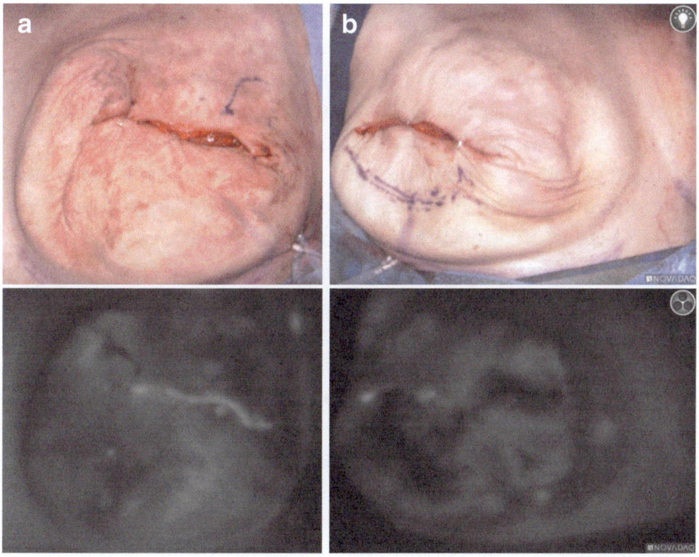

Fig. 8.1 (**a**, **b**) Intraoperative mastectomy flaps before and after SPY angiography. Areas of hypoperfusion are darker than areas of adequate perfusion

a marking pen to delineate the separation between areas of adequate perfusion and areas of hypoperfusion based on angiography image (Fig. 8.1a, b). Following dissection of perforators, dissection of the donor site flap, and microvascular anastomosis to the recipient site, SPY angiography can also be used prior to inset of the flap. At this point, trimming the areas of hypoperfusion can take place. Using this method has been associated with a significant reduction of the rates of fat necrosis. While rates of partial flap loss have been shown to be decreased in patients who underwent SPY angiography and subsequent flap trimming based on perfusion, these studies were underpowered due to low rates of occurrence [4]. In patients with breast cancer-related lymphedema (BCRL) undergoing autologous breast reconstruction with vascularized inguinal lymph node transfer, SPY angiography is a useful tool to identify sentinel lymph nodes of the groin, identify lymphatic channels, and map recipient vessels. It can be used to identify the appropriate lymph node basin when undergoing autologous breast reconstruction with lymph node transfer. SPY angiography allows surgeons to incorporate lymph nodes adjacent to the pedicle during dissection. It can then be used following dissection to assess flap and lymph node perfusion. Finally, it can be used following microvascular anastomosis to assess patency [11].

Indocyanine green angiography is also useful in patients with previous abdominal liposuction seeking to undergo autologous breast reconstruction. While previous studies have shown that abdominal-based autologous reconstruction is feasible after liposuction, it was once controversial [12]. Studies found that when performed, the surgeon typically used a method of perfusion assessment, such as Doppler, angiography, or CT angiography in addition to clinical exam. Casey et al. found that by using indocyanine green angiography intraoperatively and resecting areas of hypoperfusion, rates of partial flap loss and fat necrosis reduced from 71.4% to 0% [12]. Of note, they found no significant difference in anastomotic complications or total flap loss between patients who underwent clinical evaluation and indocyanine green laser angiography.

Complications associated with autologous breast reconstruction lead to additional surgical interventions, postoperative imaging studies, and follow-up appointments. In a 7-year single-center retrospective study of 1000 free flaps for breast reconstruction, Hembd et al. found that indocyanine green angiography was independently associated with a decrease in the odds of fat necrosis (OR, 0.38, $p = 0.004$) [13]. Per single incident of fat necrosis, the studied cohort underwent an additional 0.69 revision provisions, 1.22 imaging studies, 0.77 biopsies, and 1.7 additional oncologic office visits. They also found an 84.9 g higher weight of resected tissue without indocyanine green angiography versus with indocyanine green angiography. Therefore, patient factors may guide the use of indocyanine green angiography in breast reconstruction.

Cost-Effectiveness

While surgeons have the ability to use SPY angiography for all breast reconstruction patients, it is not without cost. The cost of successful surgery utilizing SPY angiography is dependent on the institution [9, 14]. This cost can be offset by prevention of costs associated with mastectomy necrosis or partial flap failure, especially in high-risk patients. Studies have shown that the use of SPY angiography is only cost-effective in patients who are smokers, are obese, and have larger breasts [2]. The use of indocyanine green angiography is associated with savings of $2098.80 for smokers, $5162.30 for patients with a BMI of 30 or more, and $1892.70 for patients with mastectomy weight greater than 800 g [2]. Therefore, in high-risk patients undergoing implant-based reconstruction, SPY angiography may be a useful adjunct that not only reduces postoperative complications but also controls overall costs in this patient population. In autologous breast reconstruction, cost-utility analysis by Chatterjee et al. revealed a baseline cost difference of $773.66, a gain in quality-adjusted life years of 0.22, and an incremental cost-utility ratio of $3516.64 per quality-adjusted life year [14]. Overall, SPY angiography is only cost-effective when the complication rate is 5% or greater [14]. Given that the overall complication rates are as high as 41% in autologous breast reconstruction, angiography will be cost-effective for this subset of breast reconstruction patients. Therefore, when determining the cost-effectiveness of SPY angiography, patient factors should be considered for those undergoing implant-based reconstruction. On the other hand, most patients undergoing SPY angiography for autologous reconstruction may not only reap the benefits of decreased complications but also experience less financial burden in the long run with its use.

Use in Lymphedema Surgery for Breast Reconstruction Patients

The lymphatic system has three fundamental functions, including tissue fluid homeostasis, regulation of the immunologic response, and transportation of gastrointestinal lipids. Lymphedema is a chronic, progressive disease of the lymphatic system resulting in fluid imbalance and subsequent accumulation of protein-rich interstitial fluid. This process results in swelling, inflammation, and irreversible changes of the tissue that primarily affect the upper and lower limbs. Lymphedema can be categorized as primary or secondary. Primary lymphedema is caused by intrinsic defects in the development of the lymphatic system and can occur at various stages of life (i.e., congenital lymphedema, lymphedema praecox, and lymphedema tarda). Secondary lymphedema is caused by extrinsic interruptions in the lymphatic system such as infection, malignancy, or tissue trauma. Lymph node dissection is the most common cause of tissue trauma resulting in secondary lymphedema. Of note, breast cancer-related lymphedema (BCRL) is the most common noninfectious secondary lymphedema in the United States that significantly impacts patients' quality of life [15]. Therefore, the prevention and treatment of BCRL still remains a challenge. The likelihood of developing BCRL is related to the extent of therapeutic interventions ranging from sentinel lymph node biopsy to axillary lymph node dissection (ALND) and adjunct radiation. Since the introduction of sentinel lymph node biopsy for surgical staging in 1992 by Drs. Morton and Cochran, the incidence of BCRL has been reduced to 5–7% [16]. However, among patients undergoing axillary lymph node dissection (ALND), the reported incidence of BCRL is approximately 20%. The reported incidence of BCRL is even higher among patients undergoing both ALND and radiotherapy, ranging from 25% to 40% [16].

The clinical manifestations of lymphedema and the time of presentation are variable among patients. The most common early sign is extremity swelling, but occasionally patients report pain and recurrent cellulitis as their primary complaints. Identifying a patient's stage of lymphedema begins with a thorough clinical examination. While various staging systems have been reported, the most widely accepted staging system is the International Society of Lymphology (ISL) staging system which grades lymphedema based on the clinical findings and its natural progression [17] (Table 8.1). Subclinical or stage 0 lymphedema refers to an early stage of dysfunctional lymph transport without clinical manifestations. Stage 1 is characterized by reversible edema either with extremity elevation or compression with or without pitting edema. Conversely, in stage 2, lymphedema presents as irreversible pitting edema and some tissue fibrosis, which

Table 8.1 International Society of Lymphology staging system. Executive Committee of the International Society of Lymphology. The diagnosis and treatment of peripheral lymphedema: 2020 Consensus Document of the International Society of Lymphology. Lymphology 2020; 53:3

International Society of Lymphology lymphedema staging classification			
Stage	Description	Pathophysiology	Clinical features
0	Subclinical	Impaired lymph transport	Swelling not evident
I	Spontaneously reversible	Early lymph accumulation	Swelling relieved by limb elevation Pitting may be present
II	Not spontaneously reversible	Fat hypertrophy and deposition with tissue fibrosis	Swelling not improved by limb elevation Pitting edema present with fibrosis
III	Lymphostatic elephantiasis	Chronic lymphatic stasis and inflammation, further fibrosis and fatty deposition	Swelling not improved by limb elevation Edema nonpitting and wooden hyperkeratotic and verrucous skin changes

does not improve with extremity elevation or compression. Finally, stage 3 designates lymphedema that has progressed to irreversible non-pitting edema associated with thick-wooden subcutaneous tissue and hyperkeratotic and verrucous skin changes. Additional staging systems have been proposed including Cheng's Lymphedema affected Grading System, which is based on the circumference differential between affected and unaffected limbs [18] (Table 8.2).

While lymphoscintigraphy has been the standard imaging modality for lymphedema, ICG lymphangiography has become a widely utilized tool in this patient population. ICG lymphangiography is a noninvasive test that allows precise, real-time evaluation of the superficial lymphatic drainage with the added advantage of not utilizing radioactive particles. Similar to lymphoscintigraphy, ICG lymphangiography permits a qualitative evaluation of

Table 8.2 Chang's lymphedema grading system. Patel, KM, Lin, CY, Cheng, MH. A prospective evaluation of lymphedema-specific quality-of-life outcomes following vascularized lymph node transfer. Ann Surg Oncol. 2015;22(7):2424–2430. Copyright © 2014 Society of Surgical Oncology

Grade	Symptoms	Circumferential differentiation	Lymphoscintigraphy
0	Reversible	<9	Partial occlusion
I	Mild	10–19	Partial occlusion
II	Moderate	20–29	Total occlusion
III	Severe	30–39	Total occlusion
IV	Very severe	>40	Total occlusion

the lymphatic circulation and facilitates staging. There is evidence that ICG lymphangiography is more accurate at detecting early upper extremity lymphedema when compared to lymphoscintigraphy [4]. Therefore, breast cancer patients at high risk for developing BCRL may benefit from early ICG lymphangiography after breast surgery to facilitate early detection of lymphedema prior to measurable volume changes on clinical exam.

ICG lymphangiography involves injecting a fluorescent dye intradermally into the distal hand. An infrared light source is then used to stimulate the dye, and visualization is obtained using a camera with an infrared filter allowing dynamic evaluation of lymphatic flow. Flow patterns seen on ICG lymphangiography correlate well with various clinical stages [7]. Flow patterns can be classified as either linear or dermal backflow patterns, the latter of which includes a progression from "splash," then "stardust," to finally "diffuse" subpatterns. The linear pattern refers to a linear fluorescent image produced by the ICG as it travels through normally functioning superficial lymphatic collectors. This pattern is observed in the non-affected limb and in some mild lymphedema cases. In contrast, the dermal backflow pattern describes the nonlinear images produced as the ICG dye follows the pathologic dermal backflow of the lymphatic system, which is found in the more severe lymphedema cases. This backflow pattern includes a group of three subpatterns (splash, stardust, and diffuse) that represent the natural progression of the lymphedema. The splash pattern consists of scattered areas of shining dye that changes from bright to faint in tortuous lymphatic channels. The stardust pattern demonstrates a dimly luminous background with spotted areas of higher fluorescent signals as lymphatic flow decreases. In the diffuse pattern, the dye is widely dispersed with no identifiable lymphatics. Several backflow patterns may occur at the same time. Therefore, the indicator of lymphatic function is based on the worst pattern. Recently, a "no flow" pattern was described [4]. In this case, the injected dye does not extend beyond the wrist and there is no linear or backflow pattern in the arm.

Identifying flow patterns can guide microsurgical options available. The main goal of lymphedema microsurgery is to restore drainage of excess interstitial fluid. This is in contrast to earlier surgical procedures that involved excision of the fibrotic and nonfunctional tissues, which are still useful for advanced-staged lymphedema. The main indication for lymphedema microsurgery is early stage lymphedema prior to adipose deposition and tissue fibrosis. The three main lymphatic microsurgical procedures are lymphaticovenous anastomosis (LVA), vascularized lymph node transfer (VLNT), and the combination of microsurgical breast reconstruction with lymph node transfer (known as the Barcelona Cocktail) [19]. The supermicrosurgical LVA was first described by Koshima in 2000 and became popular after the introduction of new technology and indocyanine green lymphangiography [20]. In this procedure, several remaining lymphatic channels with linear flow are anastomosed to subdermal veins. Vascularized lymph node transfer (VLNT) was developed in animal studies in the 1990s. In this procedure, a lymph node bed of tissue vascularized by a named pedicle is transferred to a distant location as a free tissue transfer. This is a surgical option that allows restoring fluid drainage once LVA is not possible in the setting of absent lymphatic vessels by bringing in new healthy lymph nodes. Commonly used donor sites for lymph node transfer include the submental nodes, supraclavicular nodes, inguinal nodes, lateral thoracic nodes, or omentum. These are then transferred using standard microsurgery techniques to the affected regions as needed. Additionally, a vascularized lymph node transfer can be combined with free flap breast reconstruction using a deep inferior epigastric artery perforator (DIEP) flap. In this procedure, the superficial inguinal lymph nodes are dissected with the DIEP flap and oriented in the axilla during free flap inset (Fig. 8.2).

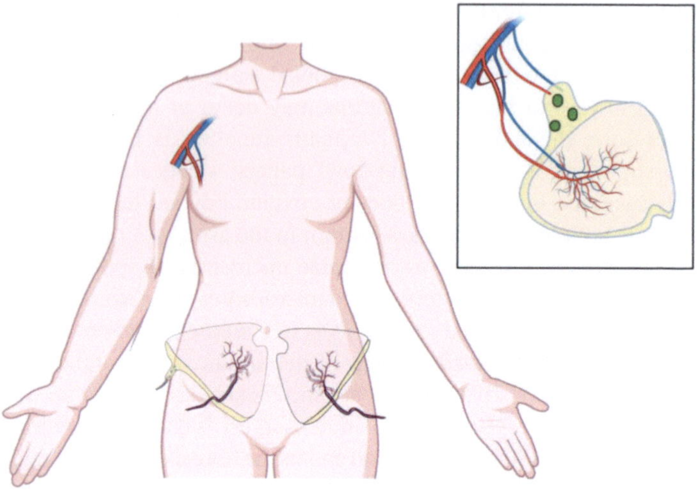

Fig. 8.2 Lymph node transfer of inguinal lymph nodes to the axilla during DIEP free flap reconstruction

Technique

The SPY Agent Green is packaged as a sterile lyophilized green powder which contains 25 mg indocyanine green in a 20 ml single-patient use vial [21]. It contains no more than 5% sodium iodide. As previously mentioned, ICG is a water-soluble tricarbocyanine dye reconstituted by mixing with sterile water to yield a 2.5 mg/ml solution. The initial injection volume is dependent upon the planned procedure. During the procedure, additional doses may be used but should not exceed 2 mg/kg total dose. A larger dose may be required in areas of increased deposits of adipose tissue. In pediatric patients, smaller doses may be used based on body weight and age. Of note, a number of psychiatric, neurologic, and cardiac drugs are associated with increased clearance and should therefore be documented and communicated with anesthesia in order to optimize dosage. These medications include phenobarbital, haloperidol, primidone, heparin, nifedipine, nitrofurantoin, and propranolol. The mixture is shaken slowly until all precipitation is resolved. ICG is unstable in aqueous solution and once reconstituted, it must be used within 6 h. It should be discarded if precipitation is noted in the vial and the precipitation does not dissolve with gentle shaking. Following injection, a normal saline bolus should be administered in order to minimize the dilution of the dye in the slow-flowing venous system. The operating room lights should then be turned down for improved visualization of images.

ICG Angiography for Breast Mastectomy Flaps

Steps for use are outlined below.

1. Prepare and drape imaging equipment in a sterile manner.
2. Reconstitute 25 mg of ICG in 10 ml of sterile water, yielding a 2.5 mg/ml solution.
3. Shake the solution gently to mix. (If precipitation is present, continue to shake gently until the ICG is dissolved. If precipitation persists, discard the solution and prepare a new solution.)
4. Inject 2 ml of the solution via peripheral IV.
5. Flush with 10 cc normal saline.
6. Turn down the operating room lights and use the imaging device to evaluate tissue perfusion of mastectomy flaps. Areas of hyperintensity have higher rates of tissue perfusion, while areas of hypointensity have poor tissue perfusion. Quantification of tissue perfusion is facilitated by percentages relative to the highest perfused areas displayed as an onlay (Fig. 8.3).
7. Use a marking pen to demarcate areas of inadequate tissue perfusion.
8. Perform surgical excision of hypoperfused areas accordingly.

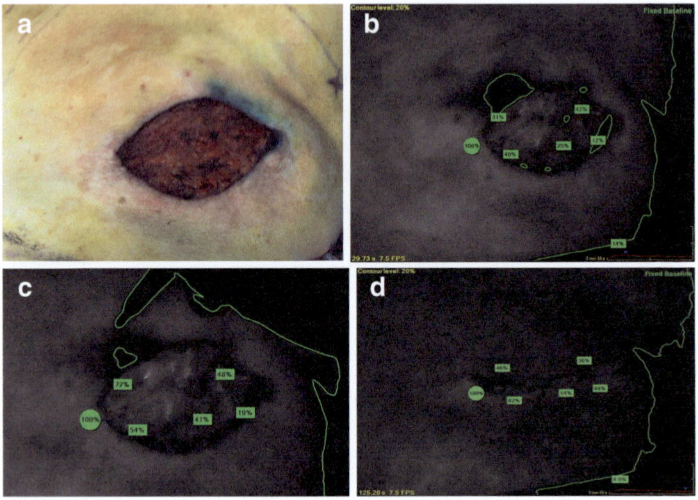

Fig. 8.3 ICG angiography perfusion assessment of a breast mastectomy flap using SPY fluorescence imaging technology (SPY Elite Fluorescence Imaging System, SPY-Q tissue perfusion quantification software, NOVADAQ, now part of Stryker). To quantify the tissue perfusion of the flap, the surgeon has placed a reference marker on healthy well-perfused tissue away from and of the same type as the surgical area (100%), and perfusion in other areas is shown as a percentage relative to this reference (e.g., 44%). A contour can be mapped to delineate the area which is less than a selected % perfusion of the reference. This information can guide surgical excision of hypoperfused areas. Use of SPY angiography to assess perfusion of mastectomy flaps. (**a**) Mastectomy flaps prior to SPY angiography. (**b**) Tissue perfusion quantified by percentage. (**c**) Use of skin marker to outline area of low tissue perfusion prior to staples. (**d**) Perfusion pattern after stapling flaps

ICG Angiography for Lymphaticovenous Anastomosis

Steps for use are outlined below.

1. Prepare and drape imaging equipment in a sterile manner.
2. Reconstitute 25 mg of ICG in 10 ml of sterile water, yielding a 2.5 mg/ml solution.
3. Shake the solution gently to mix. (If precipitation is present, continue to shake gently until the ICG is dissolved. If precipitation persists, discard the solution and prepare a new solution.)

4. Inject 0.2 ml of ICG intradermally into web spaces of the distal hand (Fig. 8.4).
5. Turn down the operating room lights and use the imaging device to evaluate the lymphatic flow pattern.
6. Mark and select the linear flow pattern segment on the skin with a skin marker.
7. Identify and mark "dark crossing areas" that may indicate crossing veins which are possible LVA locations. Injection 0.3 ml of lymphazurin blue into the dermis several centimeters distal to the incision site may assist with visualization of the lymphatic channels.
8. Prepare and drape the extremity.
9. Under the microscope, make a superficial 1.5–2 cm transverse incision over the selected lymphatic vessel, which is located in the superficial subcutaneous tissue.
10. Incise to the deep layer of the dermis using fine dissecting instruments (Fig. 8.5).
11. Once the lymphatic channel and adjacent venule have been identified, anastomosis is carried out via a variety of techniques (Fig. 8.6).
12. A new injection of lymphazurin blue or ICG lymphangiography can be used to confirm the patency of LVA.

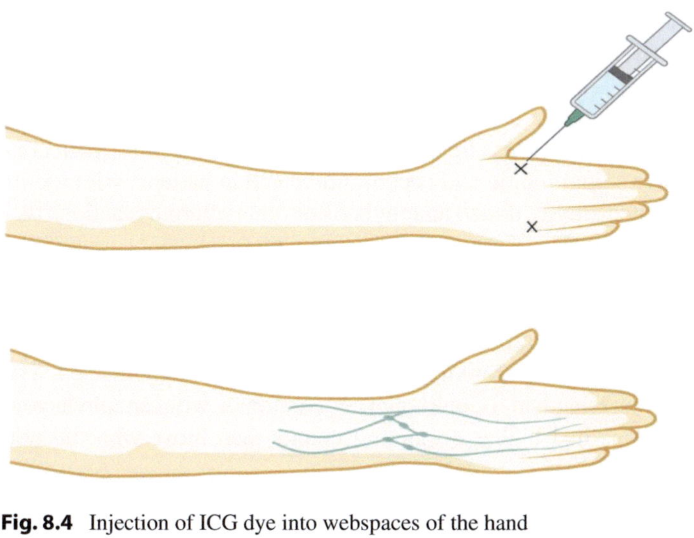

Fig. 8.4 Injection of ICG dye into webspaces of the hand

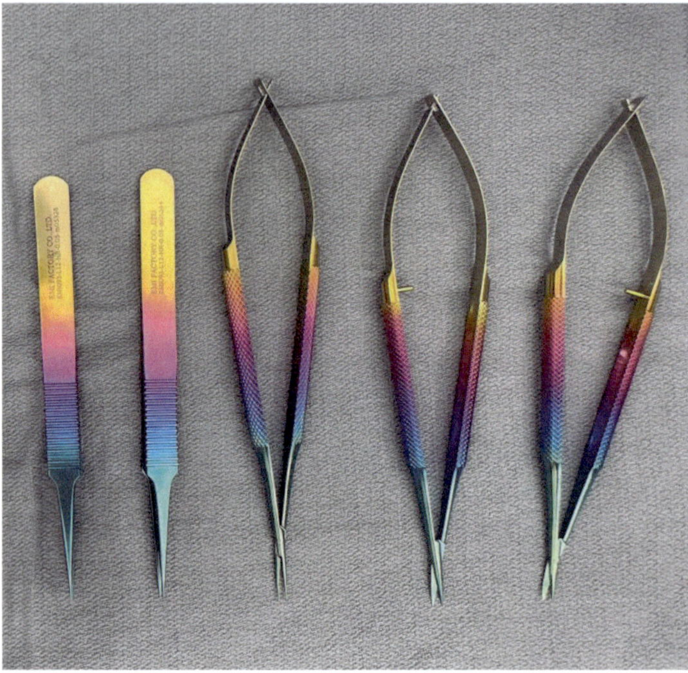

Fig. 8.5 Microsurgical instruments utilized for lymphaticovenous anastomosis

Contraindications and Adverse Reactions

Indocyanine green can be used in adults and pediatric patients, except for those less than 1 month of age. Indocyanine green contains sodium iodide and is contraindicated in patients with iodine hypersensitivity due to anaphylaxis or other allergic reactions that may occur. There are very few reports of anaphylactic reaction to ICG, with an incidence of 1 in 40,000. In patients with renal failure or uremia and those on dialysis, ICG should be used with caution due to reports of anaphylactoid reactions including dyspnea, palpitations, anxiety, nausea, edema, and hypotension. The clear mechanism is unknown, but patients with anaphylactoid reactions had higher eosinophil counts than those who did not.

While not a contraindication to ICG use, the SPY Agent Green contains iodine, and this could reduce the iodine binding capacity of thyroid tissue for at least a week after administration. Therefore, patients who are scheduled to undergo radioactive iodine uptake studies should not do so for at least 1 week following ICG administration. Finally, while there are no adverse events associated

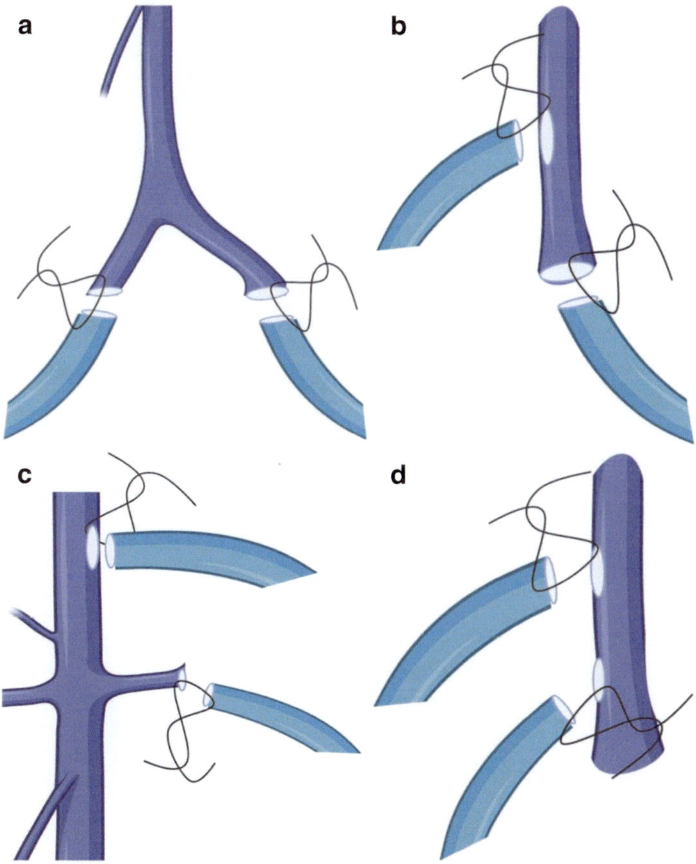

Fig. 8.6 Lymphaticovenous anastomosis techniques. (**a**) Y-shaped LVA. (**b**) Lambda-shaped LVA. (**c**) K-shaped LVA. (**d**) Pi-shaped LVA. (**e**) X-shaped LVA

Fig. 8.6 (continued)

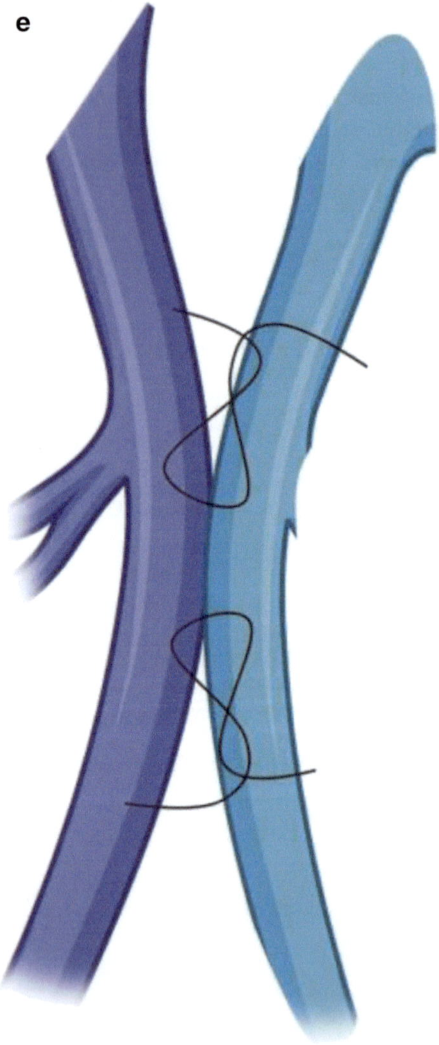

with pregnancy or breastfeeding, use of ICG in these patient populations should be used with caution. ICG is a US FDA category C drug with animal studies showing an adverse effect on the fetus. There are no well-controlled studies in humans nor is there controlled data in human pregnancy. The small studies published have not reported major birth defects, miscarriage, or adverse maternal or fetal outcomes. Additionally, there has been no report of placental transfer of ICG or detectable levels of ICG in fetal blood or umbilical vein blood after ICG administration in the pregnant mother. There is currently no data on the presence of ICG in human milk or the effects on milk production.

Adverse reactions can be mild, moderate, or severe. Mild reactions include flushing, syncope, weakness, headache, urticaria, anxiety, vomiting, and diaphoresis. Moderate reactions include edema, hypotension, erythema, wheezing, sinus tachycardia, palpitations, dyspnea, and confusion. Severe reactions include anaphylactic shock, anaphylactoid reactions, respiratory arrest, cyanosis, cardiac arrest, laryngospasm, bronchospasm, and visual impairment. There have been reports of anaphylaxis, urticaria, and death with use of this product, and therefore, careful monitoring is important and cardiopulmonary resuscitation equipment and personnel should always be available. Patients should be warned of the risks and told to seek medical attention if they develop signs of anaphylaxis such as difficulty breathing, tongue or throat swelling, hives, itching, flushed or pale skin, low blood pressure, or a weak pulse or rapid pulse [21].

Conclusion

Since the introduction of indocyanine green (ICG) angiography to medical use in the mid-1950s, it has become a reliable and popular method to assess tissue perfusion. However, it was not until 1999 that it was used in plastic surgery as a tool to assess flap perfusion in burn reconstruction. Since then, it has had multiple applications throughout plastic surgery, including the management of diabetic ulcers, assessment of flap perfusion, lymph flow reconstruction, and breast reconstruction, with experimental use in face transplant preoperative planning. This chapter serves an overview of ICG in breast reconstruction encompassing mastectomy flap perfusion, free flap viability, and breast cancer-associated lymphedema.

ICG angiography provides surgeons with objective visual evidence of poor perfusion that may not manifest clinically until several days postoperatively. Therefore, the use of ICG has been found to reduce rates of mastectomy skin necrosis, partial flap loss, and fat necrosis by guiding intraoperative decision-making, reducing patient costs associated with complications management, and improving patient satisfaction. Its short half-life enables repeated examinations via multiple injections without reaching toxic levels, vital to plastic surgery applications.

ICG lymphangiography is a noninvasive test that allows precise, real-time evaluation of superficial lymphatic drainage without utilizing radioactive particles. ICG lymphography permits a qualitative assessment of the lymphatic circulation, facilitates its staging, and guides the intraoperative restoration of the lymph flow. Moreover, there is evidence that ICG lymphangiography is more accurate at detecting early upper extremity lymphedema when compared to lymphoscintigraphy and before measurable volume changes on clinical exams.

Overall, applications of ICG in plastic surgery have expanded over the past two decades with a focus on angiography and lymphangiography. In this chapter, we have focused on its use in breast reconstruction, which has shown to be expansive. ICG enables intraoperative tissue assessment via direct visualization that improves decision-making with the goal of improving overall patient satisfaction and outcomes. While it is a relatively new technology in the field of plastic surgery, it has shown potential for improving the overall operative experience and associated outcomes.

References

1. Phillips BT, Munabi NCO, Roeder RA, Ascherman JA, Guo L, Zenn MR. The role of intraoperative perfusion assessment: what is the current state and how can i use it in my practice? Plast Reconstr Surg. 2016;137:731–41.
2. Phillips BT, Lanier ST, Conkling N, Wang ED, Dagum AB, Ganz JC, et al. Intraoperative perfusion techniques can accurately predict mastectomy skin flap necrosis in breast reconstruction: results of a prospective trial. Plast Reconstr Surg. 2012;129(5):778e–88e.

3. Rinker B. A comparison of methods to assess mastectomy flap viability in skin-sparing mastectomy and immediate reconstruction: a prospective cohort study. Plast Reconstr Surg. 2016;137:395–401.
4. Akita S, Nakamura R, Yamamoto N, Tokumoto H, Ishigaki T, Yamaji Y, et al. Early detection of lymphatic disorder and treatment for lymphedema following breast cancer. Plast Reconstr Surg. 2016;138(2):192e–202e.
5. Momeni A, Sheckter C. Intraoperative laser-assisted indocyanine green imaging can reduce the rate of fat necrosis in microsurgical breast reconstruction. Plast Reconstr Surg. 2020;145(3):507E–13E.
6. Bilezikian JA, Tenzel PL, Bebb GG, Kays CR. The broad application of Prepectoral direct-to-implant breast reconstruction with acellular dermal matrix drape and fluorescent imaging in a community setting. Plast Reconstr Surg. 2020;145(2):291–300.
7. Yamamoto T, Yamamoto N, Doi K, Oshima A, Yoshimatsu H, Todokoro T, et al. Indocyanine green–enhanced lymphography for upper extremity lymphedema: a novel severity staging system using dermal backflow patterns. Plast Reconstr Surg [Internet]. 2011;128(4):941–7. Available from: https://journals.lww.com/plasreconsurg/Fulltext/2011/10000/Indocyanine_Green_Enhanced_Lymphography_for_Upper.26.aspx.
8. Moyer HR, Losken A. Predicting mastectomy skin flap necrosis with Indocyanine green angiography: the gray area defined. Plast Reconstr Surg. 2012;129(5):1043–8.
9. Kanuri A, Liu AS, Guo L. Whom should we SPY? A cost analysis of laser-assisted indocyanine green angiography in prevention of mastectomy skin flap necrosis during prosthesis-based breast reconstruction. Plast Reconstr Surg. 2014;133(4):448e–54e.
10. Varela R, Casado-Sanchez C, Zarbakhsh S, Diez J, Hernandez-Godoy J, Landin L. Outcomes of DIEP flap and fluorescent angiography: a randomized controlled clinical trial. Plast Reconstr Surg. 2020;145(1):1–10.
11. Chattha A, Bucknor A, Chen AD, Lee BT, Lin SJ. Indocyanine green angiography use in breast reconstruction: a national analysis of outcomes and cost in 110,320 patients. Plast Reconstr Surg. 2018;141(4):825–32.
12. Casey WJ, Connolly KA, Nanda A, Rebecca AM, Perdikis G, Smith AA. Indocyanine green laser angiography improves deep inferior epigastric perforator flap outcomes following abdominal suction lipectomy. Plast Reconstr Surg. 2015;135(3):491e–7e.
13. Hembd AS, Yan J, Zhu H, Haddock NT, Teotia SS. Intraoperative assessment of DIEP flap breast reconstruction using indocyanine green angiography: reduction of fat necrosis, resection volumes, and postoperative surveillance. Plast Reconstr Surg. 2020;146(1):1e–10e.
14. Chatterjee A, Krishnan NM, Van Vliet MM, Powell SG, Rosen JM, Ridgway EB. A comparison of free autologous breast reconstruction with and without the use of laser-assisted indocyanine green angiography: a cost-effectiveness analysis. Plast Reconstr Surg. 2013;131(5):693e–701e.

15. Yamamoto T, Iida T, Yoshimatsu H, Fuse Y, Hayashi A, Yamamoto N. Lymph flow restoration after tissue replantation and transfer: importance of lymph axiality and possibility of lymph flow reconstruction without lymph node transfer or lymphatic anastomosis. Plast Reconstr Surg. 2018;142(3):796–804.
16. DiSipio T, Rye S, Newman B, Hayes S. Incidence of unilateral arm lymphoedema after breast cancer: a systematic review and meta-analysis. Lancet Oncol. 2013;14(6):500–15.
17. International Society of Lymphology. The diagnosis and treatment of peripheral lymphedema: 2013 consensus document of the International Society of Lymphology. Lymphology. 2013;46(1):1–11.
18. Patel KM, Lin C-Y, Cheng M-H. A prospective evaluation of lymphedema-specific quality-of-life outcomes following vascularized lymph node transfer. Ann Surg Oncol. 2015;22(7):2424–30.
19. Yamamoto T, Yamamoto N, Yoshimatsu H, Narushima M, Koshima I. Factors associated with lymphosclerosis: an analysis on 962 lymphatic vessels. Plast Reconstr Surg. 2017;140:734–41.
20. Pandey SK, Fahradyan V, Orfahli LM, Chen WF. Plastic and Aesthetic Research Supermicrosurgical lymphaticovenular anastomosis vs. vascularized lymph vessel transplant-technical optimization and when to perform which. Plast Aesthet Res. 2021;8:47. https://doi.org/10.20517/2347-9264.2021.61.
21. Spy Elite SNTUC. Product information.

Use of Fluorescence Guidance in Plastic and Reconstructive Surgery: Skin and Muscle Flaps

9

Zachary A. Koenig, Cristiane M. Ueno, Jack J. Gelman, and Kerri Woodberry

Introduction

Fluorescence angiography using indocyanine green is a valuable tool to assess flap viability, both for skin flaps and muscle flaps. Image-guided surgery is a technique that uses optical imaging to assess tissues during reconstructive surgery in plastic surgery. Examples of these technologies include indocyanine green (ICG) angiography, dynamic infrared thermography (DIRT), and photo-spectrometry. One of the most common methods involves the use of near-infrared (NIR) fluorescence imaging that requires an injection of a fluorescent dye that can be captured using NIR cameras. ICG is the most used dye, and it has multiple indications including utilization to identify tissue perfusion, vessels, nerves, and lymphatic drainage.

Z. A. Koenig · J. J. Gelman · K. Woodberry
Department of Surgery, Division of Plastic and Reconstructive Surgery, West Virginia University School of Medicine, Morgantown, WV, USA

C. M. Ueno (✉)
Department of Plastic and Reconstructive Surgery, Ohio State University College of Medicine, Columbus, OH, USA

N. Szoka et al. (eds.), *The SAGES Manual of Fluorescence-Guided Surgery*, https://doi.org/10.1007/978-3-031-40685-0_9

The use of image-guided technologies such as ICG angiography allows detection of areas of poor or no blood perfusion that is often not clearly visible to the human eye. Its applications have been described in evaluation of orthopedic, trauma, military, and vascular injuries as well as plastic surgery reconstructions. Traditionally, clinical judgment has been one of the most acceptable parameters to determine tissue viability. Other methods of assessment include subjective assessment of skin or tissue color, capillary refill, flap temperature, tissue bleeding, prick tests, Doppler ultrasound, and use of tactile sensation. The use of ICG angiography allows an objective measure of perfusion and tissue viability.

Images provided by NIR cameras can provide real-time information in the operating room which is an advantage for surgical planning. For example, fluorescence angiography can be used for identification of lymphatic vessels in lymphatic anastomosis, identification of lymph nodes during lymph node dissection, evaluation of patency of a vessel anastomosis, or evaluation of tissue perfusion.

According to Burns et al. (level of evidence 3), the use of NIR technologies intraoperatively has the potential to provide data that can improve intraoperative decisions about flap design with subsequent better outcomes [1]. In another study group (level of evidence 3), authors compared three technologies and their capability to "predict" tissue perfusion. Their findings showed that the intraoperative sensitivity for ICG angiography was 90.9% (95% CI: 77.5–100) with an accuracy of 98.6% (95% CI: 97.6–99.7), sensitivity for DIRT was 33% (95% CI: 11.3–64.6) with specificity of 100% (95% CI 84.9–100) and accuracy of 80% (95% CI: 71.2–89.7), and sensitivity for photo-spectrometry was 92% (95% CI: 72.4–98.6) with specificity of 100% (95% CI: 98.8–100) and accuracy of 100% (95% CI: 98.7–100) [2].

The advantages of ICG are its short half-life (3–4 min in healthy adults) which allows multiple runs in one single surgery without exceeding the maximum dosage, its efficacy in predicting clinical outcomes for partial or total tissue necrosis, and its evaluation of maximal size of a flap with delineation between the zones of poor and no perfusion [3], (level of evidence 4). The adverse reactions reported from ICG are uncommon and occur in 0.34% of patients, based on a study by Obana et al. with mild reactions of nausea, skin rash, and itchiness, and with very rare instances of anaphylactic shock (level of evidence 5) [1, 4].

Plastic surgery has benefited from systemic ICG perfusion angiography use in many aspects. One of its classic uses is for evaluation of tissue perfusion in pedicled flaps, free flaps, and perforator flaps. Holm et al. (level of evidence 2) described a first-time use of intraoperative ICG imaging in free flap tissue perfusion [1]. Patients were prospectively evaluated with ICG angiography performed intraoperatively after flap inset. Postoperatively, monitoring was done exclusively by clinical means without the use of ICG. The authors found 2/10 (20%) of complications with one partial and one total flap loss that had been detected intraoperatively by ICG imaging. The study was able to show cases of arterial spasms, venous congestion, and tissue hypoperfusion with intraoperative ICG imaging [5]. These findings are supported by other studies (level of evidence 4) investigating the use of ICG angiography in free flap operations [3, 6, 7]. However, since then, other aspects of plastic surgery have also benefited from use of ICG perfusion angiography guidance.

Indications: Use in Extremity Reconstruction

The use of NIR technologies in extremities, specially by consulting services in anticipation of tissue coverage, allows better coordination of care and preservation of tissue with subsequent improvement of post-reconstruction function (Figs. 9.1, 9.2, 9.3, and 9.4).

Dietz et al. (level of evidence 5) described the utilization of SPY-Q system technology to determine tissue viability in trauma allowing for more thoughtful debridement, especially in orthopedic surgery, when preservation of certain tissues may signify functional preservation [1, 8]. Moreover, it allows evaluation of levels of amputation and perfusion of avulsed tissues and vessels in trauma.

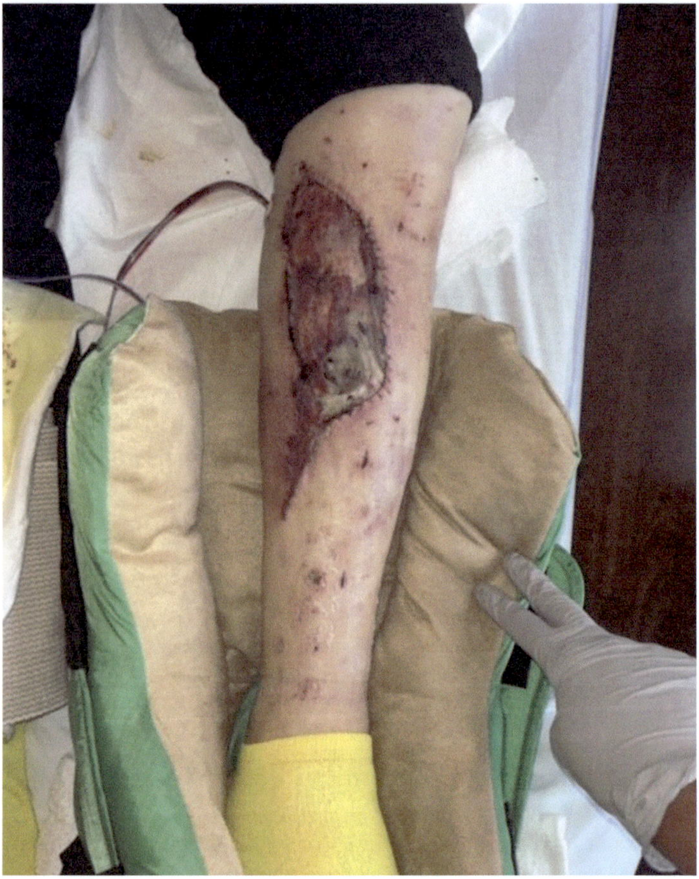

Fig. 9.1 Preoperative defect with concern for poor perfusion

As described by Green et al. (level of evidence 4), the use of SPY-Q system technology minimizes perfusion-related complications by allowing intraoperative modifications and revisions that will decrease poor tissue perfusion [1, 9]. Fluorescence angiography allows intraoperative modifications, such as excision of distal flap segments with poor perfusion, angiosome or perfisome mapping (which is especially useful in random flaps and propeller

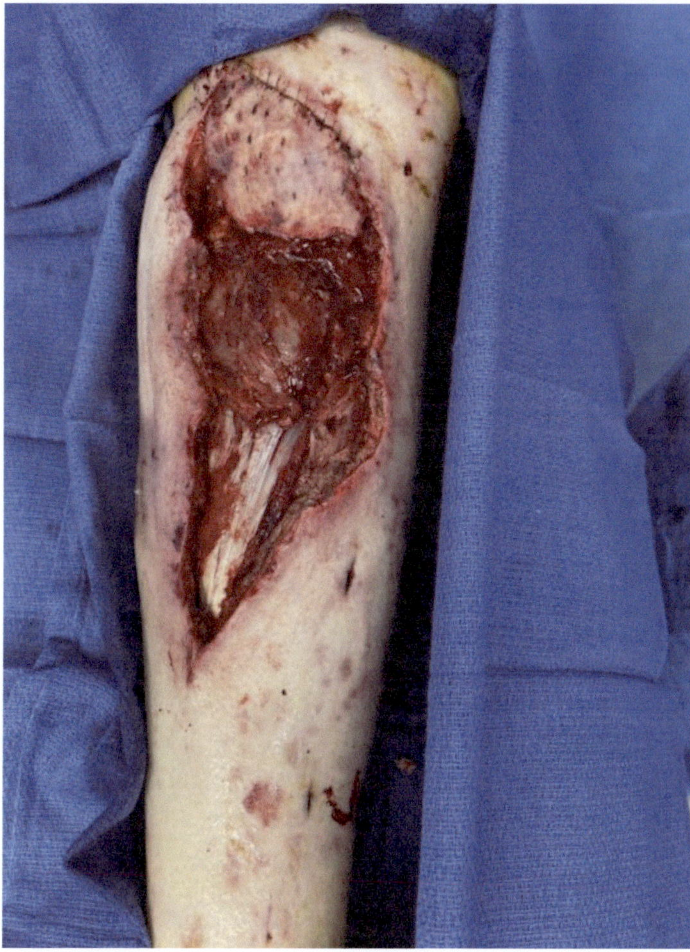

Fig. 9.2 Exposure of the underlying defect

flaps), flap inset modifications to salvage reconstruction, release of sutures during closure if the tissue is noted to be ischemic or under excess tension, and evaluation of free flap anastomosis as described by Lohman et al. These intraoperative adjustments improve reconstructive outcomes.

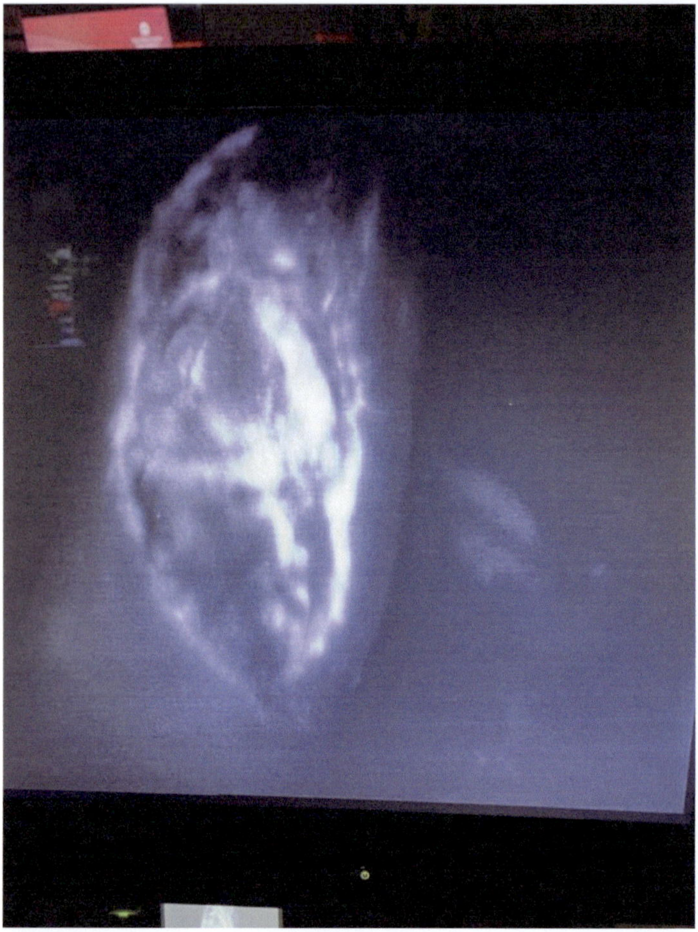

Fig. 9.3 Fluorescence angiography to identify flap regions of poor perfusion

The described decisions can be crucial in designing axial pattern flaps or pedicled flaps. These flaps, unlike free flaps, can be a challenge in extremity reconstruction due to the limited amount of available tissue, limited reach, and the need for advancement of tissue without potentially sacrificing tissue perfusion. The use of intraoperative ICG assists with tissue mapping during harvest of the flap, insetting of the flap, and the decision to delay a flap or add a second flap.

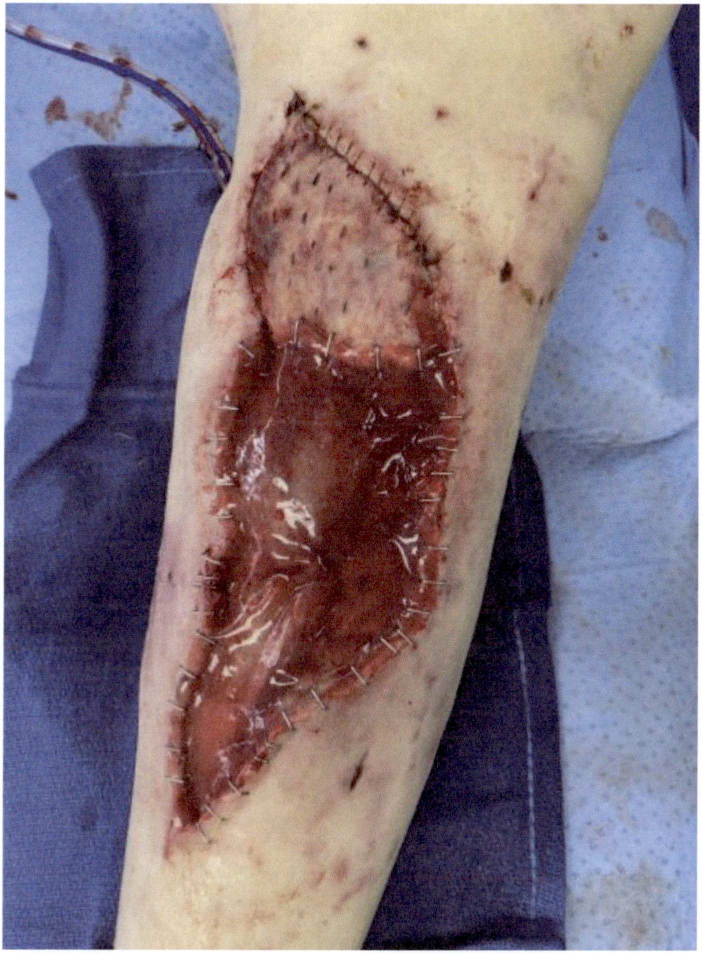

Fig. 9.4 Debridement of devitalized tissue and coverage with a skin substitute

Indications: Use in Skin Flaps

Skin flaps are utilized in plastic surgery as a primary method of reconstruction for soft tissue defects and coverage of wounds. There are many types of skin flaps based primarily on the tissue included in the flap or based on the source of blood supply to the flap.

Skin flaps may include the skin, subcutaneous fat, fascia, tendon, muscle, nerves, and bones. Flaps are often named based on the contents of the flap, such as skin flap (skin and subcutaneous tissue), fasciocutaneous flap (skin, subcutaneous fat, and fascia), myocutaneous flap (skin, subcutaneous fat, fascia, and muscle), or osteocutaneous flap (skin, subcutaneous fat, and bone). Flaps are sometimes described based on the pattern of movement of the tissue, specifically whether the tissue is rotated, advanced, or transposed to cover the defect. In addition, flaps can be described based on the pattern and source of blood supply to the flap. Random pattern flaps are based on blood supply through the subdermal plexus and do not have a named blood vessel supplying the flap, such as in axial patterned flaps. Flaps can be used to cover defects locally, regionally, and in distant locations or used as free flaps anywhere in the body.

One of the major challenges with skin flaps is maintaining adequate perfusion to tissue to ensure viability. There have been many methods to assess skin flaps, which includes axial pattern flaps and pedicled flaps, as described earlier. The use of indocyanine green has been a major asset to the armamentarium of tools used preoperatively, intraoperatively, and postoperatively to design and evaluate skin flaps. Random pattern flaps are designed based on length to width ratios typically of 2:1, and axial patterned flaps are based on known anatomical regions of perfusions surrounding the named vessels. Although several factors contribute to complications of flap healing such as nicotine, obesity, diabetes, radiation, and vascular insufficiency, fluorescence angiography allows us to assess real-time perfusion of flaps as we aim to limit tissue necrosis and improve tissue survivability and, therefore, improve outcomes.

The use of fluorescence angiography for evaluation of skin flaps in breast reconstruction has been discussed in another chapter. However, fluorescence angiography is also utilized for the evaluation of skin flaps of the head and neck, trunk, and extremities. Laser-induced fluorescence of ICG has been used by several studies to evaluate skin viability in skin flaps. Graham et al. laid the framework for use of fluorescein as an injectable marker in rats to assess random flap perfusion [10]. The first human study using ICG angiography for evaluation of pedicled skin flap perfusion was done by Still et al. (level of evidence 3), and this showed promising results in that wound healing was accurately predicted by ICG angiography [1, 11]. Another prospective study by Holm et al. (level of evidence 3) corroborated these findings by suggesting that ICG angiography is a sensitive tool for assessing nutritive blood flow in pedicled skin flaps with and without an axial vessel [1, 5]. Other studies support the findings listed above for use of fluorescence angiography in pedicled skin flaps (levels of evidence 3–5) [1, 12–14].

Indications: Use in Abdominoplasty and Panniculectomy

Abdominoplasty and panniculectomy are two common operations performed by plastic surgeons for functional and cosmetic improvements particularly in patients with excess skin. One complication of any abdominal procedure is delayed wound healing caused by poor circulation to the skin. Complications like wound dehiscence, skin necrosis, and wound infection can be related to decreased perfusion of the skin flap and are inherent to these surgical procedures secondary to undermining of large skin flaps. When compounded with underlying patient comorbidities which affect the microcirculation, the likelihood of poor perfusion to localized areas of the skin during wound healing increases exponentially. As adequate tissue perfusion is crucial for normal wound healing, a better understanding of abdominal skin perfusion after these procedures may contribute to reducing wound healing problems (Figs. 9.5, 9.6, 9.7, and 9.8).

Standard abdominoplasty and panniculectomy can have a significant impact on abdominal skin perfusion. Nergård et al. (level of evidence 2) were the first to quantify abdominal skin perfusion following abdominoplasty using DIRT where they identified the least perfusion occurring at Hager zone II near the lower transverse incision line [1, 15]. Patel et al. (level of evi-

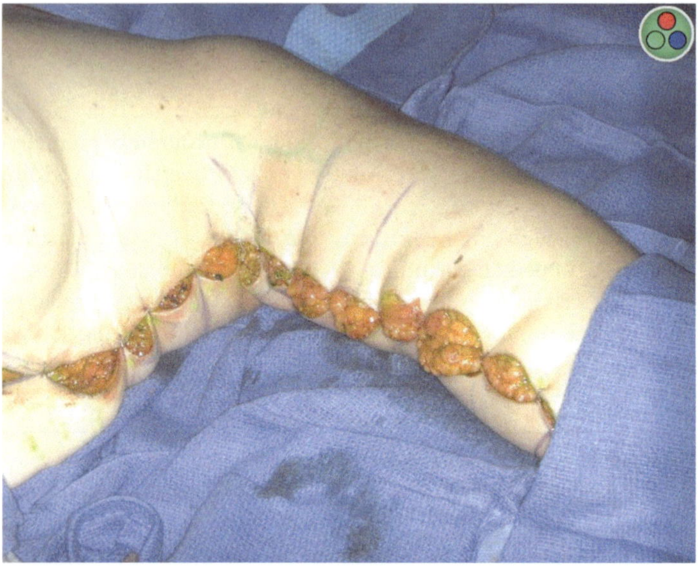

Fig. 9.5 Intraoperative angiography used during brachioplasty

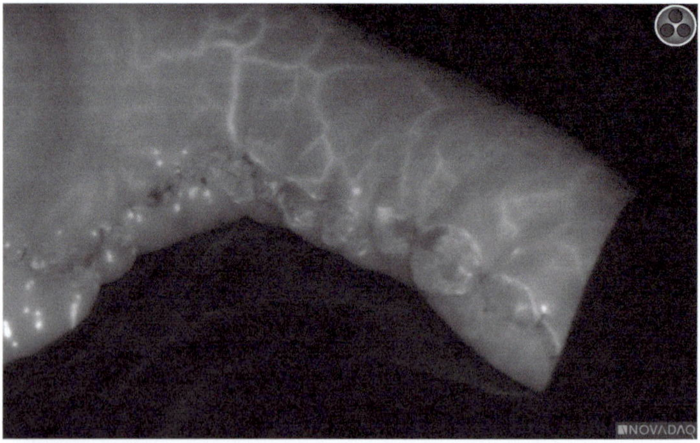

Fig. 9.6 Intraoperative angiography used during brachioplasty

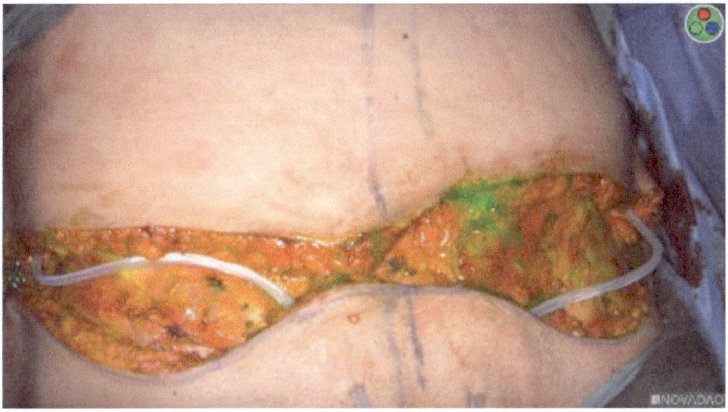

Fig. 9.7 Intraoperative image of panniculectomy, indocyanine green visible in overlay mode

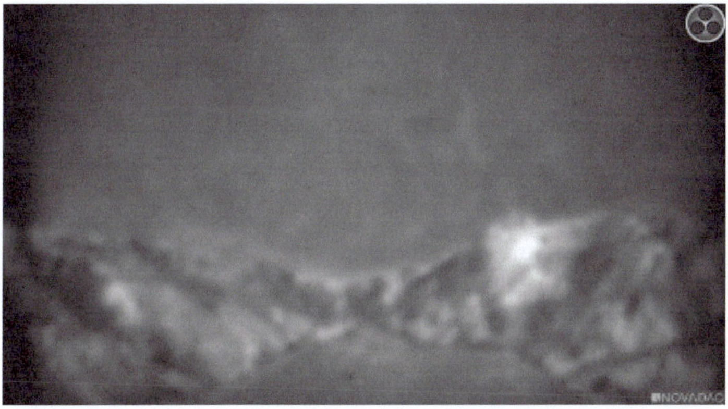

Fig. 9.8 Intraoperative angiography shows excellent perfusion of flaps in fluorescence mode

dence 4) showed that ICG angiography can accurately detect perfusion abnormalities to decrease wound healing complications in patients undergoing complex hernia repair with concomitant panniculectomy [1, 16]. Numerous other studies support the use of ICG angiography to identify perfusion abnormalities in patients with risk factors such as obesity, current tobacco use, prior wound infection, and hypertension (levels of evidence 2–5) [1, 17–19].

Technique

In our institution, we use indocyanine green (ICG) to assess tissue perfusion. ICG is a water-soluble dye that binds to plasma proteins in the blood or tissue and emits an energy in the NIR spectrum of 750–810 nm. It has been utilized for evaluation of retinal angiography, cardiovascular function, and hepatic clearance for over 50 years [8, 20]. The use of NIR fluorescence is well-known and reproducible and provides good diagnostic accuracy. It can be used with a handheld camera or a microscope. ICG can be injected systemically (angiography) when looking for flap, composite graft, or bone perfusion, or subcutaneously when looking for lymph nodes or lymphatic perfusion. When utilized systemically, the administered dose range is 0.025 to 0.50 mg/kg and 0.03 to 0.25 mg/kg when injected subcutaneously [21] (level of evidence 3). There are some differences in dosages depending on indications and surgeon's habits. As an example, for sentinel node mapping, the dosage is 25 mg ICG diluted in 5 ml of distilled water with doses of 0.4 to 1.2 ml; lymphography for lymphedema evaluation is usually 0.1 to 0.3 ml and for evaluation of tissue perfusion, the dose is 5 mg or 0.5 mg/kg [22], (level of evidence 4).

There are many laser-assisted fluorescence angiography cameras, and one of the most common NIR fluorescence tools utilizing ICG is performed with SPY-Q imaging analysis software. SPY-Q system is an analytical software that provides quantifiable data that can be used preoperatively, intraoperatively, or postoperatively. ICG can show perfusion in tissue to a depth of 1–1.5 cm. In general, a dose of 7.5 mg (ICG concentration 2.5 mg/ml) is administered systemically, and the area of interest is visualized directly with the use of a handheld camera and a screen with capability of video recording.

The images provided by SPY-Q system can be analyzed with two techniques:

- Relative percentage provides information about the fluorescence of a selected area relative to a pre-selected reference point that represents an ideal perfusion of 100%. In general, a percentage of 15–20% or less indicates poor perfusion which indicates higher chance of tissue necrosis.
- Absolute measurement utilizing a 255-level grayscale system which depends on signal intensity. The level reported ranges from 0 to 255 with a higher level indicating higher perfusion and a lower level (generally 6.0) indicating lower perfusion.

With the use of optical technologies such as ICG angiography, there has been significant improvement in the capacity of:

- Preoperative planning by identifying tissue viability (e.g., perfusion during debridement of bone, muscle perfusion before and during reconstruction)
- Intraoperative reconstruction by optimizing flap design
- Postoperative evaluation of areas of poor flap perfusion and anticipation of possible areas of subsequent tissue necrosis

Timing of Dye Administration: Preoperative Considerations

Methylene blue and lymphazurin blue will interfere with imaging. Likewise, vasoconstrictors such as epinephrine will decrease blood flow and interfere with imaging. A delay of at least 2 h after administration of epinephrine is required before imaging [23], (level of evidence 5). Factors associated with ischemia include previous surgery, previous radiation treatment, current smoking, obesity, diabetes, vasculopathy, chronic steroid use, and thin flaps [24, 25].

Timing of Dye Administration: Intraoperative Considerations

The intraoperative use of image-guided technologies such as ICG angiography at the time of flap design, flap elevation, flap inset, and final closure allows for intraoperative modifications such as angiosome mapping (especially useful in random, propeller flaps), excision of distal flap segments with poor perfusion, flap inset modifications (ischemic incision closures, especially in closures under tension, or in cases of a skin/tissue bridge), or evaluation of free flap anastomoses, which will all allow for improvement in reconstructive surgeries.

In our institution, we have been using both SPY-PHI and SPY-Elite fluorescence imaging systems by Stryker/LifeCell. SPY-PHI refers to the "Portable Handheld Imager." The imaging head is positioned prior to the anesthesiologist giving the ICG. The ICG (25 mg) is reconstituted with 10 ml of sterile water. This yields a 2.5 mg/ml solution of ICG. For plastic, reconstructive, and microsurgery cases, the volume of ICG for images which are acquired through the patient's skin is 3–4 ml [7]. ICG is administered through a peripheral IV and flushed with 10 ml of saline immediately prior to imaging. It is often given prior to closing in order to assess skin perfusion. It can also be utilized preoperatively during flap design, intraoperatively to assess flap perfusion prior to insetting, and after completion of surgery. We will sometimes use fluorescence angiography two or three times during the operation. Recordings are performed according to the owner's manual for SPY-PHI or SPY-Elite [24, 25].

Timing of Dye Administration: Postoperative Considerations

In addition to the described traditional methods for evaluation of tissue perfusion (physical examination, Doppler ultrasound, tactile feedback), technologies such as the SPY-Q system can provide objective data of tissue perfusion and vascular anastomosis patency (such as use to evaluate venous thrombosis at the anastomosis) and even allow evaluation of neovascularization of a flap to determine if a pedicled flap is ready for division and insetting [26], (level of evidence 4).

Our institutional experience and literature review shows that the use of ICG fluorescence angiography allows early detection of tissue with compromised vascularity and minimizes the risks of postoperative partial or total necrosis, which can lead to further surgeries, surgical revisions, poor outcomes, and increased morbidity.

Documentation and Medical Coding

Appropriate coding and documentation are essential for reimbursement for fluorescence angiography. The American Medical Association Current Professional Terminology (CPT) Professional Codebook 2022 lists 15,860 as the appropriate code. CPT code 15860 is defined as "intravenous injection of agent (e.g., fluorescein) to test vascular flow in flap or graft." In this case, the agent is ICG. There are no additional codes for the intraoperative laser angiography. CPT codes 99,240 and 99,242 refer to ICG angiography specifically for ophthalmology and are not appropriate for flaps elsewhere on the body [27].

According to the 2022 National Physician Fee Schedule Relative Value File, CPT code 15860 has a corresponding work relative value unit (RVU) of 1.95 and a facility total RVU of 3.14 [28]. To best ensure reimbursement, copies of intraoperative angiography images must be retained and placed in the patient's medical record.

Conclusion

The use of image-guided surgery such as SPY-Q system in extremity reconstruction, not only by plastic surgeons but also by surgeons in associated departments such as orthopedic surgery, general surgery, trauma surgery, vascular surgery, and otolaryngology, allows improvement in tissue salvage through reliable debridement, improvement in function, and better treatment planning. Such technologies are useful in all settings (preoperatively, intraoperatively, and postoperatively) and help facilitate decisions of flap design, flap assessment, and early detection of potential tissue necrosis, decreasing additional surgeries and morbidity.

Overall, the use of fluorescence angiography reduces complications and improves outcomes [29].

References

1. Burns PB, Rohrich RJ, Chung KC. The levels of evidence and their role in evidence-based medicine. Plast Reconstr Surg. 2011;128(1):305–10. https://doi.org/10.1097/PRS.0b013e318219c171.
2. Lohman RF, Ozturk CN, Ozturk C, Jayaprakash V, Djohan R. An analysis of current techniques used for intraoperative flap evaluation. Ann Plast Surg. 2015;75(6):679–85. https://doi.org/10.1097/SAP.0000000000000235.
3. Ludolph I, Horch RE, Arkudas A, Schmitz M. Enhancing safety in reconstructive microsurgery using intraoperative indocyanine green angiography. Front Surg. 2019;6:39. https://doi.org/10.3389/fsurg.2019.00039.
4. Obana A, Miki T, Hayashi K, et al. Survey of complications of indocyanine green angiography in Japan. Am J Ophthalmol. 1994;118(6):749–53. https://doi.org/10.1016/s0002-9394(14)72554-1.
5. Holm C, Tegeler J, Mayr M, Becker A, Pfeiffer UJ, Mühlbauer W. Monitoring free flaps using laser-induced fluorescence of indocyanine green: a preliminary experience. Microsurgery. 2002;22(7):278–87. https://doi.org/10.1002/micr.10052.
6. Hitier M, Cracowski JL, Hamou C, Righini C, Bettega G. Indocyanine green fluorescence angiography for free flap monitoring: a pilot study. J Craniomaxillofac Surg. 2016;44(11):1833–41. https://doi.org/10.1016/j.jcms.2016.09.001.
7. Mothes H, Dönicke T, Friedel R, Simon M, Markgraf E, Bach O. Indocyanine-green fluorescence video angiography used clinically to evaluate tissue perfusion in microsurgery. J Trauma. 2004;57(5):1018–24. https://doi.org/10.1097/01.ta.0000123041.47008.70.
8. Dietz MJ, Hare JT, Ueno C, Prud'homme BJ, Boyd JW. Laser-assisted fluorescent angiography to assess tissue perfusion in the setting of traumatic elbow dislocation. Wounds Compend Clin Res Pract. 2018;30(10):E93–7.
9. Green JM, Sabino J, Fleming M, Valerio I. Intraoperative plastic and reconstructive surgery: a review of applications and outcomes in war-related trauma. Mil Med. 2015;180(3 Suppl):37–43. https://doi.org/10.7205/MILMED-D-14-00632.
10. Graham BH, Walton RL, Elings VB, Lewis FR. Surface quantification of injected fluorescein as a predictor of flap viability. Plast Reconstr Surg. 1983;71(6):826–33. https://doi.org/10.1097/00006534-198306000-00016.
11. Still J, Law E, Dawson J, Bracci S, Island T, Holtz J. Evaluation of the circulation of reconstructive flaps using laser-induced fluorescence of

indocyanine green. Ann Plast Surg. 1999;42(3):266–74. https://doi.org/10.1097/00000637-199903000-00007.
12. Holzbach T, Taskov C, Henke J, et al. Evaluation of perfusion in skin flaps by laser-induced indocyanine green fluorescence. Handchir Mikrochir Plast Chir. 2005;37(6):396–402. https://doi.org/10.1055/s-2005-872986.
13. Krishnan KG, Schackert G, Steinmeier R. The role of near-infrared angiography in the assessment of post-operative venous congestion in random pattern, pedicled Island and free flaps. Br J Plast Surg. 2005;58(3):330–8. https://doi.org/10.1016/j.bjps.2004.10.003.
14. Yano T, Okazaki M, Tanaka K, Tsunoda A, Aoyagi M, Kishimoto S. Use of intraoperative fluorescent indocyanine green angiography for real-time vascular evaluation of pericranial flaps. Ann Plast Surg. 2016;76(2):198–204. https://doi.org/10.1097/SAP.0000000000000519.
15. Nergård S, Mercer JB, de Weerd L. Impact on abdominal skin perfusion following abdominoplasty. Plast Reconstr Surg Glob Open. 2021;9(1):e3343. https://doi.org/10.1097/GOX.0000000000003343.
16. Patel KM, Bhanot P, Franklin B, Albino F, Nahabedian MY. Use of intraoperative indocyanin-green angiography to minimize wound healing complications in abdominal wall reconstruction. J Plast Surg Hand Surg. 2013;47(6):476–80. https://doi.org/10.3109/2000656X.2013.787085.
17. Swanson E. Comparison of limited and full dissection abdominoplasty using laser fluorescence imaging to evaluate perfusion of the abdominal skin. Plast Reconstr Surg. 2015;136(1):31e–43e. https://doi.org/10.1097/PRS.0000000000001376.
18. Mayr M, Holm C, Höfter E, Becker A, Pfeiffer U, Mühlbauer W. Effects of aesthetic abdominoplasty on abdominal wall perfusion: a quantitative evaluation. Plast Reconstr Surg. 2004;114(6):1586–94. https://doi.org/10.1097/01.prs.0000138757.33998.ee.
19. Colavita PD, Wormer BA, Belyansky I, et al. Intraoperative indocyanine green fluorescence angiography to predict wound complications in complex ventral hernia repair. Hernia. 2016;20(1):139–49. https://doi.org/10.1007/s10029-015-1411-4.
20. Burnier P, Niddam J, Bosc R, Hersant B, Meningaud JP. Indocyanine green applications in plastic surgery: a review of the literature. J Plast Reconstr Aesthetic Surg. 2017;70(6):814–27. https://doi.org/10.1016/j.bjps.2017.01.020.
21. Cornelissen AJM, van Mulken TJM, Graupner C, et al. Near-infrared fluorescence image-guidance in plastic surgery: a systematic review. Eur J Plast Surg. 2018;41(3):269–78. https://doi.org/10.1007/s00238-018-1404-5.
22. Holm C, Mayr M, Höfter E, Becker A, Pfeiffer UJ, Mühlbauer W. Intraoperative evaluation of skin-flap viability using laser-induced fluorescence of indocyanine green. Br J Plast Surg. 2002;55(8):635–44. https://doi.org/10.1054/bjps.2002.3969.

23. Gurtner GC, Jones GE, Neligan PC, et al. Intraoperative laser angiography using the SPY system: review of the literature and recommendations for use. Ann Surg Innov Res. 2013;7:1. https://doi.org/10.1186/1750-1164-7-1.
24. SPY Elite imaging system (Lifecell) operator's manual. Stryker. 2013. https://www.stryker.com/us/en/endoscopy/products/spy-elite.html. Accessed 16 Feb 2022.
25. SPY Portable Hand Imaging System (PHI) operator's manual. Stryker. 2019. https://www.stryker.com/us/en/endoscopy/products/spy-phi.html. Accessed 16 Feb 2022.
26. Mandelbaum M, Lakhiani C, Lenert JJ. Is 21 days too short? Utility of indocyanine green angiography in predicting successful cross-leg flap division in the compromised lower extremity. Plast Reconstr Surg. 2021;147(5):919e–20e.https://doi.org/10.1097/PRS.0000000000007872.
27. CPT Professional 2022. American Medical Association (AMA); 2021.
28. 2022 National Physician Fee Schedule Relative Value File. Centers for Medicare and Medicaid Services. 2021. https://www.cms.gov/medicaremedicare-fee-service-paymentphysicianfeeschedpfs-relative-value-files/rvu22a. Accessed 16 Feb 2022.
29. Liu DZ, Mathes DW, Zenn MR, Neligan PC. The application of indocyanine green fluorescence angiography in plastic surgery. J Reconstr Microsurg. 2011;27(6):355–64. https://doi.org/10.1055/s-0031-1281515.

10 Use of Fluorescence Guidance in Burn Surgery

Apinut Wongkietkachorn, Palakorn Surakunprapha, Supawich Wongkietkachorn, Sarinya Boonpoapichart, and Phachara Longmeewong

Introduction

Burn injuries are a significant global public health issue because of their high frequency and potentially severe physical, emotional, and economical effects on people, households, and communities [1, 2]. Burns from fire, heat, and hot substances rank fourth among all civilian traumatic injuries in the globe, after falls, traffic accidents, and interpersonal violence [2]. According to the estimation, there are between 7 and 12 million people (up to 33,000 every

Supplementary Information The online version contains supplementary material available at https://doi.org/10.1007/978-3-031-40685-0_10.

A. Wongkietkachorn (✉)
Division of Plastic and Reconstructive Surgery, Department of Surgery, Faculty of Medicine, Mae Fah Luang University, Chiang Rai, Thailand

P. Surakunprapha · S. Boonpoapichart · P. Longmeewong
Division of Plastic and Reconstructive Surgery, Department of Surgery, Faculty of Medicine, Khon Kaen University, Khon Kaen, Thailand
e-mail: palsur@kku.ac.th; L_phachara@kkumail.com

S. Wongkietkachorn
Department of Surgery, Police General Hospital, Bangkok, Thailand

N. Szoka et al. (eds.), *The SAGES Manual of Fluorescence-Guided Surgery*, https://doi.org/10.1007/978-3-031-40685-0_10

day) suffering each year from burn injuries that necessitate medical attention, cause extended absences from work or school, or even result in death [3]. In contrast, the incidence of burn injuries is higher than the combined incidence of tuberculosis and human immunodeficiency virus (HIV/AIDS), and it is close to the incidence of all malignant neoplasms [4].

Burns result in high morbidity and cost [5]. Nonfatal burns are the main cause of morbidity, which includes extended hospital stays, disfigurement, and disability, frequently with associated rejection and social stigmata [2]. According to a recent study, burn injuries have an impact on morbidity and mortality for at least 5 to 10 years following the injury [5]. The overall cost of hospital care per patient ranged from US$ 10.58 to US$ 125,597.86 [6]. The cost of 1% of total body surface area burned varied from US$ 2.65 to US$ 11,245.04, and the cost of hospital care per day varied from US$ 24.23 to US$ 4125.50 [6].

This chapter will discuss on the knowledge of burn wound evaluation, various methods of burn determination, the limitation of burn depth determination, and a thorough review of the development, fundamentals, and evidence base for using ICGA precise marking for burn wound evaluation and excision in clinical practice.

Pathophysiology of Burn Wounds

Burn wounds result from accidental injury to the human body by various etiologies such as heat, electricity, friction, chemicals, or radiation [7]. Thermal injury is reported to be the most common [8]. The extent of thermal injury correlates with the contact time, temperature, and skin thickness of the damaged area [9]. Thermal burns can be produced by flames, hot objects, liquids, and steam [10].

The pathophysiology of burns can be classified into two levels: local changes and systemic changes [7]. Local tissues are damaged when the tissue came into contact with the thermal source resulting in heat transfer. This induces coagulative necrosis, intraepidermal separation, or dermoepidermal separation [11]. Burns lead to systemic changes when the injury reaches approximately 20% of total body surface area (TBSA) [12]. The consequences are significant hypovolemia and the release of numerous inflammatory mediators resulting in a cardiovascular insufficiency known as burn shock [12, 13]. Burn shock is a complicated circulatory and microcirculatory failure process that causes generalized edema in both injured and uninjured body parts. Although the patient is appropriately resuscitated, the burn shock remains irreversible in some severe cases.

Burn wounds are categorized based on the depth of tissue injury, which determines the burn management to be either conservative or operative. Burn depth is classified into four categories: epidermal, superficial partial-thickness, deep partial-thickness, and full-thickness skin loss [14, 15]. Epidermal burns involve only the epidermis. The typical etiology is sunburn. The wounds appear erythematous, painful, and blanch with pressure. Superficial partial-thickness burns affect the superficial part of the dermis, with scald burn being the most frequent etiology. These wounds are erythematous and tender, and blisters can appear up to 24 h after the injury. Deep partial-thickness burns involve the deep part of the dermis, where hair follicles and glandular tissue are located. This kind of burn wound is not painful unless the burn area is pressured with significant force. These wounds contain variously mottled colorization from patchy white to red, and they were not blanched with the pressure. Finally, full-thickness burns, the deepest degree, involve the epidermis and all layers of the dermis. A diverse wound color can be observed, such as waxy white, leathery gray, charred, and dark black. The wound is dry, inelastic, and painless. It does not blanched with pressure.

There are several factors affecting the treatment of burn wounds. Inflammatory and anti-inflammatory medications can disturb the healing process [16, 17]. Inflammation is the early phase of wound healing. When the inflammatory mediators are released, they stimulate immune signals, causing the engagement of leukocytes and macrophages, which primarily start the proliferation phase of inflammation [16]. These cytokines from the inflammatory process activate keratinocytes and fibroblasts to migrate from the hair follicles to the injury area, consequently aiding wound reepithelialization [18]. Thus, inflammation is vital for the success of burn wound healing. Anti-inflammatory treatments can worsen the wound healing mechanism and prolong the healing process [17]. For example, conventional anti-inflammatory therapy, such as nonsteroidal anti-inflammatory drugs or steroids, inhibits prostaglandin synthesis, which inevitably impairs wound healing [19].

Infection can also impair burn wound healing [20]. The skin is a vital organ, which serves as a barrier to protect the external environment, maintain body temperature and homeostasis, provide sensory detection, and provide metabolic and immunological support. Destruction of this vital organ damages the innate immunological response and increases the risk of infection [20]. Therefore, burn patients are certainly at a higher risk of infection [21]. When burn patients are hospitalized long enough to get infected by drug-resistant organisms, the infection process prolongs the hospital stay, delays the wound healing, increases hospital cost, and increases mortality [22, 23].

Nutrition contributes to proper burn wound healing [24]. Minimizing the consequence of hypermetabolism and supplying adequate nutritional support are the main components that contribute to the appropriate wound healing process and recovery [25].

The following health factors can also impact burn severity and the burn recovery process: diabetes, obesity, and geriatric status. Diabetes mellitus significantly affects burn patients [26]. It impairs the body's ability to deal with stress due to glucose-related cell, end-organ, and vascular damage, which deteriorates clinical outcomes in admitted patients [27]. The hyperglycemic state injures the immune cells causing their function to be impaired. This distinctly leads to a greater risk of infection in diabetic patients [28], which is one of the lethal complications in burns [20].

Patients with excessive adiposity can also have altered physiological responses in burns, thus are considered a challenge in burn treatment [29]. Burn patients with obesity usually have multiple comorbidities, including diabetes mellitus, hypertension, cardiovascular disease, and lung disease [29]. Even with a burn assessment tool, for example, the Lund-Browder chart, the body surface area can be misinterpreted due to the deviated body mass distribution in obesity [30].

The elderly population possesses a unique burn characteristic [31]. Most burn events accidentally occur at home, frequently in a kitchen and a bathroom, owing to sluggish alertness, decreased reaction time, and slower mobility [32]. The reduction of metabolism and the fragility of the skin contribute to the increased depth of burn extent, which consistently elevates mortality [33].

Burn Wound Assessment

The following is a review of current modalities available to assess burn wound depth. There are various techniques starting from simple clinical assessment and tissue biopsy to more advanced modalities such as thermography, ultrasound, laser Doppler imaging, and ICGA [34].

Clinical Assessment

Clinical assessment is easy, simple, and inexpensive; however, its accuracy has significant limitations [35]. The principle of this method mainly depends on a subjective evaluation of wound characteristics such as wound surface, capillary refill, and pain sensitivity [36]. Therefore, it is possible to differentiate between very deep and very shallow burns with decent reliability [35]. However, the clinical assessment is significantly less accurate for burns with intermediate depth, which was equal to 50–75%, even though this was performed by burn experts [37–40]. Moreover, the validity of the clinical assessment was noted to be unreliable [35]. Clinical evaluation of burn depth based on appearance can vary between surgeons [41]. The significant factors of this variation depend on differences in surgeon experience as well as the evolution of tissue damage that occurs in the hours following burn injury [42, 43]. For this reason, a more accurate burn depth assessment method is essential to aid burn depth evaluation.

Pathological Study

Although pathologic evaluation of burn tissue is considered the gold standard to clarify the depth of burn wounds, it is an invasive and time-consuming method [34, 35]. Punch biopsy has to be performed on the indeterminate burn area and sent for tissue fixation with hematoxylin and eosin staining, which is later reported by the pathologist [44]. The burn depth interpretation is identified by the level of destruction and denaturation of cellular structures damaged by burns [44]. Five factors are generally described to clarify the depth of burn wounds, including collagen discoloration, intercollagen basophilic material, endothelial cell necrosis, epithelial cell necrosis, and mesenchymal cell necrosis [45]. It is suggested that the microvascular damage indicates a partial-thickness burn, while collagen denaturation indicates a full-thickness burn [46]. Computing the most superficial patent and the deepest blocked vessels can also increase precision [47].

Pathologic tissue study has several great disadvantages. First, it is invasive to obtain a tissue biopsy, which may leave unnecessary scars in the superficial burn and is not practical for clinical application [48]. Second, pathologic assessment represents structural damage of the burn tissue rather than functional loss [44, 49]. Furthermore, burn wounds can deteriorate post biopsy due to their progressive nature [49]. Third, sampling error can occur because the selected biopsy area may not accurately represent the entire burn area [47]. Finally, biopsy interpretation can be subjective and requires an experienced pathologist [44].

Thermography

Thermography measures the temperature in a burn wound to determine its depth [50]. Deep burns yield less heat than the unburned area due to decreased blood flow to the wound surface [51]. The accuracy of thermography has been reported to be as high as 90% [52], but is limited by evaporative heat loss, granulation tissue, and sensitive timing [53]. These drawbacks discourage the use of thermography after 72 h from onset of injury [53].

Ultrasound

Ultrasound has been proven to provide accurate burn assessment [54, 55]. Ultrasound is operated by scanning the burn wound structure to measure the thickness of each layer, which is divided into the epidermis, dermis, and subcutaneous tissue [55]. However, the ultrasound device requires its probe to be contacted with the burn wound during an assessment. This can cause pain to the patient. Hence, its clinical application is also restricted [55, 56].

Laser Doppler Imaging

Laser Doppler imaging (LDI) is a promising burn diagnostic tool with few drawbacks. It is the sole modality approved by the American Food and Drug Administration (FDA) for burn depth evaluation [34]. Its accuracy is very high, approaching 97% with an excellent long-term predictive ability [57]. LDI assesses the tissue perfusion of a burn wound by detecting the red blood cell movement and illustrates the results as two-dimensional photos [58]. The disadvantages include the need for immobilization of the scanned area, a long scanning time (up to 5 min), and a limitation on the depth of penetration [59]. These disadvantages limit the use of LDI. However, ICGA can solve some of these problems.

Indocyanine Green Angiography (ICGA)

ICGA works by detecting vascular perfusion within the wound area [60, 61]. A single 0.5 mg/kg dose of indocyanine green (ICG) is administered intravenously to the patient and will bind to albumin to form a protein complex. Then, the ICGA imaging machine can detect the protein complex through the infrared (840–850 nm) fluorescence emission [62]. Percentage of maximal perfusion was reported and can differentiate between superficial and deep burn wounds [60, 63–65]. The cut point is the value of less than 33% and this number represents an excellent predictive value for nonviable tissue [63]. Thus, an amount of greater than 33% indicates that the burn wound is superficial [38, 63]. The accuracy of ICGA is remarkably better than the clinical evaluation to analyze the indeterminate burn wounds. ICGA has been reported to provide almost 100% accuracy in clarifying the depth indeterminate burn wounds, compared to only 50% accuracy by the clinical assessment [66]. The number needed to treat of using ICGA was only 2 [66].

ICGA is an excellent adjunct for a burn assessment, particularly in critical areas such as the face, palms, and soles [66]. ICGA equipment is commonly an available resource in hospitals because of its various applications in other fields such as neurosurgery, ophthalmology, general surgery, and plastic surgery [66]. Therefore, further use of ICGA in burn wound evaluation can be applicable and cost-effective [66, 67].

Nevertheless, ICGA has a few limitations. First, it requires the intravenous injection of ICG to the patient, which can be considered invasive [66]. Second, a patient who is allergic to iodine or shellfish prohibits the use of ICGA [66, 68]. Third, there can be a possible misinterpretation in unburned skin with intact melanin because melanin can absorb the wavelength detected by ICGA equipment which consequently mislead as a deep burn wound [38, 65, 69]. Thus, ICGA must be used in conjunction with clinical evaluation.

Table 10.1 summarizes the advantages and disadvantages of important modalities of burn assessment.

Use of Indocyanine Green Angiography for Burn Wound Assessment

ICGA works by detecting vascular perfusion within the wound area and has several preferable features for clinical applications compared to other modalities: results are objective and reliable, providing nearly 100% accuracy in the diagnosis of indeterminate burns, compared to only 50% accuracy of the clinical assessment [36, 60, 61, 66]. No tissue biopsy is required in ICGA, which overcomes the weakness of the pathological study [48]. Additionally, the ICGA does not need the probe applied to the

Table 10.1 A summary of the advantages and disadvantages of important modalities of burn assessment

Burn assessment modalities	Method of assessment	Advantages	Disadvantages
1. Clinical assessment	A subjective evaluation of wound characteristics	Easy, simple, commonly used and cheap	Significantly less accurate for burns of intermediate depth
2. Pathological study	Punch biopsy, tissue fixation, and hematoxylin and eosin staining	Gold standard of burn diagnosis	Invasive and time-consuming
3. Thermography	Detection of the difference between temperatures of viable and nonviable tissue	Reported accuracy as high as 90%	Limited by evaporative heat loss, granulation tissue, and sensitive timing
4. Ultrasound	Scan the burn wound structure and measure the thickness of each dermal layer	Good accuracy, noninvasive	Probe contacting to the burn wound, which could cause pain to the patient
5. Laser Doppler imaging	Assessment of tissue perfusion by detecting the red blood cell movement and illustrating results as two-dimensional photos	Reported accuracy as high as 97% with an excellent long-term predicting ability	Requires immobilization of the scanned area, a long scanning time which could take as long as 5 min, and limited depth of penetration
6. Indocyanine green angiography	Detecting vascular perfusion within the wound area	Almost 100% accuracy in diagnosing indeterminate burns	Requires intravenous injection of ICG, contraindicated in patients with iodine allergy

wound, unlike thermography and ultrasound [53, 55, 56]. The patient motion does not affect the working of ICGA which is superior to laser Doppler imaging [59].

ICGA illustrates real-time imaging without the need for immobilization, and its depth of penetration is 2.5 cm which is sufficient for scanning the entire layer of the dermis [70]. Moreover, the number needed to treat of using ICGA is 2 [34]. However, ICGA has some disadvantages, which are the need for ICG intravenous injection, a contraindication with iodine allergy, and a short available period of an assessment (5–10 min after injection). However, allergy of ICGA is reported to be small [68] and 5–10 min is considered adequate for recording the images of the investigated burn area [66].

Quantitative Interpretation of Indocyanine Green Angiography

There was a systematic review reporting the use of ICGA to evaluate burn depth in 2019 [71]. This review described the development of ICGA from animal experiments to human studies which eventually demonstrated it as a promising tool for assessing burn depth [71]. However, the review pointed out that there were two major pitfalls found in these previous trials, which were a lack of quantitative measurement when using ICGA to interpret burn depth and the need for a comparative study focusing on indeterminate burn wounds [71]. Recently, there has been one significant study [66] that can unlock these two significant pitfalls. The study disclosed the quantitative assessment and the cut point primarily in the indeterminate burn wounds [66, 72]. This prospective, multicentered, diagnostic trial showed that the accuracy of ICGA was as high as 100.0%, compared to 50.0% accuracy in clinical evaluation [66]. The study presented a quantitative measuring method using a percentage of maximal perfusion for determining burn depth. Hence, the ICG angiography interpretation was precisely reproducible in the clinical setting [66]. The percentage of maximal perfusion can distinguish a superficial burn from the deep burn [60, 63–65]. As a result, the 33% was the appropriate cut point [66]. The result of less than 33% was reported to have an excellent predictive value for nonviable tissue [63], while the number greater than 33% indicated the burn wound to be superficial [38, 63].

Use of Indocyanine Green Angiography for Burn Excision

During burn excision, a decision whether to excise or not excise the area with indeterminate burn depth can be difficult [73]. Indeterminate burn wounds are defined as burn wounds that cannot be distinguished clinically between the superficial and deep second-degree burns. The accuracy of clinical assessment was reported to be as low as 50–75%, even performed by burn experts [37–40]. In some institutions, these inconclusive wounds are debrided to decrease the morbidity, infection, length of stays, and healthcare cost [73]. However, this management causes the patients to be operated on for unnecessary debridement. Therefore, any adjunct modality that can provide a more precise evaluation of indeterminate burn wounds would be advantageous.

Although there is considerable evidence showing the potency of ICGA for burn wound evaluation, the documentation on how to use ICGA in burn surgery is lacking [71]. There was a recent study that demonstrated how to use ICGA for precise wound marking before burn wound excision [74]. A patient was injected with 0.5 mg/kg of ICG (Diagnogreen Injection; Daiichi Sankyo Propharma, Japan). The Fluobeam 800 clinical system was utilized, and simultaneously the wound was evaluated by the operator.

The 33% criteria, which was previously reported with high accuracy [66], was applied [74]. The superficial second-degree burn appears as a bright area, while the deep second-degree burn appears as a dark area [63, 66]. Unlike other healthy tissue, the superficial burn wounds were hyperemic due to their pathophysiology [75]. Consequently, the percent of maximal perfusion is significantly different between superficial and deep burn wounds, which aids the evaluation of burn wounds [76]. The junction of superficial and deep areas can be marked during the application of ICGA [74]. The ink from markers does not disturb ICGA interpretation [74]. Eventually, the wounds can be debrided appropriately following the marking [74]. The demonstration of the burn wound marking and the clinical outcomes is shown in Video 10.1 [77].

Association of Pathologic Tissue Evaluation, ICG Interpretation, and Clinical Outcomes

There is an association between pathological study, ICGA interpretation criteria, and clinical outcomes. Based on a previous study that compared the pathological study to the ICGA objective criteria [66], five parameters were used to determine pathologic tissue, including collagen discoloration, intercollagen basophilic substance, endothelial cell necrosis, epithelial cell necrosis, and mesenchymal cell necrosis [45]. If these parameters were injured greater than the midpoint of the dermis or deep skin adnexal structures were destroyed, this tissue was considered a deep burn wound and was found to be associated with the maximal perfusion of less than 33% in the ICGA interpretation [44, 45, 47, 61]. On the contrary, if these parameters were injured not greater than the midpoint of the dermis or there was lymphocytic infiltration in the dermis without destroyed deep adnexal structures, this tissue was considered superficial burn wound and was found to be associated with the maximal perfusion of greater than 33% in the ICGA interpreting criteria [44, 45, 47, 61].

The long-term wound outcomes and ICGA interpretation criteria were also investigated and yielded a 95% correction rate [78]. If the wound had less than 33% of maximal perfusion, the wound was found to be unhealed 21 days after the injury; thus, it should be excised [78]. If the wound had greater than 33% of maximal perfusion, it was found to be healed within 21 days after the injury [78].

The summary of the association between pathological study, ICGA interpretation criteria, and clinical outcomes is illustrated in Fig. 10.1.

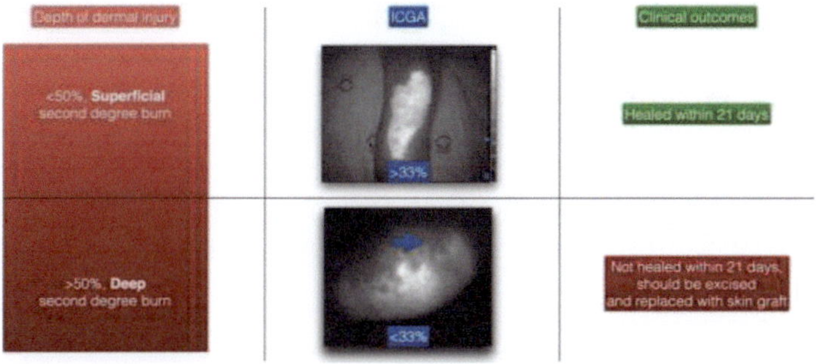

Fig. 10.1 The summary of the association between pathological study, ICGA interpretation criteria, and clinical outcomes

ICGA Technique for Burns

We would like to share our technique in using ICGA in burn surgery, which was supported by a prospective, multicentered, double-blinded, interventional one group study.

Candidate for the Intervention

Inclusion criteria required that patients be admitted to the hospital with indeterminate burn wounds on any body area. They were older than 18 and showed no signs of hemodynamic instability (mean arterial pressure ≥65 mmHg, urine output of 0.5–1 mL/kg/h, and adequate consciousness).

Exclusion criteria included an allergy to ICG and iodides, pregnancy, bleeding tendency, and psychiatric disorder. Patients are also excluded if they have comorbidities that could impair wound healing, such as diabetes mellitus, malnutrition, current active infection, immunocompromised host, obesity, old age (>65 years old), and anti-inflammatory medications. In addition, areas with indeterminate wounds with scars, moles, or tattoos were excluded.

Intervention

The study flow diagram is shown in Fig. 10.2. Indeterminate burn wounds were clinically evaluated. The definition of indeterminate burn wounds was second-degree burn wounds in which distinguishing between superficial and deep dermal extent could not be recognized by clinical judgment alone. Superficial partial-

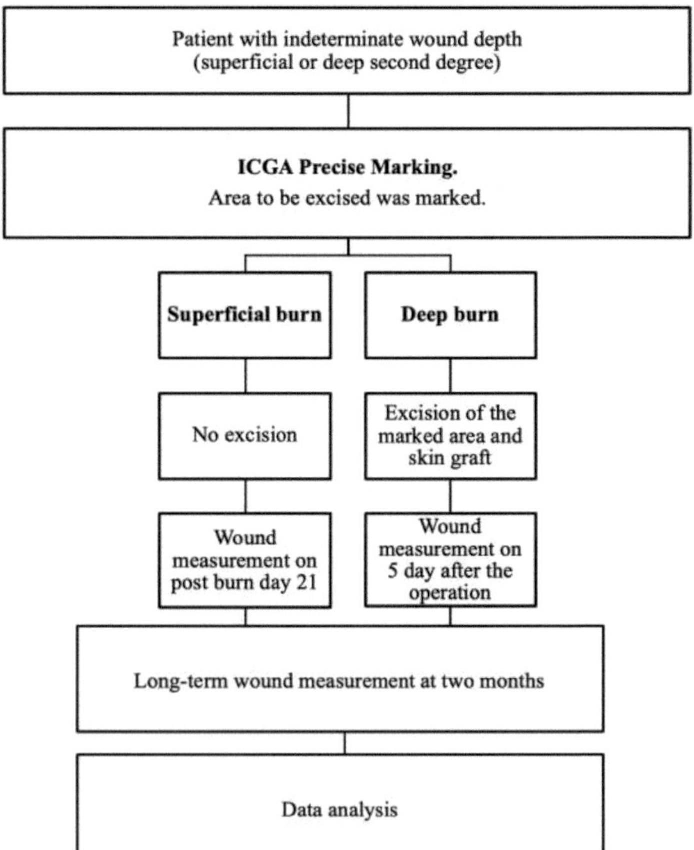

Fig. 10.2 Study flow diagram

thickness burns involved the superficial part of the dermis; the wounds were erythematous and tender and usually became blistered within 24 h [79]. Deep partial-thickness burns extended deeper into the deep part of the dermis, which contains hair follicles and glandular tissue; they were not painful unless pressure is applied to the affected area. These wounds contained variously mottled colorization from patchy white to red, and they did not blanch with pressure [79].

ICGA precise marking was performed as shown in Video 10.2 [80]. A single 0.5 mg/kg dose of ICG (Diagnogreen® Injection, Daiichi Sankyo Propharma, Japan) was injected intravenously to the patient. The Fluobeam® 800 clinical system was utilized. Figure 10.3 depicts the indocyanine green dye. Figure 10.4 illustrated the use of Fluobeam® 800 clinical system in a burn patient. The room's lights were turned off during the procedure. The viewer of the machine was held approximately 30 cm perpendicularly to the wound. It took 5–10 seconds after the injection for the image to appear on the monitor, and the illustration of ICGA on the monitor lasted approximately 5–10 min per single injection.

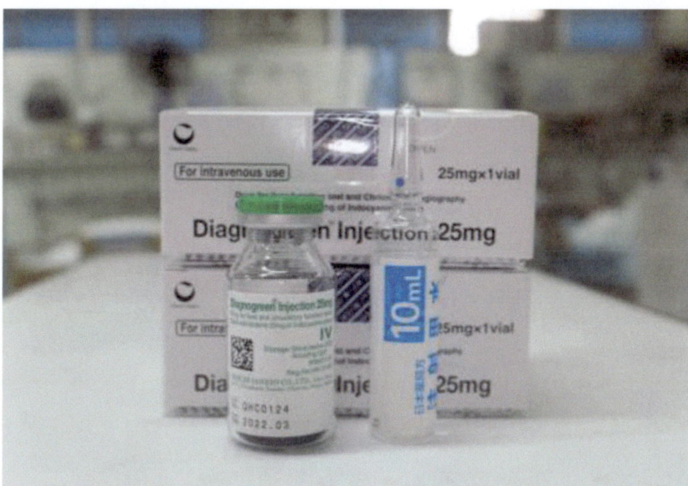

Fig. 10.3 Indocyanine green dye. (Diagnogreen® Injection, Daiichi Sankyo Propharma, Japan) was injected intravenously

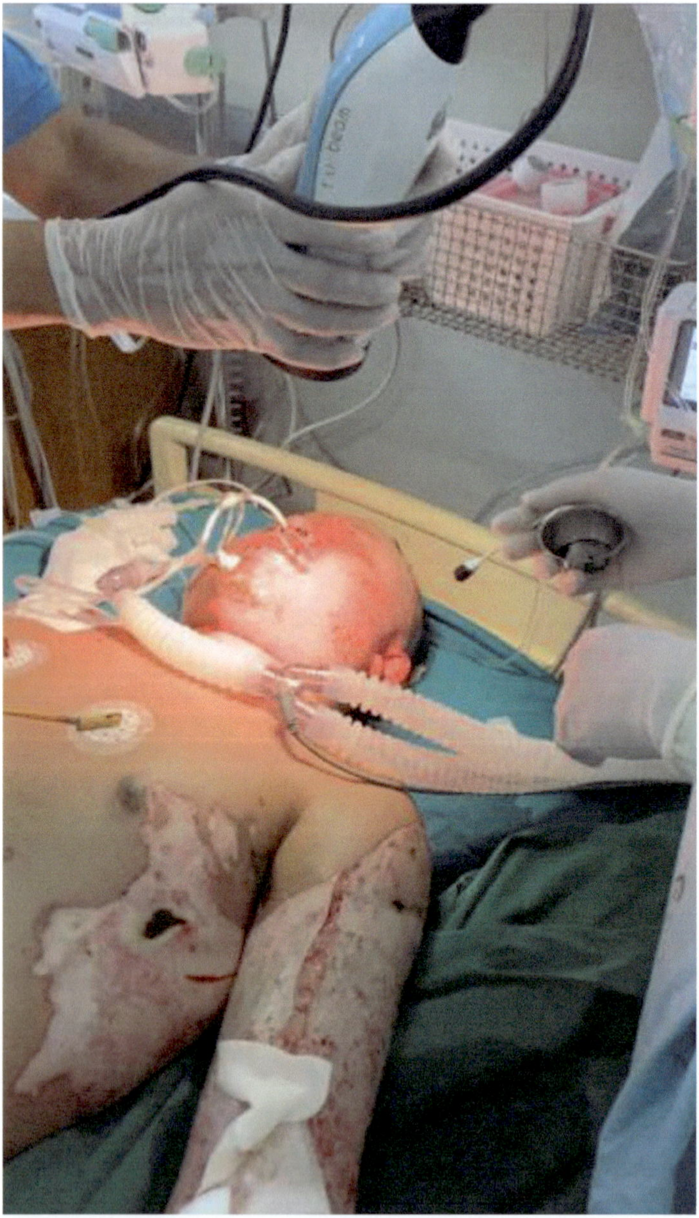

Fig. 10.4 The Fluobeam® 800 clinical system

The Fluobeam® 800 clinical system was approved by the US Food and Drug Administration (FDA), and its penetrating depth was reported to be 2.5 cm, which was adequate to evaluate the full thickness of the skin [62, 70].

ICGA Objective Interpretation Criteria

Thirty-three percent of maximal perfusion was applied as a cut point between superficial and deep second-degree burns [60, 63–65]. Fig. 10.5 depicts the objective interpretation of ICGA. Superficial second-degree burns were defined as burns with maximal perfusion of more than 33% that were bright and diffuse, showing patency of small vessels of the subpapillary and dermal plexuses [38, 63]. Deep second-degree burns were defined as burns with maximal perfusion of less than 33% or the dark area yielding mottled yet diffuse fluorescence showing partial patency of the dermal plexus [38, 63]. As a result, the deep second-degree burns were methylene blue-painted to determine the area to be excised in the operating room.

Following the ICGA, the painted wounds, which were deemed to be deep burn wounds, were excised and covered with skin grafts. Five days following the operation, the grafted area was checked for wound closure. Unmarked areas, which were consid-

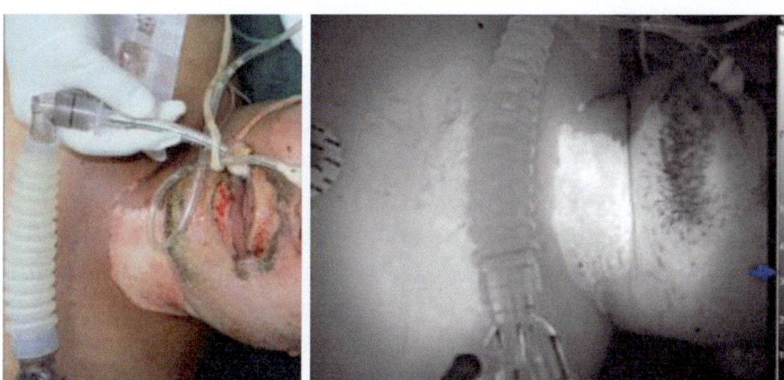

Fig. 10.5 How to objectively interpret ICGA. The blue arrow indicates 33% of maximal perfusion as a cut point between superficial and deep second-degree burns

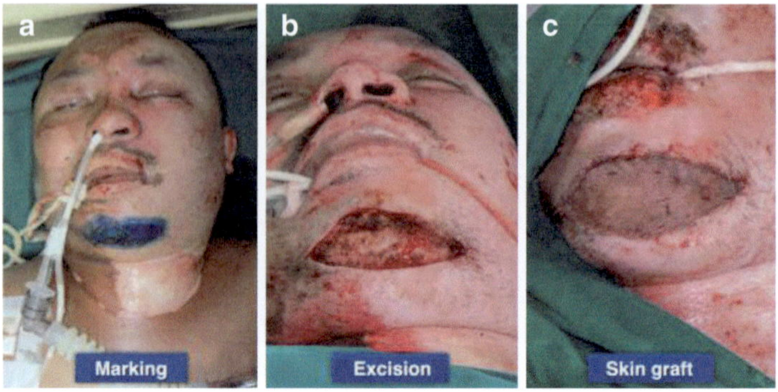

Fig. 10.6 An example of ICGA precise marking results. (**a**) ICGA precise marking, (**b**) excision along the marking, (**c**) skin graft placement

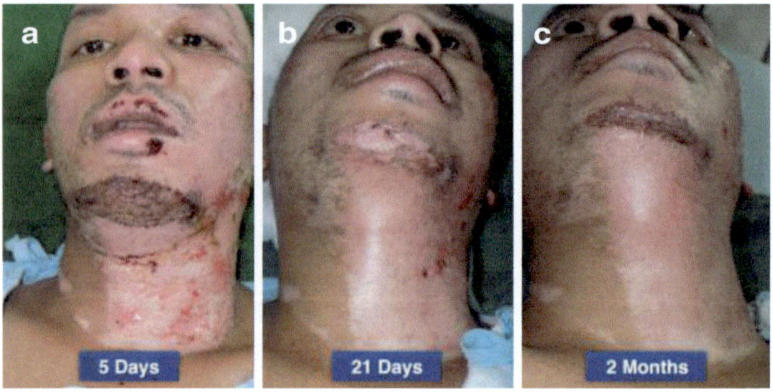

Fig. 10.7 An example of ICGA precise marking results. (**a**) Five days after the operation to confirm the complete wound closure. (**b**) The unmarked area was measured on post-burn day 21 to determine the complete wound closure (**c**) The patient wound was followed up at 2 months after the injury

ered superficial burn wounds, were covered with silver-contained hydrofiber (Aquacel® Ag + Extra™; Convatec, UK). On post-burn day 21, the unmarked region was measured to evaluate complete wound closure, which also confirmed the superficial nature of the wounds. All wounds were followed up at 2 months after the injury.

Figures 10.6, 10.7, 10.8, and 10.9 illustrate an example of ICGA marking accuracy. The summary of the findings is shown in

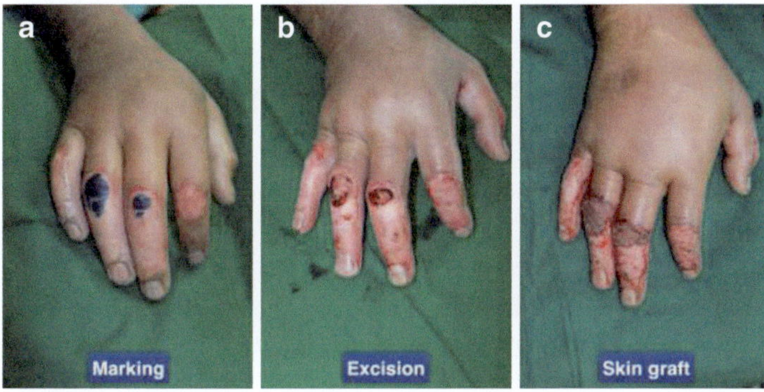

Fig. 10.8 Another example of ICGA precise marking results on the right hand. (**a**) ICGA precise marking, (**b**) excision along the marking, (**c**) skin graft placement

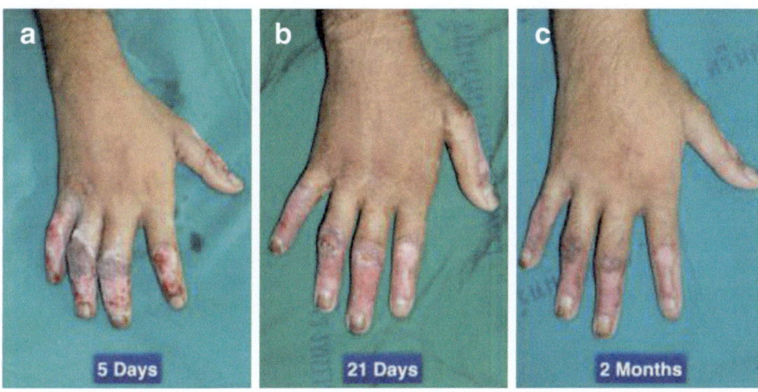

Fig. 10.9 Another example of ICGA precise marking results on the right hand. (**a**) Five days after the operation to confirm the complete wound closure. (**b**) The unmarked area was measured on post-burn day 21 to determine the complete wound closure (**c**) The patient wound was followed up at 2 months after the injury

Table 10.2. Using ICGA precise marking, the overall rate of short-term complete wound closure, which included both superficial and deep burns, was reported to be as high as 96.7% (29/30). This high rate of complete wound closure was significantly higher than the expected rate of 80%, $p = 0.01$. The long-term complete

Table 10.2 Summary of results

Wounds	Wound closure on Day 5 or day 21	Wound closure at 2 months	*P*-value
Superficial group	17	18	>0.999
Deep group	12	12	>0.999
Overall	29	30	>0.999

wound closures at 2 months confirmed the short-term result and achieved 100% of complete wound closure. There were no significant differences between the short-term and long-term wound closure rates ($p > 0.999$).

Post hoc analysis was conducted. In the superficial group, the short-term complete wound closure rate was 94.4% (17/18), while the long-term complete wound closure rate at 2 months was 100.0% (18/18). There was no significant difference between short-term and long-term wound closures ($p > 0.999$). On the other hand, the deep burn achieved both short-term and long-term complete wound closures of 100% (12/12). There was also no difference between short-term and long-term wound closures ($p > 0.999$).

Discussion

Interpretation

The study demonstrated that employing ICGA precise marking to guide indeterminate burn excision led to a remarkable rate of complete wound closure. In some centers, indeterminate burns were early excised, with deep burns to prevent infection and encourage early wound closure [81]. In our study that included 30 indeterminate burns, it was found that 18 (60%) were superficial second-degree burns. Up to 94.4% (17/18) healed within 21 days without any need for excision. This demonstrates the benefit of ICGA in sparing tissue areas. If the wound is located in a critical area, such as the face, hand, sole, or joints, ICGA could significantly save the patient's function.

The intervention occurred as early as 2.4 days. This clearly shows the advantage of employing ICGA in indeterminate burns. One of the obstacles found in burn excision was that the indeterminate burn made surgeons delay the surgery for the well-defined depth of the wound [82, 83]. Moreover, the debridement of indeterminate burn in the early phase could also result in unnecessary excision of the viable tissue if the tissue was later found to be superficial burn [84]. Utilizing ICGA precise marking has the further benefit of allowing for the minimally invasive excision of indeterminate burns and the safe early debridement of other distinctive types of wounds, including deep second and third burns. The skin graft could be applied after the excision, while the other superficial parts of the wound would heal in 21 days. This adequate and precise surgery not only helps burn patients to get cured faster but also helps them begin rehabilitation, recover function, and get back to work quicker [85].

The slight difference between short-term and long-term wound results revealed that the ICGA precise marking procedure could promote quicker wound healing with persistent results. Without using ICGA, some deep burns may recover in the short term, but later on could progress to unstable scars, as such the wound may become weak and trend to recur [86]. Consequently, this difficulty may require further wound dressings or even secondary surgery and closure with a skin graft [86, 87].

The Appropriate Time to Perform ICGA Marking

The appropriate time for ICGA marking is important. This study performed ICGA about 2.4 days following injury. First, the patients gain more benefits if the ICGA is performed early, and patients could have earlier excision than the standard treatment. Conventionally, surgeons need to wait for the indeterminate wound to become more distinct as either superficial or deep burn before making excision because the features of the wound (superficial or deep) become more significant when the wound is clinically assessed late [36]. Second, ICGA should be conducted on the day that the patient is sufficiently stable to undergo further early excision. Commonly, it was reported that the time of early excision was within 1–6 days [88]. The mean of 2.4 days in this study was suitable in the 6-day limit [88]. Third, performing ICGA at a single time point in the first 5 days after burn injury is sufficient to differentiate between superficial and deep burn [65]. There was a case series that the ICGA was conducted daily on the burn area for the first 5 days after burn injury [65]. It was found that the percent of perfusion changed over time, but the difference between superficial and deep burn was still obvious [65].

The Importance of Adequate Measurements for Complete Wound Closure

This study examined complete wound closures at two time periods, including short-term and long-term assessments, to be appropriately characterized as complete wound closure in the global standard and utilized in future analytical studies [89]. The US Food and Drug Administration (FDA) currently defines complete wound closure as achieving 100% epithelialization without drainage or dressing requirements confirmed at two consecutive study visits at least 2 weeks apart [89]. A literature review that studied healing rates of chronic wounds found that among 53 RCTs and comparative studies that assessed wound closure, 19 (35.8%) studies did not adequately define complete wound closure [90]. It was suggested the widespread adoption of a standard complete wound closure definition would allow more robust comparisons of treatment effects across studies to improve the evidence base and enhance the treatment decision-making process in clinical practice [91]. This study measured the short-term complete wound closure at 5 or 21 days and the long-term measurement at 2 months, which was greater than the minimum requirement of 2 weeks. As a result, the study findings were adequately defined as complete wound closure.

Passing Through the Difficulty of How to Mark the Burn Wounds

The most complex challenge in the study, and one that deserves attention, was how to mark the burn wounds. Conventionally, the surgical wound or skin is marked with the commercial marking pen or gentian violet [74]. However, there were a lot of obstacles if the conventional marking method was used to mark the burn wounds. First, the tip of the commercial pen was hard and could cause pain during the marking when the pen's tip was pressed to the burn wound. Second, the commercial ink and gentian violet were easy to be erased when facing with the nature of the burn wound, which could produce secretion, and when contacting with the ointment of the dressing. Third, the tip of the pen may cease functioning after a few inches of marking because of the secretion of the wound or the remnant of dressing ointment obstructing the tip of the pen. These were obstacles to the conventional method of burn wound marking.

There were a lot of attempts to solve the pain and easy-to-erase problems. The majority of the available markers were purchased and appraised. Aside from the markers' brands, several techniques of marking were also tested. A number of different brush sizes were sterile and examined, which might be an ideal match. Finally, it was discovered that using methylene blue as the ink and a sterile cotton bud as the painting instrument was the easiest and simplest technique that could be generalized throughout several hospitals. These two materials already are available in most hospitals.

Generalizability

Using ICGA is simple, which makes it appropriate to be generalized. The 33% of maximal perfusion cut point utilized is objective interpretation, which is uncomplicated to reproduce [66]. The described study was also among the very few studies [63, 66, 71, 76, 92], in which the objective criteria were applied in executing ICGA. Superficial and deep burn wounds are significantly different and simple to distinguish using ICGA [76] because the superficial burns tend to have a high perfusion area due to vasodilatation caused by an inflammatory response in the pathophysiology of burns [76, 92, 93]. In addition, the described study only included second-degree burns, whose pathophysiology consisted of partial dermal injury where venous drainage was not significantly involved [94]. The high intensity in burn may not be restricted in the same way with using ICGA in flap reconstruction, which high perfusion could be a sign of venous congestion and may progress to flap necrosis [95].

Limitations

Some conditions limit the use of ICGA. Firstly, ICGA requires the injection of indocyanine green. Although the allergic rate of ICGA was low [68], the use of ICGA precise marking in patients with iodine allergies is contraindicated. Secondly, the availability of the ICGA investigating period is 5–10 min after injection. The team needs to be well prepared for this limited time of the investigation, which was found to be adequate to perform precise marking. If the time runs out, an additional injection with the similar dose could be achieved. Thirdly, ICGA is limited in some areas of the body. ICGA generates pictures by detecting infrared (840–850 nm) fluorescence emission from the complex of albumin and ICG [62]. Any obstacles such as hair, tattoo, and mole could block the interpretation of ICGA and, therefore, were excluded in this study. Lastly, the marking requires a short learning curve of two to three cases because of the eye-hand coordination between the real marking and the ICGA monitor. Nevertheless, the marking is simple, and the marking's outcomes are worth the price of the practice.

Regarding the use of the ICGA, there seems to be minimal uncertainty in the diagnosis of remaining indeterminate burns. This is evidenced by the superficial burn wound that did not heal within 21 days, as confirmed by the ICGA. The explanation might lie in the ICGA interpreted cut point. It was discovered that the diagnostic of ICGA had a gray zone in indeterminate areas between 25% and 45% of maximal perfusion [63]. The use of 33% cut point was suggested to handle this problem [63] and was selected for this study. The 33% cut point was found to yield as high as 88% positive predictive value of removing non-viable tissue and as low as 16% negative predictive value of removing viable tissue [63]. Furthermore, the overall rate of short-term complete wound closure reported was 96.7%, which demonstrates that this cut point delivers favorable results but is not flawless. Further research should explore more on the diagnostic criteria used in interpreting ICGA in burn to perfect this method.

Conclusion

Using ICGA precise marking to guide indeterminate burn excision resulted in an excellent rate of complete wound closure and an improvement in short-term and long-term wound outcomes. Therefore, ICGA is an effective method to aid decision-making in burn surgeries of the indeterminate areas. The current level of evidence in using ICGA in burn excision is III. The future direction should pursue in the randomization of using versus not using ICGA in the treatment of burn.

References

1. Forjuoh SN. Burns in low- and middle-income countries: a review of available literature on descriptive epidemiology, risk factors, treatment, and prevention. Burns. 2006;32(5):529–37.
2. Peck MD, Kruger GE, van der Merwe AE, Godakumbura W, Ahuja RB. Burns and fires from non-electric domestic appliances in low and middle income countries Part I. The scope of the problem. Burns. 2008;34(3):303–11.
3. James SL, Lucchesi LR, Bisignano C, Castle CD, Dingels ZV, Fox JT, et al. Epidemiology of injuries from fire, heat and hot substances: global, regional and national morbidity and mortality estimates from the Global Burden of Disease 2017 study. Inj Prev. 2020;26(Supp 1):i36–45.
4. Peck MD. Epidemiology of burns throughout the world. Part I: distribution and risk factors. Burns. 2011;37(7):1087–100.
5. Jeschke MG, van Baar ME, Choudhry MA, Chung KK, Gibran NS, Logsetty S. Burn injury. Nat Rev Dis Primers. 2020;6(1):11.
6. Saavedra PAE, De Oliveira Leal JV, Areda CA, Galato D. The costs of burn victim hospital care around the world: a systematic review. Iran J Public Health. 2021;50(5):866–78.
7. Kaddoura I, Abu-Sittah G, Ibrahim A, Karamanoukian R, Papazian N. Burn injury: review of pathophysiology and therapeutic modalities in major burns. Ann Burns Fire Disasters. 2017;30(2):95–102.
8. Rowan MP, Cancio LC, Elster EA, Burmeister DM, Rose LF, Natesan S, et al. Burn wound healing and treatment: review and advancements. Crit Care. 2015;19:243.
9. Orgill DP, Solari MG, Barlow MS, O'Connor NE. A finite-element model predicts thermal damage in cutaneous contact burns. J Burn Care Rehabil. 1998;19(3):203–9.

10. Cheng W, Shen C, Zhao D, Zhang H, Tu J, Yuan Z, et al. The epidemiology and prognosis of patients with massive burns: a multicenter study of 2483 cases. Burns. 2019;45(3):705–16.
11. Uzun I, Akyildiz E, Inanici MA. Histopathological differentiation of skin lesions caused by electrocution, flame burns and abrasion. Forensic Sci Int. 2008;178(2–3):157–61.
12. Robins EV. Burn shock. Crit Care Nurs Clin North Am. 1990;2(2): 299–307.
13. Aulick LH, Wilmore DW, Mason AD Jr, Pruitt BA Jr. Influence of the burn wound on peripheral circulation in thermally injured patients. Am J Phys. 1977;233(4):H520–6.
14. Mertens DM, Jenkins ME, Warden GD. Outpatient burn management. Nurs Clin North Am. 1997;32(2):343–64.
15. Neligan PC. Plastic surgery. 4th ed. Toronto, ON: Elsevier; 2018.
16. Singer AJ, Clark RA. Cutaneous wound healing. N Engl J Med. 1999;341(10):738–46.
17. Tabas I, Glass CK. Anti-inflammatory therapy in chronic disease: challenges and opportunities. Science. 2013;339(6116):166–72.
18. Claudinot S, Nicolas M, Oshima H, Rochat A, Barrandon Y. Long-term renewal of hair follicles from clonogenic multipotent stem cells. Proc Natl Acad Sci U S A. 2005;102(41):14677–82.
19. Franz MG, Steed DL, Robson MC. Optimizing healing of the acute wound by minimizing complications. Curr Probl Surg. 2007;44(11): 691–763.
20. Church D, Elsayed S, Reid O, Winston B, Lindsay R. Burn wound infections. Clin Microbiol Rev. 2006;19(2):403–34.
21. Coban YK. Infection control in severely burned patients. World J Crit Care Med. 2012;1(4):94–101.
22. Branski LK, Al-Mousawi A, Rivero H, Jeschke MG, Sanford AP, Herndon DN. Emerging infections in burns. Surg Infect. 2009;10(5):389–97.
23. Shupp JW, Pavlovich AR, Jeng JC, Pezzullo JC, Oetgen WJ, Jaskille AD, et al. Epidemiology of bloodstream infections in burn-injured patients: a review of the national burn repository. J Burn Care Res. 2010;31(4): 521–8.
24. Hart DW, Wolf SE, Chinkes DL, Beauford RB, Mlcak RP, Heggers JP, et al. Effects of early excision and aggressive enteral feeding on hypermetabolism, catabolism, and sepsis after severe burn. J Trauma. 2003;54(4):755–61; discussion 61–4.
25. Andel H, Kamolz LP, Horauf K, Zimpfer M. Nutrition and anabolic agents in burned patients. Burns. 2003;29(6):592–5.
26. Dolp R, Rehou S, Pinto R, Trister R, Jeschke MG. The effect of diabetes on burn patients: a retrospective cohort study. Crit Care. 2019;23(1):28.
27. Goutos I, Nicholas RS, Pandya AA, Ghosh SJ. Diabetes mellitus and burns. Part I-basic science and implications for management. Int J Burns Trauma. 2015;5(1):1–12.

28. Casqueiro J, Casqueiro J, Alves C. Infections in patients with diabetes mellitus: a review of pathogenesis. Indian J Endocrinol Metab. 2012;16(Suppl 1):S27–36.
29. Goutos I, Sadideen H, Pandya AA, Ghosh SJ. Obesity and burns. J Burn Care Res. 2012;33(4):471–82.
30. Neaman KC, Andres LA, McClure AM, Burton ME, Kemmeter PR, Ford RD. A new method for estimation of involved BSAs for obese and normal-weight patients with burn injury. J Burn Care Res. 2011;32(3): 421–8.
31. Keck M, Lumenta DB, Andel H, Kamolz LP, Frey M. Burn treatment in the elderly. Burns. 2009;35(8):1071–9.
32. Lewandowski R, Pegg S, Fortier K, Skimmings A. Burn injuries in the elderly. Burns. 1993;19(6):513–5.
33. Hunt JL, Purdue GF. The elderly burn patient. Am J Surg. 1992;164(5):472–6.
34. Monstrey S, Hoeksema H, Verbelen J, Pirayesh A, Blondeel P. Assessment of burn depth and burn wound healing potential. Burns. 2008;34(6): 761–9.
35. Heimbach D, Engrav L, Grube B, Marvin J. Burn depth: a review. World J Surg. 1992;16(1):10–5.
36. Devgan L, Bhat S, Aylward S, Spence RJ. Modalities for the assessment of burn wound depth. J Burns Wounds. 2006;5:e2.
37. Güler Gürsu K. An experimental study for diagnosis of burn depth. Burns. 1977;4(2):97–103.
38. Still JM, Law EJ, Klavuhn KG, Island TC, Holtz JZ. Diagnosis of burn depth using laser-induced indocyanine green fluorescence: a preliminary clinical trial. Burns. 2001;27(4):364–71.
39. Jaskille AD, Ramella-Roman JC, Shupp JW, Jordan MH, Jeng JC. Critical review of burn depth assessment techniques: part II. Review of laser doppler technology. J Burn Care Res. 2010;31(1):151–7.
40. Sharma VP, O'Boyle CP, Jeffery SL. Man or machine? The clinimetric properties of laser Doppler imaging in burn depth assessment. J Burn Care Res. 2011;32(1):143–9.
41. Mileski WJ, Atiles L, Purdue G, Kagan R, Saffle JR, Herndon DN, et al. Serial measurements increase the accuracy of laser Doppler assessment of burn wounds. J Burn Care Rehabil. 2003;24(4):187–91.
42. Grunwald TB, Garner WL. Acute burns. Plast Reconstr Surg. 2008;121(5):311e–9e.
43. Johnson RM, Richard R. Partial-thickness burns: identification and management. Adv Skin Wound Care. 2003;16(4):178–87; quiz 88–9.
44. Kahn AM, McCrady VL, Rosen VJ. Burn wound biopsy. Multiple uses in patient management. Scand J Plast Reconstr Surg. 1979;13(1):53–6.
45. Singer AJ, Berruti L, Thode HC Jr, McClain SA. Standardized burn model using a multiparametric histologic analysis of burn depth. Acad Emerg Med. 2000;7(1):1–6.

46. Chvapil M, Speer DP, Owen JA, Chvapil TA. Identification of the depth of burn injury by collagen stainability. Plast Reconstr Surg. 1984;73(3):438–41.
47. Watts AM, Tyler MP, Perry ME, Roberts AH, McGrouther DA. Burn depth and its histological measurement. Burns. 2001;27(2):154–60.
48. Saranto JR, Rubayi S, Zawacki BE. Blisters, cooling, antithromboxanes, and healing in experimental zone-of-stasis burns. J Trauma. 1983;23(10):927–33.
49. Robson MC, Kucan JO, Paik KI, Eriksson E. Prevention of dermal ischemia after thermal injury. Arch Surg. 1978;113(5):621–5.
50. Mladick R, Georgiade N, Thorne F. A clinical evaluation of the use of thermography in determining degree of burn injury. Plast Reconstr Surg. 1966;38(6):512–8.
51. Lawson RN, Gaston JP. Temperature measurements of localized pathological processes. Ann N Y Acad Sci. 1964;121:90–8.
52. Cole RP, Jones SG, Shakespeare PG. Thermographic assessment of hand burns. Burns. 1990;16(1):60–3.
53. Liddington MI, Shakespeare PG. Timing of the thermographic assessment of burns. Burns. 1996;22(1):26–8.
54. Goans RE, Cantrell JH Jr, Meyers FB. Ultrasonic pulse-echo determination of thermal injury in deep dermal burns. Med Phys. 1977;4(3):259–63.
55. Brink JA, Sheets PW, Dines KA, Etchison MR, Hanke CW, Sadove AM. Quantitative assessment of burn injury in porcine skin with high-frequency ultrasonic imaging. Investig Radiol. 1986;21(8):645–51.
56. Foster FS, Zhang MY, Zhou YQ, Liu G, Mehi J, Cherin E, et al. A new ultrasound instrument for in vivo microimaging of mice. Ultrasound Med Biol. 2002;28(9):1165–72.
57. Pape SA, Skouras CA, Byrne PO. An audit of the use of laser Doppler imaging (LDI) in the assessment of burns of intermediate depth. Burns. 2001;27(3):233–9.
58. Essex TJ, Byrne PO. A laser Doppler scanner for imaging blood flow in skin. J Biomed Eng. 1991;13(3):189–94.
59. Holloway GA Jr, Watkins DW. Laser Doppler measurement of cutaneous blood flow. J Invest Dermatol. 1977;69(3):306–9.
60. Green HA, Bua D, Anderson RR, Nishioka NS. Burn depth estimation using indocyanine green fluorescence. Arch Dermatol. 1992;128(1):43–9.
61. Meyerholz DK, Piester TL, Sokolich JC, Zamba GK, Light TD. Morphological parameters for assessment of burn severity in an acute burn injury rat model. Int J Exp Pathol. 2009;90(1):26–33.
62. DSouza AV, Lin H, Henderson ER, Samkoe KS, Pogue BW. Review of fluorescence guided surgery systems: identification of key performance capabilities beyond indocyanine green imaging. J Biomed Opt. 2016;21(8):080901.

63. Moyer HR, Losken A. Predicting mastectomy skin flap necrosis with indocyanine green angiography: the gray area defined. Plast Reconstr Surg. 2012;129(5):1043–8.
64. Jerath MR, Schomacker KT, Sheridan RL, Nishioka NS. Burn wound assessment in porcine skin using indocyanine green fluorescence. J Trauma. 1999;46(6):1085–8.
65. Dissanaike S, Abdul-Hamed S, Griswold JA. Variations in burn perfusion over time as measured by portable ICG fluorescence: a case series. Burns Trauma. 2014;2(4):201–5.
66. Wongkietkachorn A, Surakunprapha P, Winaikosol K, Waraasawapati S, Chaiwiriyakul S, Eua-Angkanakul K, et al. Indocyanine green dye angiography as an adjunct to assess indeterminate burn wounds: a prospective, multicentered, triple-blinded study. J Trauma Acute Care Surg. 2019;86(5):823–8.
67. Alander JT, Kaartinen I, Laakso A, Patila T, Spillmann T, Tuchin VV, et al. A review of indocyanine green fluorescent imaging in surgery. Int J Biomed Imaging. 2012;2012:940585.
68. Hope-Ross M, Yannuzzi LA, Gragoudas ES, Guyer DR, Slakter JS, Sorenson JA, et al. Adverse reactions due to indocyanine green. Ophthalmology. 1994;101(3):529–33.
69. Fourman MS, Phillips BT, Crawford L, McClain SA, Lin F, Thode HC Jr, et al. Indocyanine green dye angiography accurately predicts survival in the zone of ischemia in a burn comb model. Burns. 2014;40(5):940–6.
70. Hirche C, Engel H, Kolios L, Cognie J, Hunerbein M, Lehnhardt M, et al. An experimental study to evaluate the Fluobeam 800 imaging system for fluorescence-guided lymphatic imaging and sentinel node biopsy. Surg Innov. 2013;20(5):516–23.
71. McUmber H, Dabek RJ, Bojovic B, Driscoll DN. Burn depth analysis using indocyanine green fluorescence: a review. J Burn Care Res. 2019;40(4):513–6.
72. Wongkietkachorn A, Surakunprapha P, Winaikosol K, Eua-Angkanakul K, Wongkietkachorn N, Punyavong P, et al. Quantitative burn depth analysis using indocyanine green angiography. J Burn Care Res. 2019;40(5):725.
73. Engrav LH, Heimbach DM, Reus JL, Harnar TJ, Marvin JA. Early excision and grafting vs. nonoperative treatment of burns of indeterminant depth: a randomized prospective study. J Trauma. 1983;23(11):1001–4.
74. Wongkietkachorn A, Surakunprapha P, Winaikosol K, Wongkietkachorn N, Wongkietkachorn S. Precise marking for burn excision by using indocyanine green angiography. Plast Reconstr Surg. 2020;145(1):229e–30e.
75. Arturson G. Pathophysiology of the burn wound. Ann Chir Gynaecol. 1980;69(5):178–90.
76. Wongkietkachorn A, Surakunprapha P, Jenwitheesuk K, Winaikosol K, Punyavong P, Chowchuen B, et al. Improvement in interpretation of indocyanine green angiography. J Plast Reconstr Aesthet Surg. 2019;73:608.

77. Wongkietkachorn A, Surakunprapha P, Jenwitheesuk K, Eua-Angkanakul K, Winaikosol K, Punyavong P, et al. An inconvenient truth of clinical assessment and indocyanine green angiography precise marking for indeterminate burn excision. Plast Reconstr Surg Glob Open. 2021;9(3):e3497.
78. Wongkietkachorn A, Surakunprapha P, Jenwitheesuk K, Eua-angkanakul K, Winaikosol K, Punyavong P, et al. An inconvenient truth of clinical assessment of indeterminate burns and indocyanine green dye angiography precise marking for burn excision: a prospective, multicentered, triple-blinded study. Plast Reconstr Surg Glob Open. 2020;8(9 Suppl):145–6. https://doi.org/10.1097/01.GOX.0000721084.58676.5d.
79. Cubison TC, Pape SA, Parkhouse N. Evidence for the link between healing time and the development of hypertrophic scars (HTS) in paediatric burns due to scald injury. Burns. 2006;32(8):992–9.
80. Wongkietkachorn A, Surakunprapha P, Jenwitheesuk K, Eua-Angkanakul K, Winaikosol K, Punyavong P, et al. Indocyanine Green angiography precise marking for indeterminate burn excision: a prospective, multicentered, double-blinded study. Plast Reconstr Surg Glob Open. 2021;9(4):e3538.
81. Tenenhaus M, Bhavsar D, Rennekampff HO. Treatment of deep partial thickness and indeterminate depth facial burn wounds with water-jet debridement and a biosynthetic dressing. Injury. 2007;38(Suppl 5):S39–45.
82. Karim AS, Shaum K, Gibson ALF. Indeterminate-depth burn injury-exploring the uncertainty. J Surg Res. 2020;245:183–97.
83. Israel JS, Greenhalgh DG, Gibson AL. Variations in burn excision and grafting: a survey of the American Burn Association. J Burn Care Res. 2017;38(1):e125–e32.
84. Gurfinkel R, Rosenberg L, Cohen S, Cohen A, Barezovsky A, Cagnano E, et al. Histological assessment of tangentially excised burn eschars. Can J Plast Surg. 2010;18(3):e33–6.
85. Esselman PC. Burn rehabilitation: an overview. Arch Phys Med Rehabil. 2007;88(12 Suppl 2):S3–6.
86. Goel A, Shrivastava P. Post-burn scars and scar contractures. Indian J Plast Surg. 2010;43(Suppl):S63–71.
87. Tredget EE, Levi B, Donelan MB. Biology and principles of scar management and burn reconstruction. Surg Clin North Am. 2014;94(4):793–815.
88. Ong YS, Samuel M, Song C. Meta-analysis of early excision of burns. Burns. 2006;32(2):145–50.
89. Singer AJ, Boyce ST. Burn wound healing and tissue engineering. J Burn Care Res. 2017;38(3):e605–e13.
90. Gottrup F, Apelqvist J, Price P. Outcomes in controlled and comparative studies on non-healing wounds: recommendations to improve the quality of evidence in wound management. J Wound Care. 2010;19(6):237–68.

91. Gould L, Li WW. Defining complete wound closure: closing the gap in clinical trials and practice. Wound Repair Regen. 2019;27(3):201–24.
92. Muntean MV, Ardelean F, Strilciuc S, Pestean C, Georgescu AV, Muntean V. Flap warming improves intraoperative indocyanine green angiography (ICGA) assessment of perfusion. An experimental study. J Plast Reconstr Aesthet Surg. 2019;72(7):1150–6.
93. Hettiaratchy S, Dziewulski P. ABC of burns: pathophysiology and types of burns. BMJ. 2004;328(7453):1427–9.
94. Nielson CB, Duethman NC, Howard JM, Moncure M, Wood JG. Burns: pathophysiology of systemic complications and current management. J Burn Care Res. 2017;38(1):e469–e81.
95. Gurtner GC, Jones GE, Neligan PC, Newman MI, Phillips BT, Sacks JM, et al. Intraoperative laser angiography using the SPY system: review of the literature and recommendations for use. Ann Surg Innov Res. 2013;7(1):1.

Use of Fluorescence Guidance in Acute Care Surgery and Trauma

11

Elwin Tham, Jennifer Knight, and Nova Szoka

Introduction

Fluorescence-guided surgery (FGS) is a medical imaging technique that uses a fluorescent dye or a near-infrared-emitting light source to identify anatomic structures during surgical procedures. The present chapter will describe the history and mechanism of action of indocyanine green (ICG) dye as well as review the use of fluorescence guidance in acute care surgery (ACS) and trauma surgery. Two of the primary applications of FGS in ACS are ICG cholangiography during cholecystectomy to define anatomic

Supplementary Information The online version contains supplementary material available at https://doi.org/10.1007/978-3-031-40685-0_11.

E. Tham · N. Szoka (✉)
Department of Surgery, West Virginia University, Morgantown, WV, USA
e-mail: elwinjennhui.tham@hsc.wvu.edu; nova.szoka@hsc.wvu.edu

J. Knight
Department of Surgery, The Ohio State University, Werner Medical Center, Columbus, OH, USA
e-mail: Jennifer.knightdavis@osumc.edu

N. Szoka et al. (eds.), *The SAGES Manual of Fluorescence-Guided Surgery*, https://doi.org/10.1007/978-3-031-40685-0_11

structures and ICG angiography to evaluate bowel perfusion. In addition, an evolving area of use for fluorescence guidance in acute care surgery is in the management of wounds and soft tissue infections. In trauma surgery, the primary application of ICG is for evaluating tissue perfusion following traumatic injury; however, there are evolving applications for the assessment of other types of traumatic injuries. ICG dosing and administration, as well as coding and reimbursement, will be discussed for each respective procedure.

History and Physiology of Indocyanine Green Dye

Originally employed for the quantitative measurement of hepatic and cardiac function as early as the mid-1950s, indocyanine green (ICG) is a nontoxic, fluorescent iodide dye with rapid hepatic clearance. In the initial studies, research centered around the measurement of serum ICG levels as a method to assess hepatic and cardiac function. Later studies in the 1970s expanded the use of ICG to the field of ophthalmology for macular hole surgery. Due to technological limitations, the development of ICG into ICG fluorescence angiography did not occur until the mid-1990s. With further technological advancement in the early 2000s, the development of improved digital imaging resolution that paralleled film-based photography resulted in the widespread acceptance of ICG angiography [1]. Since then, the utility of ICG angiography for assessing tissue perfusion has been studied, with numerous ongoing studies assessing other applications of this compound [1].

ICG is an amphiphilic, tricarbocyanine iodide dye that can be reconstituted into an aqueous solution of pH 6.5 for intravenous injection in patients. Once injected, ICG binds to plasma proteins taken up by the liver and later excreted in bile. Typically, 98% of injected ICG is plasma protein-bound, while the remaining 2% remains free in the serum. Free ICG is then transported into the bile via the enzyme glutathione S-transferase, while bound ICG remains in the intravascular space for a longer period of time [2–6].

Due to its well-tolerated biopharmacological profile, ICG can be used in a wide variety of medical applications and has a low incidence of adverse reactions [7]. Adverse reactions from ICG are commonly mild, with nausea and urticaria being the most common. The main contraindication to ICG use is iodine allergy. Typical dosing of ICG varies with the procedure, with standard vials containing 25 mg of ICG that are reconstituted in 10 ml sterile water and each single milliliter containing 2.5 mg of ICG. Individual doses range in size from 2.5 to 15 mg. Standard dosing is far below the lethal dose (LD50) for this drug, which is 50–80 mg/kg [2–8].

Once injected, ICG fluorescence has high contrast and sensitivity as the near-infrared light used to measure fluorescence makes tissues appear more translucent allowing visualization through several millimeters of tissue compared to visible light wavelengths. This is achieved by the excitation of the molecule via an external laser or light source, causing it to fluoresce at near-infrared wavelengths (750–800 nm with a maximum peak of 832 nm) [2, 3]. The near-infrared camera then captures the images and reveals real-time perfusion in the tissue assessed by quantifying the dye's fluorescence, providing objective information regarding which regions have the best blood supply. Real-time viewing of these images via video angiography also allows clinicians to make decisions immediately without the need for additional studies [2, 9].

ICG is cleared by the liver at a rate of 18–24% per min. With a half-life of 3 to 4 min, the dye is cleared from the intravascular space in the first 10 to 20 min after application. The rapid clearance rate allows ICG to be used for multiple injections during a procedure yielding significant benefits over other analogous substances. Following initial metabolism, the drug clearance rate slows, allowing trace amounts of ICG to remain in the plasma for more than an hour [2, 3, 10]. Due to ICG's hepatic clearance and excretion into bile, ICG can effectively be used to visualize biliary anatomy in cholecystectomy [11, 12].

Fluorescence Guidance in Acute Care Surgery

ICG in Laparoscopic Cholecystectomy

ICG is being applied as an adjunct to many procedures due to its ability to improve visualization of surgical anatomy via augmented reality; one such area is minimally invasive cholecystectomy [13]. In the field of acute care surgery, laparoscopic cholecystectomies are frequently performed. In the United States alone, approximately 20 million people have gallstones. Of this group, approximately 300,000 cholecystectomies are performed annually [14]. In the advanced laparoscopy era, a retrospective review of 217,774 cases from the National Surgical Quality Improvement Program (NSQIP) reported bile duct injury incidence of 0.19% [15]. In addition, cholecystectomy performed on patients with acute cholecystitis has a higher risk of complications based on disease severity [16].

Many techniques can be performed to assess hepatobiliary anatomy during a cholecystectomy. Intraoperative cholangiogram (IOC) remains the historical standard of care technique for bile duct clarification. With an odds ratio for bile duct injury of 0.60 (95% confidence interval = 0.52–0.70) based on a forest plot of the six largest population-based studies assessing IOC, the association between reduced risk of bile duct injury and use of IOC has been shown convincingly [17, 18]. IOC, however, can be difficult to interpret, is associated with higher costs, prolongs operative time by 10 to 23 minutes, and requires additional medical specialists and equipment. ICG fluorescence cholangiography, on the other hand, does not prolong operating time, uses radiation, or requires additional medical specialists, and cannot cause bile duct injury, yielding significant benefits as an adjunct for optimizing visualization of hepatobiliary anatomy (Fig. 11.1) [19].

ICG use for intraoperative fluorescence cholangiography as an adjunct to better delineate hepatobiliary anatomy (Fig. 11.2, Video 11.1) was first described in 2010 [20]. It was initially proposed to be an alternative to traditional radiographic IOC in a cohort of patients that underwent elective cholecystectomy [21]. From that study, the authors proposed that ICG fluorescence cholangiography could improve visualization of hepatobiliary anatomy (Fig. 11.3), especially in patients who were unable to be cannulated for IOC [23]. A more recent study by Broderick et al. examined outcomes in 1389 patients who underwent laparoscopic cholecystectomy with (28.8%) and without (71.2%) fluorescence guidance and found that ICG use significantly reduced operative time, rate of conversion to open operation, and hospital length of

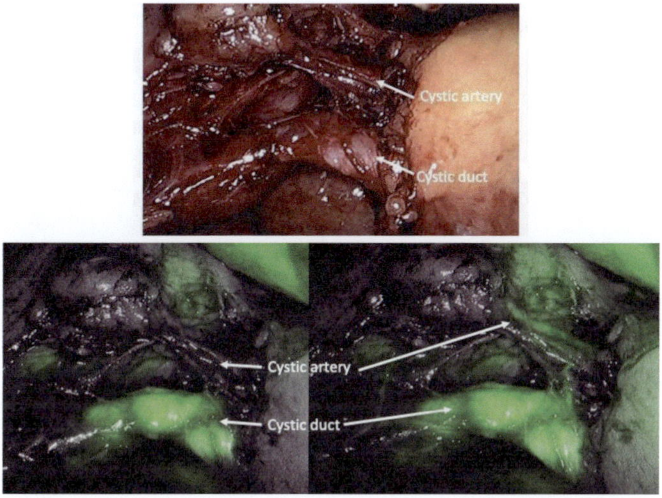

Fig. 11.1 ICG cholangiography during a robotic cholecystectomy, white light view (top image), initial near-infrared view of cystic duct (bottom left image), near-infrared view illuminating cystic artery (bottom right image). (Image source Nova Szoka MD FACS)

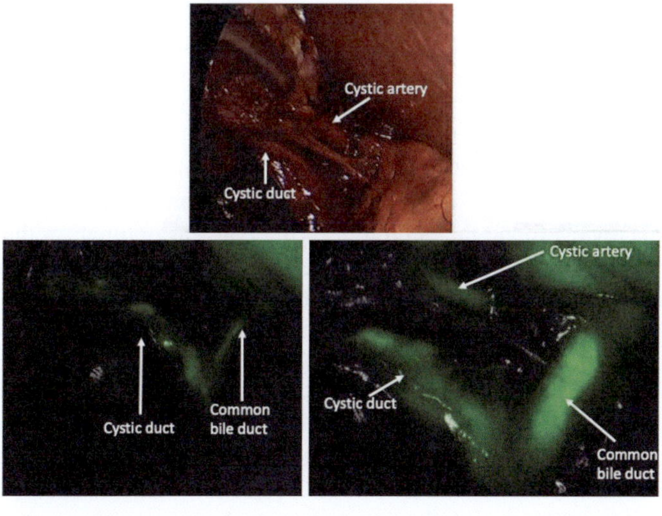

Fig. 11.2 ICG cholangiography during a laparoscopic cholecystectomy, white light view (top image), initial near-infrared view of cystic duct and common bile duct (bottom left image), near-infrared view illuminating cystic artery (bottom right image). (Image source Nova Szoka MD FACS)

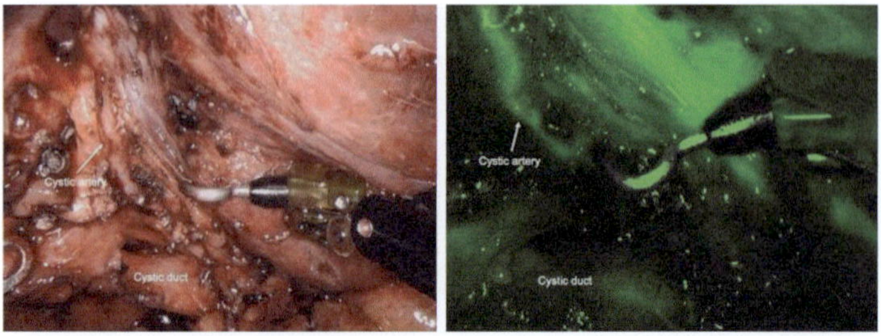

Fig. 11.3 ICG cholangiography during a robotic cholecystectomy, with images of cystic duct and cystic artery, shown with white light (left) and near-infrared light (right). Cystic artery is scarred to the liver. (Image source Nova Szoka MD FACS, citation [22])

stay. The ICG group also had decreased Strassburg classification biliary ductal injuries, decreased common bile duct injury, and decreased mortality [24]. Although many studies have been performed to assess ICG use for elective cholecystectomy, few studies address the utility and benefits of ICG use in the acute surgical patient population [21–26].

For laparoscopic cholecystectomy, 5 mg of ICG is typically injected intravenously 1 h prior to intubation in our institution to allow accumulation of the fluorescent dye within the hepatobiliary structures. In a systematic review of the optimal techniques to administer ICG for laparoscopic cholecystectomy, the authors found that patients undergoing laparoscopic hepatic or biliary operations received ICG doses ranging between 0.02 and 0.25 mg/kg, typically 10 to 180 minutes prior to fluorescence imaging. This review found that a prolonged interval was optimal for fluorescence cholangiography but could not identify specific time intervals for the best visualization of biliary anatomy [19, 27]. Regarding the timing of ICG administration, one study found that administration of ICG 24 h prior to cholecystectomy led to better discrimination of bile ducts. Despite this, administration of ICG 24 h prior to surgery is not usually feasible, especially in the acute setting [27]. In another study, the authors found that a prolonged interval (at least 3 h) between ICG injection and intraoperative ICG fluorescence cholangiography resulted in better contrast between bile ducts and liver tissue.

In ICG fluorescence cholangiography, the binding of ICG to plasma proteins allows intraoperative identification of bile duct vasculature. This, in combination with a short half-life, makes ICG an excellent contrast agent for perfusion angiography. As the fluorescence is visualized only under near-infrared wavelengths, a near-infrared capable camera must be utilized. The system typically consists of an infrared fluorescence light source, light cable, camera control unit (CCU), camera head, coupler, 0° and 30° 10 mm laparoscopes, and surgical display unit. At the specific wavelength emitted by the light source (visible and near-infrared wavelength), excitation of the molecules allows for several millimeter penetration through the tissue to visualize the underlying biliary structures which the camera captures. Image signals captured by the camera are then transmitted from the laparoscope to the CCU for processing, and a final image is displayed on the monitor. A button on the camera head can be used to toggle from visible light to near-infrared image, and many recent camera platforms now display an overlay mode that combines white light and near-infrared images [21]. Following the appropriate equipment setup, the laparoscopic cholecystectomy should be performed in a standard fashion adhering to principles described by Strasberg [28] with the benefit of ICG fluorescence cholangiography to better visualize the biliary structures.

Although ICG fluorescence cholangiography has demonstrated feasibility and safety as an adjunct for identifying biliary anatomy, there are several challenges that surgeons commonly face. Due to hepatic clearance, the liver background remains a significant problem in ICG fluorescence cholangiography. One method to reduce the liver background signal while maintaining CBD signal stability is to inject the ICG 24 h prior to surgery. However, this is not feasible for same-day surgical patients or patients with acute cholecystitis where early surgical intervention is preferred [26]. Another limitation is the inability of ICG fluorescence cholangiography to detect common bile duct (CBD) stones. Additionally, due to limited depth of penetration (approximately 1 cm of light in the near-infrared spectrum) of ICG fluorescence cholangiography, patients (especially patients with obesity) with biliary structures that lay beneath a layer of (periductal) fat are more difficult to identify [26].

The utility of ICG fluorescence cholangiography to assess biliary anatomy has been studied extensively. With a goal for ICG to reduce bile duct injuries, the low incidence of bile duct injury makes the definitive determination of biliary injury risk reduction challenging. Additionally, comparisons between ICG fluorescence cholangiography and other modalities that visualize biliary anatomy have been assessed in multiple studies. Most notably, ICG utility for biliary visualization has been compared with IOC. In a meta-analysis comparing ICG fluorescence cholangiography and IOC, the authors reported that ICG led to improved visualization of the cystic duct (CD), CBD, CD-CBD junction, and common hepatic duct compared to IOC [29]. ICG fluorescence cholangiography can also be performed in addition to IOC if necessary. In another study aiming to assess the clinical impact of ICG fluorescence cholangiography, the authors interestingly found that the use of ICG in the acute care surgery population did not decrease operative time or need for change in operative plan (i.e., conversion to open, subtotal cholecystectomy) compared to patients who did not undergo ICG fluorescence cholangiography (6.7% vs. 4.3%, $P = 0.468$). This, however, is the first series looking at the use of ICG fluorescence cholangiography specifically in an acute care surgery population [30]. Although ICG has demonstrated the ability to optimize hepatobiliary anatomical visualization in a time- and cost-effective manner in elective settings, further well-powered, randomized, multicenter studies are necessary to determine the clinical impact of ICG use in cholecystectomy for both elective and acute care surgical populations.

ICG Dosing and Administration for Cholecystectomy

For use during cholecystectomy, after determining the patient has no contraindications to ICG such as an iodine allergy, we recommend intravenously injecting 2 ml of ICG 1 h prior to starting the operation; this provides sufficient time for the dye to be excreted into the bile and enable visualization of the bile ducts. To confirm the identification of the cystic artery, once the critical view of safety is obtained, injecting 3 ml of ICG will illuminate the vasculature approximately 30–45 s after IV administration (Video 11.1).

Coding for ICG Cholangiography

The current procedural terminology (CPT) code we use for coding ICG cholangiography is 47563.

Indocyanine Green Use in Mesenteric Ischemia

Accounting for approximately 1 in 1000 hospital admissions [31, 32], acute mesenteric ischemia (AMI) is a surgical emergency that is associated with very high in-hospital mortality rates of up to 63% [33]. The etiology of AMI can be classified into thrombotic and non-thrombotic causes. Thrombotic causes include arterial thromboembolism and venous thrombosis, while non-thrombotic causes, termed non-occlusive mesenteric ischemia (NOMI), result from low flow states, i.e., hypovolemia, cardiogenic shock, heart failure, or drugs that cause spasm of the vessels [33]. In a meta-analysis assessing mortality after acute primary mesenteric infarction, the authors reported that patients with arterial mesenteric infarction or NOMI are over three times more likely to die during the first hospital admission than those with venous mesenteric infarction [31–33]. Regardless of etiology, the lack of perfusion leads to intestinal ischemia causing transmural necrosis of the bowel wall, resulting in an overwhelming inflammatory response and death. Management of AMI includes gastrointestinal decompression, fluid resuscitation, antibiotics, and frequently, operative intervention. In the operating room, the goal of the intervention centers around assessment of bowel perfusion, restoration of blood flow to compromised bowel segments, and resection of nonviable bowel while leaving viable bowel intact to prevent short gut syndrome. One of the biggest challenges associated with surgery is the intraoperative assessment of bowel viability to determine the extent of resection. Patients who survive the initial operative intervention often

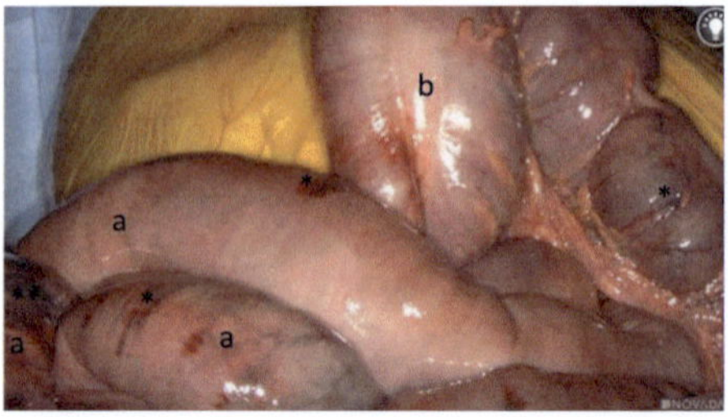

Fig. 11.4 White light view of small intestines (a) and large intestines (b) with patchy ischemia (*) and necrosis (**) present (Image source Nova Szoka MD FACS [34])

undergo multiple and extended bowel resections, which causes up to 30% of surviving patients to develop short gut syndrome, requiring permanent parenteral nutrition [32].

Traditionally, the assessment of bowel viability is performed with the surgeon's hands and eyes. The extent and severity of intestinal ischemia are determined through evaluation of the appearance of the bowel (color, distension), peristalsis, arterial pulsation of mesenteric arcades, and bleeding from cut surfaces. Bowel that appears dark compared to surrounding healthy bowel is presumed to be nonviable or ischemic and is often resected. Additionally, bowel loops that are distended with thinning of the bowel wall or perforated are also considered nonviable and are resected. In cases where the bowel is frankly necrotic, the decision to resect is obvious. However, bowel appearance does not definitively determine viability, i.e., "patchy," "dusky" bowel, causing surgeon hesitation when deciding on resection (Fig. 11.4). In situations where a significant portion of the bowel has already been removed, the fear of causing complications associated with extensive bowel resections (short gut syndrome, electrolyte derangements, intestinal failure, undernutrition) and the lack of objective information in assessing bowel viability create a dilemma for the surgeon. Often, this results in a damage control approach with temporary abdominal closure with the return to the intensive care unit (ICU) for further resuscitation and a plan for second-look laparotomy in 24–48 h to reassess bowel viability. Second-look laparotomies have the benefit of reducing morbidity and mortality in select patients, though they are also associated with risks including enteroatmospheric fistula formation, fascial

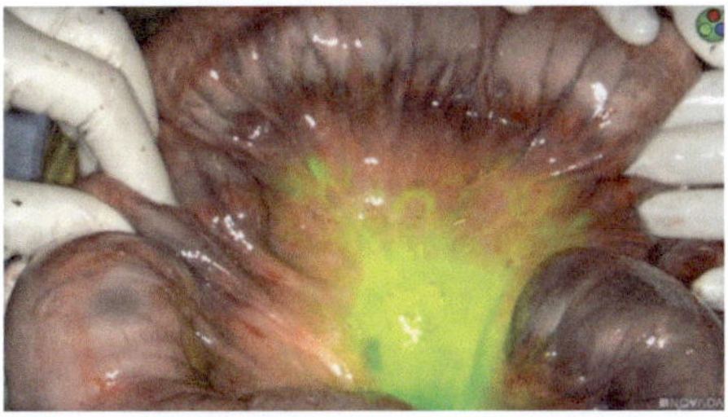

Fig. 11.5 Indocyanine green perfusion to the edge of small bowel mesentery but not beyond; no perfusion is present to the small bowel serosa. (Image source Nova Szoka MD FACS [34])

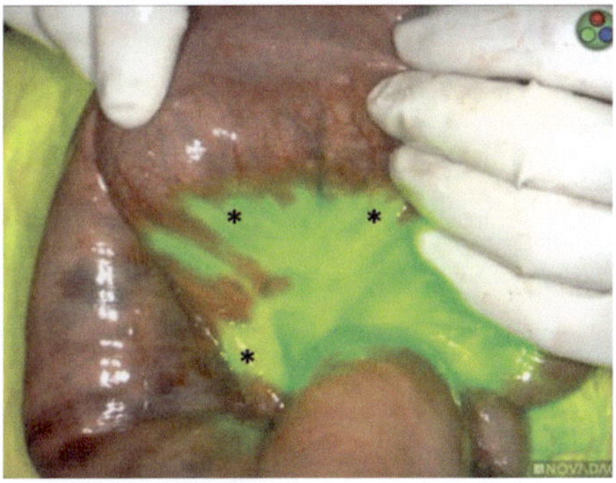

Fig. 11.6 Perfusion to the edge of small bowel mesentery but not beyond (*); the small bowel serosa has no perfusion to either micro- or macrovasculature. (Image source Nova Szoka MD FACS [34])

retraction, and hernia formation. With that said, several techniques, such as ICG fluorescence angiography, have been assessed to aid in the objective assessment of bowel viability (Figs. 11.5 and 11.6, Video 11.2).

ICG fluorescence angiography involves visualization of perfusion using intravenous administration of ICG, typically at doses of 2.5 to 7.5 mg. This is typically injected intravenously, after which a near-infrared camera system is utilized to assess vascular perfusion of the tissue. Perfusion of the bowel can typically be assessed approximately 45 s after ICG is injected (Figs. 11.7, 11.8, and 11.9). Although studies have been performed to quantitatively assess colonic perfusion using ICG angiography, a definitive criterion stratifying fluorescence intensity with different levels of perfusion or bowel viability has not been defined [35]. However, ICG angiography, despite being a qualitative assessment of bowel viability, provides the surgeon with more informa-

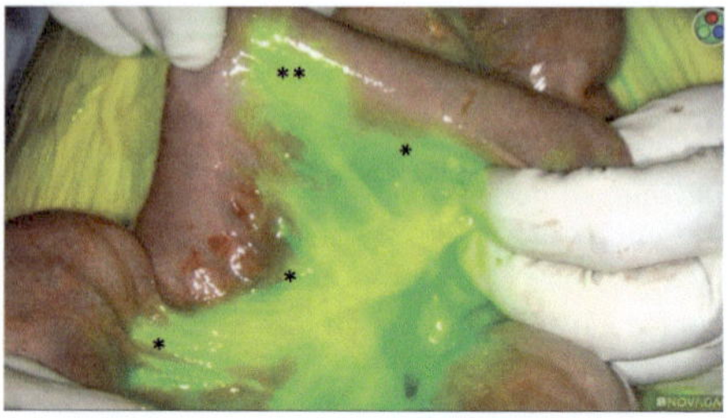

Fig. 11.7 Perfusion to the edge of small bowel mesentery but not beyond (*) and one focal area of small bowel perfusion (**). (Image source Nova Szoka MD FACS [34])

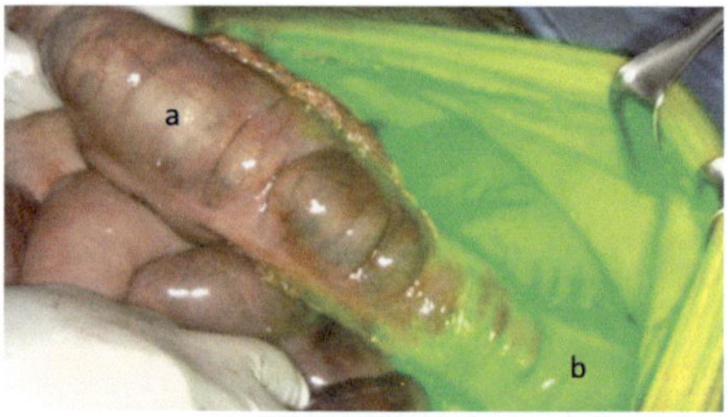

Fig. 11.8 Non-perfused/ischemic colon (a) proximal to the splenic flexure and well-perfused colon (b) distal to splenic flexure. (Image source Nova Szoka MD FACS [34])

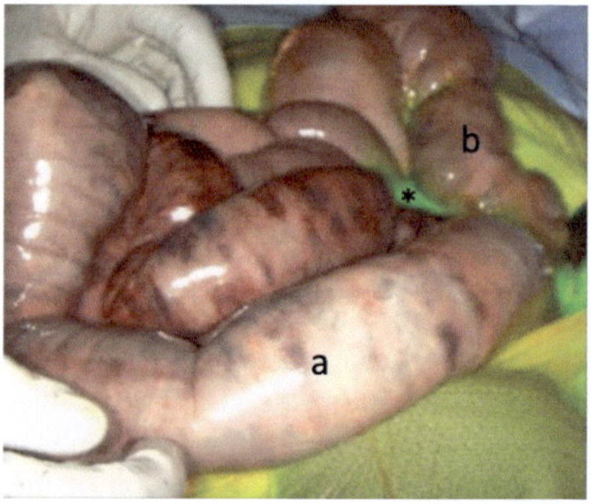

Fig. 11.9 Perfusion to the edge of mesentery but not beyond (*) indicating nonperfusion to the serosa and mucosa of small intestines (**a**) and large intestine (**b**). (Image source Nova Szoka MD FACS [34])

tion regarding microvascular tissue perfusion that is not available using traditional clinical assessment. In the setting of NOMI (i.e., small bowel obstructions (SBO), strangulated hernias, and volvulus), several case reports and studies have demonstrated the utility of ICG fluorescence angiography as an adjunct to evaluate bowel viability and perfusion of anastomosis [36–42]. In a retrospective analysis of 52 patients who underwent ICG fluorescence angiography during operative intervention for AMI, the authors report that ICG led to a major change in operative strategy in 11.5% of the patients resulting in a clinically significant benefit [43]. Albeit a retrospective study with small sample size, ICG fluorescence angiography use as an adjunct to optimize visualization and assessment of bowel viability yields significant potential in improving overall patient outcomes in a significantly morbid disease. Development of a definitive criterion, such as percent of maximal perfusion, to assist in quantitative analysis of bowel viability would synergistically contribute to the utility of ICG in the assessment of bowel viability in AMI [44].

Indocyanine Green Use in Small Bowel Obstruction

Small bowel obstructions (SBO) account for approximately 3% of emergency surgical admission. With significant morbidity and financial cost due to the recurrent nature of the disease, the etiology of SBO ranges from adhesive disease to hernias and malignancy [45]. In 2018, the American Association for the Surgery of Trauma (AAST) proposed a grading criteria for SBO ranging from grade I to V. Depending on the grading, management ranges from nonoperative management with gastrointestinal decompression, fluid and electrolyte resuscitation, and hypertonic contrast to expeditious surgery for higher grades of SBO [46, 47].

During operative intervention for SBO, assessment of bowel is essential to determine viability and extent of resection if indicated just as in mesenteric ischemia. The role of ICG in assessing bowel viability in SBO remains limited, with only a few case reports and series reporting its use [40, 48, 49]. The studies assessing the utility of ICG as an adjunct to laparoscopic surgery for SBO found that selective use of ICG in patients with concerns about vascular impairment provides a direct, objective tool for assessing bowel viability and supports the surgeon in the intraoperative decision-making process. The authors reported that the technique is reliable in determining bowel viability, assessing both vascular inflow and outflow, and permitting detection of the presence of irreversible ischemia and adequacy of venous drainage. Especially in laparoscopic surgery, the use of ICG overcomes limitations of laparoscopic assessment, which includes the lack of hand-eye inspection of mesenteric pulsation and a three-dimensional view [48–51]. ICG may also widen the proportion of procedures that can be completed minimally invasively by reducing the number of conversions due to the inability to fully assess compromised bowel; furthermore, it is proposed that the ability of ICG to aid in objective decision-making could translate into reduced medicolegal actions [50]. However, these studies were limited by a sample size of seven and 14 patients, respectively. The use of ICG for SBO in the emergent setting must also consider that arterial perfusion may be diminished during acute SBO due to splanchnic hypoperfusion resulting from shock, metabolic acidosis, and sepsis [52]. Therefore, the decision to resect bowel in borderline vascularity cases should depend not only on local bowel viability factors such as perfusion, pulsation, color, and peristalsis but also on general systemic factors such as the patient's overall condition.

Similarly, the use of ICG in the setting of SBO for prediction of bowel survival [53] and development of delayed ischemic small bowel stricture [54] has only been reported in animal studies and case reports, respectively. Due to the limited reports and lack of human studies, further studies are required to define the role of ICG in clinical practice and establish more objective perfusion thresholds to support intraoperative use in the SBO.

ICG Dosing and Administration for Evaluation of Bowel Perfusion

For use to assess bowel perfusion, after determining the patient has no contraindications to ICG such as an iodine allergy, the authors recommend injecting 2 ml (5 mg) of ICG, which will illuminate the vasculature approximately 30–45 seconds after IV administration. For open operations, near-infrared cart-based imaging systems, such as the Stryker SPY Elite System, or handheld imaging systems, such as the Stryker SPY-Portable Handheld

Imaging (PHI) system, can be used (Video 11.2). For laparoscopic or robotic operations, a minimally invasive camera system capable of near-infrared imagining can be used.

Coding for ICG Angiography

The current procedural terminology (CPT) codes that the authors' use for coding ICG angiography are CPT 44799 [unlisted procedure, small intestine] to evaluate the small bowel in an inpatient open surgery and CPT 44238 [unlisted laparoscopy procedure, intestine (except rectum)] to evaluate bowel in an inpatient laparoscopic surgery.

Indocyanine Green Use in Trauma

Trauma and traumatic injuries are a major cause of mortality and injury around the world. Injury results in over 150,000 deaths and over three million nonfatal injuries in the USA each year. Trauma is the third largest contributor to the global burden of disease around the world [55].

Reviewing the literature, the use of fluorescence guidance and ICG in trauma has been described in small case series for the diagnosis and treatment of various traumatic injuries of the following areas: ophthalmic injury [56], bowel trauma [57], and skin/soft tissue wounds [58]. Additionally, investigational research is being performed to better understand the use of contrast-enhanced near-infrared spectroscopy (NIRS) with indocyanine green (ICG) as a continuous, noninvasive bedside neuromonitoring tool for patients with traumatic brain injuries [59, 60]. However, large prospective studies on ICG use in trauma patients are warranted.

After ocular contusion, indocyanine green angiography allowed the analysis of various degrees of choroidal vascular damage, even in eyes that had no abnormality revealed by fluorescein angiography [56]. Following abdominal injury with bowel trauma, ICG angiography to evaluate bowel perfusion and anastomotic perfusion is described in a small case series. Specifically, ICG was used to evaluate the vascular perfusion in bowel segments with mesenteric lacerations and guide appropriate repair by assessing the viability of the anastomotic edges, as well as to diagnose microvascular injury in a segment of bowel that appeared macroscopically perfused under white light but was ischemic when viewed with ICG and near-infrared light.

In the setting of soft tissue wounds from high-energy mechanisms like ballistic or blast injuries or low-energy crush injuries, the ability to determine the zone of injury and thus establish initial debridement can be difficult when using the naked eye alone. Upon initial inspection, the area surrounding a traumatic wound may appear viable. These wounds often require repeated debridement and monitoring of the tissues to determine timing of reconstruction.

Fluorescence angiography has been described as a tool to assess skin flap necrosis in postmastectomy and breast reconstruction [61, 62]. However, little is reported on trauma patients, although its application in the assessment of skin perfusion can provide additional information compared to standard clinical evaluation. A review of traumatic and reconstruction cases at Walter Reed National Military Medical Center over a three-year period found that intraoperative fluorescence angiography modified the operative plan in almost 19% of cases. These modifications were seen with extremity flap reconstructions, avulsions, amputations and revisions, pedicle and free flap reconstructions, and gastrointestinal operations [63]. Another case series by Kamolz et al. examined the clinical impact of ICG video angiography to determine the extent of skin injury in a cohort of 40 patients [58]. The various injury mechanisms included mechanical crush, degloving, burn, and snakebite. Qualitative and quantitative analysis of the videos and images (evaluation of ICG uptake, steady-state distribution, and clearance of dye-marked blood from the injured area), in combination with the clinical assessment, provided additional information regarding the vascular patency of injured skin and allowed for more precise treatment plans.

With regard to the available literature, some of the most compelling data regarding the use of ICG and wound treatment comes from recent burn research [64, 65]. In their 2019 publication, Wongkietkachorn et al. conducted a prospective, multicentered, triple-blinded study to compare the accuracy of ICG angiography to that of clinical assessment of indeterminate burn wounds and whether said wounds were superficial second-degree versus deep second-degree burns. In the 30 burn sites that were assessed, the accuracy of ICG angiography was 100.0%, compared with 50.0% for clinical assessment ($p < 0.001$) [64]. In subsequent work, the same group used ICG assessment to recharacterize indeterminate depth burns as superficial second-degree burns or deep second-degree burns and mark the latter for excision; the deep second-degree burns were then excised in the operating room. Using ICG angiography for precise marking, the overall rate of short-term complete wound closure was 96.7%, and long-term complete wound closures at 2 months yielded 100.0% [65].

The following two clinical cases further demonstrate the use of ICG to evaluate tissue perfusion following traumatic injury. Figure 11.10 shows the skin of the forehead of an elderly female who fell while on anticoagulation. Fluorescence angiography was used in the operating room to assess the perfusion of her skin before (Fig. 11.11) and after (Fig. 11.12) the hematoma was evacuated. The use of fluorescence angiography in this case confirmed there was no need to resect the skin, and the patient made a full recovery with a good cosmetic result.

Morel-Lavallee lesions are an internal degloving of the superficial skin and subcutaneous fat from the fascial layers. High-

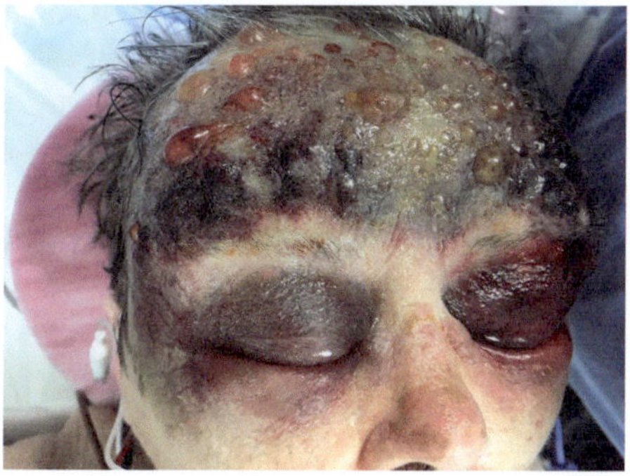

Fig. 11.10 Skin necrosis from a forehead hematoma with ecchymosis and blistering

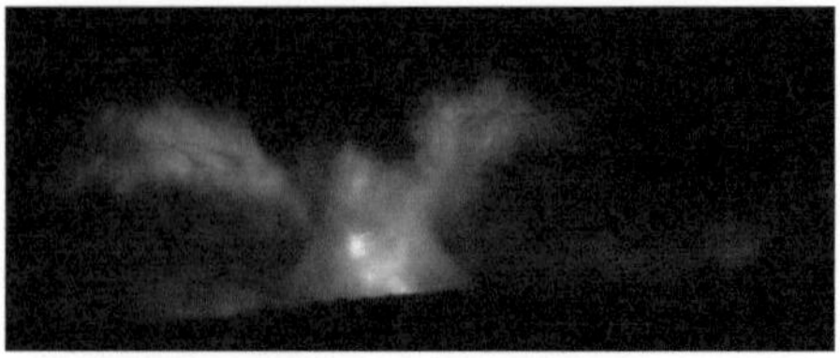

Fig. 11.11 Fluorescence angiography with perfusion evident to the skin on the eyes and but no skin perfusion above eyebrows prior to evacuation of the hematoma

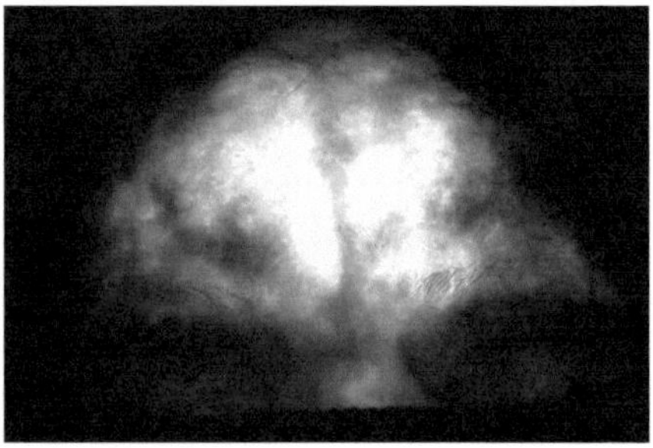

Fig. 11.12 Fluorescence angiography after evacuation of the forehead hematoma with restoration of perfusion

energy, blunt force trauma, or crush injuries are the leading causes of such defects, which commonly occur in the lower extremities but can occur anywhere on the body. Their management is varied and includes compression, drainage, and resection. Operative drainage and debridement are recommended for large lesions [66].

When debridement is required, ICG can guide the resection on devitalized tissue. A Morel-Lavallee lesion in a young patient ejected from a motor vehicle crash was managed operatively due to significant skin and fat necrosis present that required multiple operative takebacks and resections. The initial injury (Figs. 11.13 and 11.14) can be compared to subsequent resections (Fig. 11.15) and the final resection that was guided with ICG fluorescence angiography (Figs. 11.16, 11.17, and 11.18).

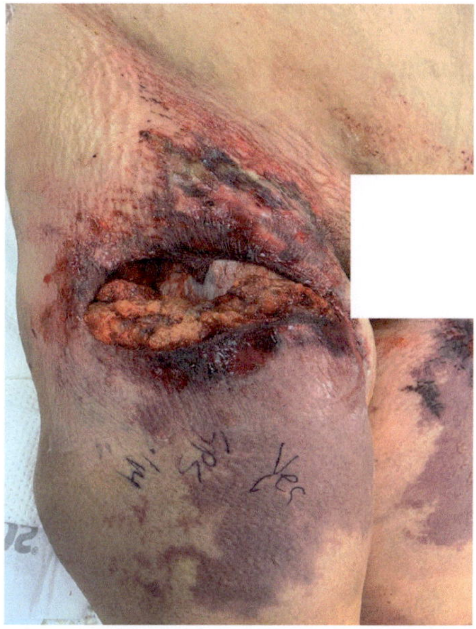

Fig. 11.13 A Morel-Lavallee lesion of the right lower extremity with disruption of the anterior skin and subcutaneous fat from the muscles of the thigh from the inguinal ligament to the knee

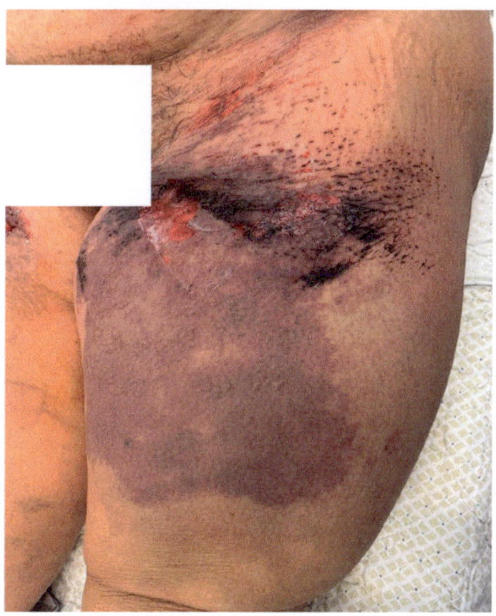

Fig. 11.14 A Morel-Lavallee lesion of the left lower extremity with disruption of the anterior skin and subcutaneous fat from the muscles of the thigh from the inguinal ligament to the knee

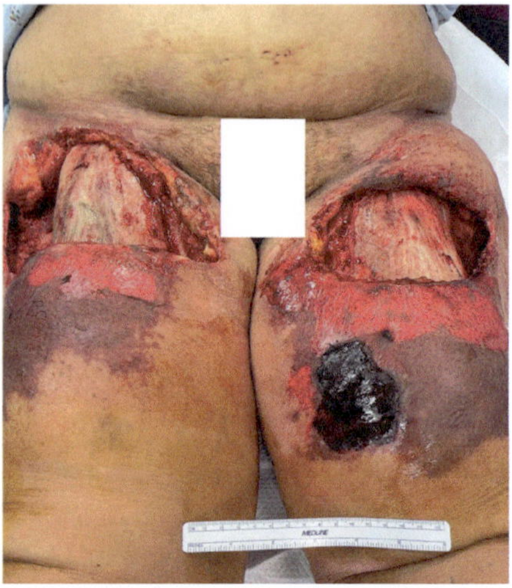

Fig. 11.15 Further demarcation of a Morel-Lavallee lesion of bilateral lower extremities prior to the use of fluorescence angiography

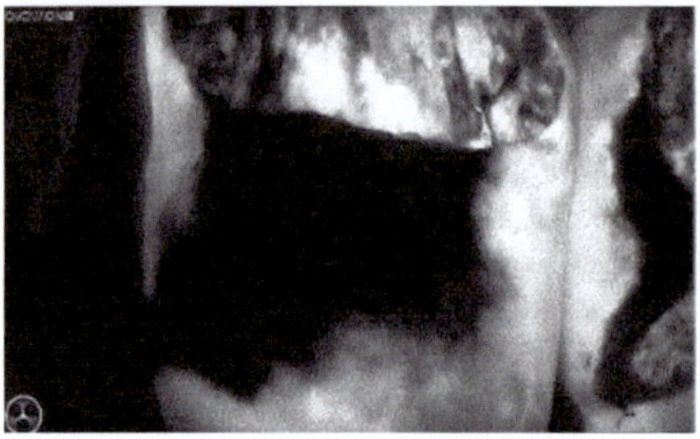

Fig. 11.16 Fluorescence angiography of the right lower extremity of a Morel-Lavallee lesion

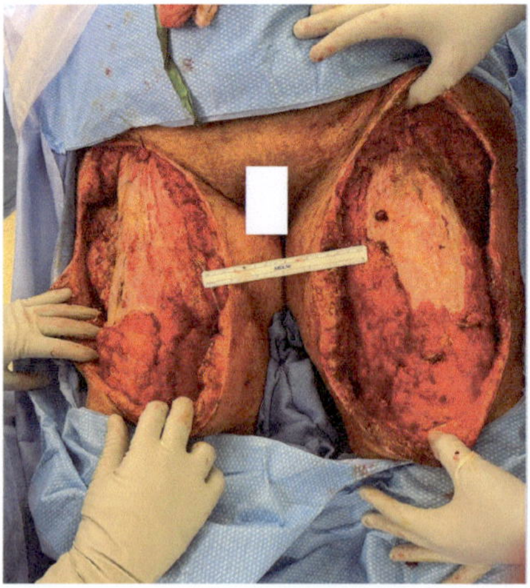

Fig. 11.17 Final resection to healthy tissue with the use of fluorescence angiography

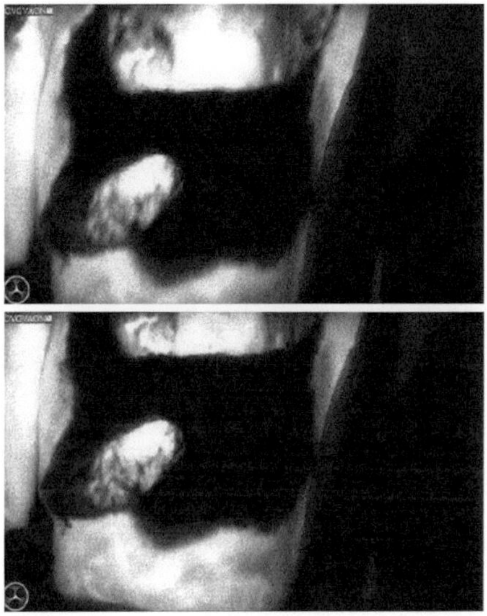

Fig. 11.18 Fluorescence angiography of a Morel-Lavallee lesion of the left lower extremity

ICG Dosing and Administration for Evaluation of Flap Perfusion

For use to assess skin flap perfusion, after determining the patient has no contraindications to ICG such as an iodine allergy, the authors recommend injecting 2 ml of ICG, which will illuminate the tissue flap for approximately 30–45 s after IV administration. As discussed above, for open operations, near-infrared cart-based imaging systems (Stryker SPY Elite) or handheld imaging systems (Stryker SPY-PHI) can be used.

Coding for ICG Evaluation of Skin and Soft Tissue

The current procedural terminology (CPT) code that the authors' use for coding ICG evaluation of skin and soft tissue as an inpatient procedure is CPT 15860 [intravenous injection of agent (e.g., fluorescein) to test vascular flow in flap or graft].

Fluorescence Guidance and Wound Care

Additional areas within acute care surgery where the use of fluorescence guidance is being actively studied include the evaluation of wound depth in chronic wounds, as well as assessment of tissue necrosis [67, 68]. With the profound angiothrombotic effects in necrotizing fasciitis and necrotizing soft tissue infection, the ability of ICG fluorescence to assess perfusion may aid in establishing the diagnosis and be used as an adjunct to help guide the extent of debridement. Although there are currently no published studies examining the use of ICG in necrotizing infection, there is an ongoing clinical trial (NCT04839302) assessing the use of ICG as a noninvasive modality for the diagnosis of necrotizing fasciitis. This study hypothesizes that ICG should demonstrate reduced fluorescence compared to the patient's unaffected tissues. If ICG fluorescence voids are characteristic of NF, ICG use could lead to a more accurate diagnosis of NF, leading to improved management and patient management outcomes.

Conclusion

The role of ICG in acute care and trauma surgery varies depending on the operative case and the patient. With regard to laparoscopic cholecystectomies, ICG has proven to be a time- and cost-effective adjunct to delineate biliary structures, though definitive benefit to prevent biliary injuries has yet to be identified. In the setting of mesenteric ischemia and bowel pathologies, ICG fluorescence video angiography yields significant potential as an adjunct to optimize visualization and assessment of bowel viability compared to the human eye and decrease the need for multiple returns to the operating room to evaluate bowel viability. Due to the high variability in the assessment of viability and the impact of physiologic derangements in these patients, further studies are required to refine the utility of ICG in these settings. In the setting of trauma patients, many case reports have proven the utility of ICG for assessing tissue viability. This has been further reinforced by research in burn patients, which is discussed in a separate chapter of this manual. Nevertheless, additional research with well-designed and appropriately powered studies is required to further validate the use of fluorescence guidance in the fields of acute care and trauma surgery.

Source of Funding None.

Conflict of Interest Dr. Szoka is the founder of Endolumik Inc.

References

1. Reinhart MB, Huntington CR, Blair LJ, Heniford BT, Augenstein VA. Indocyanine green: historical context, current applications, and future considerations. Surg Innov. 2016;23(2):166–75. https://doi.org/10.1177/1553350615604053.
2. Desmettre T, Devoisselle JM, Mordon S. Fluorescence properties and metabolic features of indocyanine green (ICG) as related to angiography. Surv Ophthalmol. 2000;45(1):15–27. https://doi.org/10.1016/s0039-6257(00)00123-5.
3. Cherrick GR, Stein SW, Leevy CM, Davidson CS. Indocyanine green: observations on its physical properties, plasma decay, and hepatic extraction. J Clin Invest. 1960;39:592–600. https://doi.org/10.1172/JCI104072.
4. Boni L, David G, Mangano A, Dionigi G, Rausei S, Spampatti S, et al. Clinical applications of indocyanine green (ICG) enhanced fluorescence in laparoscopic surgery. Surg Endosc. 2015;29(7):2046–55. https://doi.org/10.1007/s00464-014-3895-x.
5. van Manen LA-OX, Handgraaf HJM, Diana M, Dijkstra J, Ishizawa T, Vahrmeijer AA-O, et al. A practical guide for the use of indocyanine green and methylene blue in fluorescence-guided abdominal surgery. J Surg Oncol. 2018;118(2):283–300.
6. Alander JT, Kaartinen I, Laakso A, Patila T, Spillmann T, Tuchin VV, et al. A review of indocyanine green fluorescent imaging in surgery. Int J Biomed Imaging. 2012;2012:940585. https://doi.org/10.1155/2012/940585.
7. Benya R, Quintana J, Brundage B. Adverse reactions to indocyanine green: a case report and a review of the literature. Catheter Cardiovasc Diagn. 1989;17(4):231–3. https://doi.org/10.1002/ccd.1810170410.
8. Yamamoto M, Orihashi K, Nishimori H, Wariishi S, Fukutomi T, Kondo N, et al. Indocyanine green angiography for intra-operative assessment in vascular surgery. Eur J Vasc Endovasc Surg. 2012;43(4):426–32. https://doi.org/10.1016/j.ejvs.2011.12.030.

9. Holm C, Mayr M, Höfter E, Becker A, Pfeiffer UJ, Pfeiffer Mühlbauer W. Intraoperative evaluation of skin-flap viability using laser-induced fluorescence of indocyanine green. Br J Plast Surg. 2002;55(8):635–44.
10. Wirts CW, Cantarow A. A study of the excretion of bromsulphthalein in the bile. Am J Dig Dis. 1942;9(3):101–6. https://doi.org/10.1007/BF02996980.
11. Paumgartner G, Vasella DL, Herz R, Reichen J, Preisig R. Hepatic extraction of taurocholate and indocyanine green in patients with liver disease (author's transl). Z Gastroenterol. 1979;17(11):753–61.
12. Rowell LB, Blackmon JR, Bruce RA. Indocyanine green clearance and estimated hepatic blood flow during mild to maximal exercise in upright man. J Clin Invest. 1964;43:1677–90. https://doi.org/10.1172/JCI105043.
13. Marano A, Priora F, Lenti LM, Ravazzoni F, Quarati R, Spinoglio G. Application of fluorescence in robotic general surgery: review of the literature and state of the art. World J Surg. 2013;37(12):2800–11. https://doi.org/10.1007/s00268-013-2066-x.
14. Blythe J, Herrmann E, Faust D, Falk S, Edwards-Lehr T, Stockhausen F, et al. Acute cholecystitis - a cohort study in a real-world clinical setting (REWO study, NCT02796443). Pragmat Obs Res. 2018;9:69–75. https://doi.org/10.2147/POR.S169255.
15. Mangieri CW, Hendren BP, Strode MA, Bandera BC, Faler BJ. Bile duct injuries (BDI) in the advanced laparoscopic cholecystectomy era. Surg Endosc. 2019;33(3):724–30. https://doi.org/10.1007/s00464-018-6333-7.
16. Madni TD, Nakonezny PA, Imran JB, Taveras L, Cunningham HB, Vela R, et al. A comparison of cholecystitis grading scales. J Trauma Acute Care Surg. 2019;86(3):471–8. https://doi.org/10.1097/TA.0000000000002125.
17. Buddingh KT, Nieuwenhuijs VB, van Buuren L, Hulscher JB, de Jong JS, van Dam GM. Intraoperative assessment of biliary anatomy for prevention of bile duct injury: a review of current and future patient safety interventions. Surg Endosc. 2011;25(8):2449–61. https://doi.org/10.1007/s00464-011-1639-8.
18. Flum DR, Flowers C, Veenstra DL. A cost-effectiveness analysis of intraoperative cholangiography in the prevention of bile duct injury during laparoscopic cholecystectomy. J Am Coll Surg. 2003;196(3):385–93. https://doi.org/10.1016/S1072-7515(02)01806-9.
19. Vlek SL, van Dam DA, Rubinstein SM, de Lange-de Klerk ESM, Schoonmade LJ, Tuynman JB, et al. Biliary tract visualization using near-infrared imaging with indocyanine green during laparoscopic cholecystectomy: results of a systematic review. Surg Endosc. 2017;31(7):2731–42. https://doi.org/10.1007/s00464-016-5318-7.
20. Aoki T, Murakami M, Yasuda D, Shimizu Y, Kusano T, Matsuda K, et al. Intraoperative fluorescent imaging using indocyanine green for liver

mapping and cholangiography. J Hepatobiliary Pancreat Sci. 2010;17(5):590–4. https://doi.org/10.1007/s00534-009-0197-0.

21. Osayi SN, Wendling MR, Drosdeck JM, Chaudhry UI, Perry KA, Noria SF, et al. Near-infrared fluorescent cholangiography facilitates identification of biliary anatomy during laparoscopic cholecystectomy. Surg Endosc. 2015;29(2):368–75. https://doi.org/10.1007/s00464-014-3677-5.
22. Bronikowski D, Lombardo D, DeLa OC, Szoka N. Robotic subtotal cholecystectomy in a geriatric acute care surgery patient with super obesity. Case Rep Surg. 2021;2021:9992622. https://doi.org/10.1155/2021/9992622.
23. Ambe PC, Plambeck J, Fernandez-Jesberg V, Zarras K. The role of indocyanine green fluoroscopy for intraoperative bile duct visualization during laparoscopic cholecystectomy: an observational cohort study in 70 patients. Patient Saf Surg. 2019;13:2. https://doi.org/10.1186/s13037-019-0182-8.
24. Broderick RC, Lee AA-O, Cheverie JN, Zhao B, Blitzer RR, Patel RJ, et al. Fluorescent cholangiography significantly improves patient outcomes for laparoscopic cholecystectomy. Surg Endosc. 2021;35(10):5729–39.
25. Ankersmit M, van Dam DA, van Rijswijk AS, van den Heuvel B, Tuynman JB, Meijerink W. Fluorescent imaging with indocyanine green during laparoscopic cholecystectomy in patients at increased risk of bile duct injury. Surg Innov. 2017;24(3):245–52. https://doi.org/10.1177/1553350617690309.
26. Boogerd LSF, Handgraaf HJM, Huurman VAL, Lam HD, Mieog JSD, van der Made WJ, et al. The best approach for laparoscopic fluorescence cholangiography: overview of the literature and optimization of dose and dosing time. Surg Innov. 2017;24(4):386–96. https://doi.org/10.1177/1553350617702311.
27. Verbeek FP, Schaafsma BE, Tummers QR, van der Vorst JR, van der Made WJ, Baeten CI, et al. Optimization of near-infrared fluorescence cholangiography for open and laparoscopic surgery. Surg Endosc. 2014;28(4):1076–82. https://doi.org/10.1007/s00464-013-3305-9.
28. Strasberg SM, Brunt LM. Rationale and use of the critical view of safety in laparoscopic cholecystectomy. J Am Coll Surg. 2010;211(1):132–8.
29. Lim SH, Tan HTA, Shelat VG. Comparison of indocyanine green dye fluorescent cholangiography with intra-operative cholangiography in laparoscopic cholecystectomy: a meta-analysis. Surg Endosc. 2021;35(4):1511–20. https://doi.org/10.1007/s00464-020-08164-5.
30. Turcotte J, Leydorf SD, Ali M, Feather C, Klune JR. Indocyanine green does not decrease the need for bail-out operation in an acute care surgery population. Surgery. 2021;169(2):227–31. https://doi.org/10.1016/j.surg.2020.05.045.

31. Bryski MG, Frenzel Sulyok LG, Kaplan L, Singhal S, Keating JJ. Techniques for intraoperative evaluation of bowel viability in mesenteric ischemia: a review. Am J Surg. 2020;220(2):309–15. https://doi.org/10.1016/j.amjsurg.2020.01.042.
32. Tilsed JV, Casamassima A, Kurihara H, Mariani D, Martinez I, Pereira J, et al. ESTES guidelines: acute mesenteric ischaemia. Eur J Trauma Emerg Surg. 2016;42(2):253–70. https://doi.org/10.1007/s00068-016-0634-0.
33. Adaba F, Askari A, Dastur J, Patel A, Gabe SM, Vaizey CJ, et al. Mortality after acute primary mesenteric infarction: a systematic review and meta-analysis of observational studies. Color Dis. 2015;17(7):566–77. https://doi.org/10.1111/codi.12938.
34. Szoka N, Kahn M. Acute-on-chronic mesenteric ischemia: the use of fluorescence guidance to diagnose a nonsurvivable injury. Case Rep Surg. 2022;2022:5459774. https://doi.org/10.1155/2022/5459774.
35. Son GM, Kwon MS, Kim Y, Kim J, Kim SH, Lee JW. Quantitative analysis of colon perfusion pattern using indocyanine green (ICG) angiography in laparoscopic colorectal surgery. Surg Endosc. 2019;33(5):1640–9. https://doi.org/10.1007/s00464-018-6439-y.
36. Mehdorn M, Ebel S, Kohler H, Gockel I, Jansen-Winkeln B. Hyperspectral imaging and indocyanine green fluorescence angiography in acute mesenteric ischemia: a case report on how to visualize intestinal perfusion. Int J Surg Case Rep. 2021;82:105853. https://doi.org/10.1016/j.ijscr.2021.105853.
37. Nakagawa Y, Kobayashi K, Kuwabara S, Shibuya H, Nishimaki T. Use of indocyanine green fluorescence imaging to determine the area of bowel resection in non-occlusive mesenteric ischemia: a case report. Int J Surg Case Rep. 2018;51:352–7. https://doi.org/10.1016/j.ijscr.2018.09.024.
38. Irie T, Matsutani T, Hagiwara N, Nomura T, Fujita I, Kanazawa Y, et al. Successful treatment of non-occlusive mesenteric ischemia with indocyanine green fluorescence and open-abdomen management. Clin J Gastroenterol. 2017;10(6):514–8. https://doi.org/10.1007/s12328-017-0779-3.
39. Nitori N, Deguchi T, Kubota K, Yoshida M, Kato A, Kojima M, et al. Successful treatment of non-occlusive mesenteric ischemia (NOMI) using the HyperEye Medical System™ for intraoperative visualization of the mesenteric and bowel circulation: report of a case. Surg Today. 2014;44(2):359–62. https://doi.org/10.1007/s00595-013-0503-y.
40. Guerra F, Coletta D, Greco PA, Eugeni E, Patriti A. The use of indocyanine green fluorescence to define bowel microcirculation during laparoscopic surgery for acute small bowel obstruction. Color Dis. 2021;23(8):2189–94. https://doi.org/10.1111/codi.15680.
41. Ryu S, Hara K, Goto K, Okamoto A, Kitagawa T, Marukuchi R, et al. Fluorescence angiography vs. direct palpation for bowel viability evaluation with strangulated bowel obstruction. Langenbeck's Arch Surg. 2021;407:797. https://doi.org/10.1007/s00423-021-02358-8.

42. Daskalopoulou D, Kankam J, Plambeck J, Ambe PC, Zarras K. Intraoperative real-time fluorescence angiography with indocyanine green for evaluation of intestinal viability during surgery for an incarcerated obturator hernia: a case report. Patient Saf Surg. 2018;12:24. https://doi.org/10.1186/s13037-018-0173-1.
43. Karampinis IA-O, Keese M, Jakob J, Stasiunaitis V, Gerken A, Attenberger U, et al. Indocyanine green tissue angiography can reduce extended bowel resections in acute mesenteric ischemia. J Gastrointest Surg. 2018;22(12):2117–24.
44. Wongkietkachorn A, Surakunprapha P, Winaikosol K, Waraasawapati S, Chaiwiriyakul S, Eua-Angkanakul K, Wongkietkachorn N, et al. Indocyanine green dye angiography as an adjunct to assess indeterminate burn wounds: a prospective, multicentered, triple-blinded study. J Trauma Acute Care Surg. 2019;86(5):823–8.
45. Miller G, Boman J, Shrier I, Gordon PH. Etiology of small bowel obstruction. Am J Surg. 2000;180(1):33–6. https://doi.org/10.1016/s0002-9610(00)00407-4.
46. Pekmezci S, Saribeyoglu K, Korman U. Guidelines for management of small bowel obstruction. J Trauma. 2009;66(4):1262. https://doi.org/10.1097/TA.0b013e318198d6a2.
47. Hernandez MC, Haddad NN, Cullinane DC, Yeh DD, Wydo S, Inaba K, et al. The American Association for the Surgery of Trauma Severity Grade is valid and generalizable in adhesive small bowel obstruction. J Trauma Acute Care Surg. 2018;84(2):372.
48. Nakashima KA-O, Ryu S, Okamoto A, Hara K, Ishida K, Ito R, et al. Intestinal blood flow evaluation using the indocyanine green fluorescence imaging method in a case of incarcerated obturator hernia: a case report. Asian J Endosc Surg. 2021;14(3):565–9.
49. Nakashima K, Ryu S, Okamoto A, Hara K, Ishida K, Ito R, et al. Usefulness of blood flow evaluation with indocyanine green fluorescence imaging during laparoscopic surgery for strangulated bowel obstruction: a cohort study. Asian J Surg. 2021;45:867. https://doi.org/10.1016/j.asjsur.2021.08.020.
50. Urbanavičius L, Pattyn P, de Putte DV, Venskutonis D. How to assess intestinal viability during surgery: a review of techniques. World J Gastrointest Surg. 2011;3(5):59–69. https://doi.org/10.4240/wjgs.v3.i5.59.
51. Choudhry AJ, Haddad NN, Rivera M, Morris DS, Zietlow SP, Schiller HJ, et al. Medical malpractice in the management of small bowel obstruction: a 33-year review of case law. Surgery. 2016;160(4):1017–27. https://doi.org/10.1016/j.surg.2016.06.031.
52. Mathew R. Caution warranted in use of indocyanine green fluorescence in laparoscopic evaluation of microcirculation in acute small bowel obstruction. Color Dis. 2021;23(9):2472. https://doi.org/10.1111/codi.15757.

53. Matsui A, Winer JH, Laurence RG, Frangioni JV. Predicting the survival of experimental ischaemic small bowel using intraoperative near-infrared fluorescence angiography. Br J Surg. 2011;98(12):1725–34. https://doi.org/10.1002/bjs.7698.
54. Iinuma Y, Hirayama Y, Yokoyama N, Otani T, Nitta K, Hashidate H, et al. Intraoperative near-infrared indocyanine green fluorescence angiography (NIR-ICG AG) can predict delayed small bowel stricture after ischemic intestinal injury: report of a case. J Pediatr Surg. 2013;48(5):1123–8. https://doi.org/10.1016/j.jpedsurg.2013.03.067.
55. Trauma TAAftSo: AAST - trauma facts. 2022. https://www.aast.org/resources/trauma-facts. Accessed 2022.
56. Kohno T, Miki T, Hayashi K. Choroidopathy after blunt trauma to the eye: a fluorescein and indocyanine green angiographic study. Am J Ophthalmol. 1998;126(2):248–60. https://doi.org/10.1016/s0002-9394(98)00153-6.
57. Afifi I, Abdelrahman H, El-Faramawy A, Mahmood I, Khoschnau S, Al-Naimi N, et al. The use of Indocyanine green fluorescent in patients with abdominal trauma for better intraoperative decision-making and less bowel anastomosis leak: case series. J Surg Case Rep. 2021;2021(6):rjab235. https://doi.org/10.1093/jscr/rjab235.
58. Kamolz L-P, Andel H, Auer T, Meissl G, Frey M. Evaluation of skin perfusion by use of indocyanine green video angiography: rational design and planning of trauma surgery. J Trauma Acute Care Surg. 2006;61(3):635.
59. Ganau M, Iqbal M, Ligarotti GKI, Syrmos N. Breakthrough in the assessment of cerebral perfusion and vascular permeability after brain trauma through the adoption of dynamic indocyanine green-enhanced near-infrared spectroscopy. Quant Imaging Med Surg. 2020;10(11):2081–4. https://doi.org/10.21037/qims-20-905.
60. Forcione M, Chiarelli AM, Davies DJ, Perpetuini D, Sawosz P, Merla A, et al. Cerebral perfusion and blood–brain barrier assessment in brain trauma using contrast-enhanced near-infrared spectroscopy with indocyanine green: a review. J Cereb Blood Flow Metab. 2020;40(8):1586–98. https://doi.org/10.1177/0271678X20921973.
61. Pruimboom T, Schols RM, Van Kuijk SMJ, Van der Hulst R, Qiu SS. Indocyanine green angiography for preventing postoperative mastectomy skin flap necrosis in immediate breast reconstruction. Cochrane Database Syst Rev. 2020;4:CD013280. https://doi.org/10.1002/14651858.CD013280.pub2.
62. Liu EH, Zhu SL, Hu J, Wong N, Farrokhyar F, Thoma A. Intraoperative SPY reduces post-mastectomy skin flap complications: a systematic review and meta-analysis. Plast Reconstr Surg Glob Open. 2019;7(4):e2060-e. https://doi.org/10.1097/GOX.0000000000002060.
63. Green JM 3rd, Sabino J, Fleming M, Valerio I. Intraoperative fluorescence angiography: a review of applications and outcomes in war-related

trauma. Mil Med. 2015;180(3 Suppl):37–43. https://doi.org/10.7205/MILMED-D-14-00632.

64. Wongkietkachorn A, Surakunprapha P, Winaikosol K, Waraasawapati S, Chaiwiriyakul S, Eua-angkanakul K, et al. Indocyanine green dye angiography as an adjunct to assess indeterminate burn wounds: a prospective, multicentered, triple-blinded study. J Trauma Acute Care Surgery. 2019;86(5):823.
65. Wongkietkachorn A, Surakunprapha P, Jenwitheesuk K, Eua-Angkanakul K, Winaikosol K, Punyavong P, et al. Indocyanine green angiography precise marking for indeterminate burn excision: a prospective, multicentered, double-blinded study. Plast Reconstr Surg Glob Open. 2021;9(4):e3538. https://doi.org/10.1097/GOX.0000000000003538.
66. Singh R, Rymer B, Youssef B, Lim J. The Morel-Lavallee lesion and its management: a review of the literature. J Orthop. 2018;15(4):917–21. https://doi.org/10.1016/j.jor.2018.08.032.
67. Sen CK, Ghatak S, Gnyawali SC, Roy S, Gordillo GM. Cutaneous imaging technologies in acute burn and chronic wound care. Plast Reconstr Surg. 2016;138(3 Suppl):119S–28S. https://doi.org/10.1097/PRS.0000000000002654.
68. Fang C, Wang K, Zeng C, Chi C, Shang W, Ye J, et al. Illuminating necrosis: from mechanistic exploration to preclinical application using fluorescence molecular imaging with indocyanine green. Sci Rep. 2016;6:21013. https://doi.org/10.1038/srep21013.

12 Use of Fluorescence Guidance in Pediatric Surgery

Stefan Scholz, Hannah Rinehardt, Ranjeet S. Kalsi, Jillian C. Jacobson, and Samir Pandya

S. Scholz (✉)
Division of Pediatric General and Thoracic Surgery, Department of Surgery, University of Pittsburgh School of Medicine, UPMC Children's Hospital of Pittsburgh, Pittsburgh, PA, USA
e-mail: stefan.scholz@chp.edu

H. Rinehardt
Department of Surgery, University of Pittsburgh School of Medicine, Pittsburgh, PA, USA
e-mail: Rinehardthn@upmc.edu

R. S. Kalsi
Division of Pediatric General and Thoracic Surgery, Department of Surgery, University of Pittsburgh Medical Center/Children's Hospital of Pittsburgh, Pittsburgh, PA, USA
e-mail: rkalsi@myhealthsystem.org

J. C. Jacobson
Department of Surgery, UT Southwestern Medical Center, Dallas, TX, USA
e-mail: Jillian.Jacobson@UTSouthwestern.edu

S. Pandya
Division of Pediatric Surgery, Department of Surgery, UT Southwestern Medical Center, Dallas, TX, USA
e-mail: Samir.Pandya@UTSouthwestern.edu

N. Szoka et al. (eds.), *The SAGES Manual of Fluorescence-Guided Surgery*, https://doi.org/10.1007/978-3-031-40685-0_12

Introduction

Fluorescence-guided surgery (FGS) is a medical imaging technique used to detect fluorescently labeled structures during surgery. Camera systems that detect near-infrared (NIR) light not visible to the human eye guide can provide information about anatomy or tissue viability to the surgeon through real-time visualization in the operating field. Indocyanine green (ICG) is the only NIR fluorescent agent currently approved for human use. ICG is a safe, water-soluble compound that received FDA approval in the 1950s. Despite the bright green color of the reagent to the human eye, its use as a contrast agent is based on its robust fluorescence in the NIR range. Applications for ICG in the pediatric world are emerging. ICG can be used for arteriogram, venogram, or general perfusion assessment of tissues such as intestinal perfusion before anastomosis or soft tissue pedicles or flaps during plastic surgery. ICG is exclusively cleared by the liver and the bile duct and is applied in fluorescence cholangiography. When administered as an intradermal, ICG gets protein-bound and confined to clearance via the lymphatic system, which is used to facilitate sentinel lymph node detection and biopsy.

Scientific Basis

Indocyanine green (ICG) is the only NIR fluorescent agent currently approved for human use. ICG is a water-soluble, anionic, amphiphilic tricarbocyanine (776 Da) that rapidly binds to plasma proteins in the body. ICG was first produced in 1955 by Kodak Research Laboratories and received FDA approval for retinal angiography in 1959. Historically, it has been used to measure cardiac output and hepatic function and for retinal angiography. After intravenous application, ICG remains largely protein-bound in the intravascular space and is cleared exclusively by the liver. ICG allows multiple uses due to its short intravascular half-life of 150 to 180 s. From the vasculature, ICG undergoes uptake by hepatocytes and hepatic clearance. The dye can then be detected within minutes, peaks over the course of hours, and continues for over a day after typical dosing. When administered intradermally, ICG gets protein-bound and confined to clearance via the lymphatic system, which is used to facilitate sentinel lymph node detection and biopsy.

ICG is excited using 780–810 nm near-infrared (NIR) radiation and emits fluorescence at 830–840 nm. The specific wavelength of light emitted is visualized with a specialized camera system [1]. The emitted fluorescence can also be detected by a photodynamic eye system or SPY portable handheld imager by Stryker® (Kalamazoo, MI) in open operations. The da Vinci robot (Intuitive Surgical®, Sunnyvale, CA) is equipped with a NIR camera called Firefly Mode to visualize ICG fluorescence. The half-life of ICG is 3–5 min. It can be injected locally (for urologic or lymphatic indications) or intravenously. The usual dose is 0.25–0.5 mg/kg and can be re-dosed with caution. ICG is safe with rare adverse events. ICG should not be used in patients with an iodine or shellfish allergy given the risk for anaphylaxis. IV ICG circulates in the bloodstream, is taken up by the liver, is excreted into the bile, and then travels into the bowel loops. ICG can offer real-time identification of cancer tissues, insight into intestinal viability, and visualization of lymphatic structures and assist with fine dissection around biliary structures to prevent injury. Fluorescence visualizes ICG up to a depth of 5–10 mm deep. Structures deeper than 10 mm cannot be visualized with ICG alone [1]. ICG offers a great deal of promise for a variety of indications. In pediatric patients, ICG is still an emerging technology with mounting evidence that will be reviewed here. A review of ICG in the pediatric population was published in 2021 in *Frontiers in Pediatrics* with analysis of 64 articles including a total of 664 pediatric patients [2]. There were no major adverse reactions reported from any of the studies related to ICG, and the individual studies lacked power due to low sample size. Additional details of some of the articles will be discussed here. ICG has been shown to be safe in pediatric patients, but more investigation is needed to evaluate the risks and benefits of using this technology in each operation where it may offer utility.

Side Effects and Complications

Fluorescence-guided surgery (FGS) has been used across multiple fields with significantly improved outcomes and decreased complications. Throughout its history, ICG has maintained a high safety index with a favorable side effect profile and severe complications are infrequent. Albeit rare, adverse reactions to ICG have been reported throughout the literature. These include dyspnea, wheezing, cough, cyanosis, headache, urticaria, nausea, pruritus, hypotension, cough, anxiety, laryngospasm, laryngobronchospasm, pulmonary congestion, facial edema, anaphylactic shock, and death [3, 4]. More recently, Shafy et al. evaluated intraoperative administration of ICG in 100 patients, who ranged in age from 5 days old to 31 years old, with a median age of 12 years. Procedures included laparoscopic cholecystectomy, colorectal surgery, sagittal anorectovaginourethroplasty, transanal pull-through for Hirschsprung's disease, perineal reconstruction, exploratory laparotomy, and renal procedures. ICG was administered IV to all patients with a median dose of 1.1 mL (2.5 mg/mL ICG solution). In this cohort, they found no hemodynamic or respiratory alterations due to ICG usage. None of these patients needed treatment with an anticholinergic drug, a vasoactive drug, or a drug to treat bronchospasm [5]. Recent literature continues to describe uncommon adverse reactions such as anaphylactic shock to ICG [6, 7]. ICG contains sodium iodide and there are rare reports about anaphylaxis or urticarial reactions (1:10,000, as reported by the manufacturer). Iodine uptake studies should not be performed for a week following its use. Lastly, there is no data to support or contraindicate use in pregnant or nursing mothers.

Overall, the present incidence of side effects and complications of ICG in the pediatric population is low, and FGS is an asset to the surgeon.

Dosing and Timing Guide for Pediatric Applications

Summary of doses and timing of indocyanine green by indication.

Application	Dose (concentration)	Timing
Laparoscopic cholecystectomy	Children: 2.5 mg (2.5 mg/mL) Infants: 0.1 mg/kg mg (2.5 mg/mL)	Just prior to trocar placement to 18 h prior[a]
Biliary atresia	0.5 mg/kg (2.5 mg/mL)	24 h prior to operation
Bowel viability/tissue perfusion	Small children: 0.05–0.1 mg/kg (0.125–0.25 mg/mL) Older children: 5 mg (2.5 mg/mL)	Just prior to assessment
Hepatoblastoma primary	0.5 mg/kg (not specified)	4 days prior to procedure
Hepatoblastoma lung metastases	0.5 mg/kg (not specified)	24 h prior to procedure
Identification of pulmonary segment	0.5 mg/kg (not specified)	Following ligation of segmental artery
Thoracic duct	0.5 mg/kg (5 mg/mL)	Injection into inguinal lymph node 60 min prior
Ureter localization	2.5 mg/mL 2 mL per ureter	Cystoscopic-guided retrograde intraureteral ICG

[a]There is a variation in reports. Earlier injection may lead to increased fluorescence of the biliary tree at time of operation

Fluorescence-Guided Surgery Best Practices

After initial government regulatory clearances, growth of a new technology is industry-driven with training being peer-to-peer or industry-to-user, often without significant professional society guidance but rather with an approach driven by local or individual best practice principles. The intraoperative use of ICG and fluorescence imaging is growing exponentially. Many variations continue to exist in how ICG is dosed and administered, and in many other technical aspects of its use. Numerous other issues remain, such as indications and contraindications for its use, whether it still should be considered experimental, or whether specific patient consent is required.

No current consensus guidelines exist regarding a wide spectrum of, partly very basic, areas important for fluorescence-guided surgery: indications for use, ICG dose and concentration, administration route and timing, re-administration and timing, status as a routine versus still experimental procedure, patient education and consent, physician training, and other technical considerations. Professional societies such as the International Society for Fluorescent Guided Surgery (ISFGS) should play a role helping to ensure that standards are established and met, and the future interventional procedures continue to be done with safe and effective technology or systems, also for pediatric patients. Standards for outcomes and data-driven applications should lead to established best practices in the field.

Pediatric Surgery Clinical Applications

Hepatobiliary Surgery

Hepatobiliary surgery in pediatric patients offers the most obvious use of ICG given its excretion into bile and resultant immunofluorescence of the biliary tree. Hepatobiliary surgery using ICG can be limited by bowel interference if given intraoperatively. Due to this concern, ICG is given at least 72–96 h prior to the hepatic procedure operation and 2 to 4 h prior to ICG fluorescence cholangiography (ICG-FC). This allows the biliary structures to strongly fluoresce without concurrent bowel fluorescence. ICG-FC has utility in the pediatric population for cholecystectomy, Kasai portoenterostomy, and hepatic resection for hepatoblastoma or other liver tumors. As with other uses of ICG in pediatric patients, the evidence is limited to mostly case series. We will review the current evidence and discuss techniques in using ICG for hepatobiliary surgery in the pediatric population.

Laparoscopic Cholecystectomy

ICG-FC is of particular interest for use in laparoscopic cholecystectomy in pediatric patients. As in adult patients undergoing cholecystectomy, the major complication surgeons aim to avoid is common bile duct (CBD) injury. Attaining the critical view of safety (CVS) helps avoid error traps leading to CBD injury and is successful at preventing CBD injury in most cases. The rate of CBD injury in pediatric laparoscopic cholecystectomy remains at approximately 0.5% despite widespread use of laparoscopy and CVS [8]. ICG-FC is of particular interest as it allows for visualization of the extrahepatic biliary tree including the common hepatic duct (CHD), cystic duct, and CBD. The CHD and CBD are not dissected out in a routine laparoscopic cholecystectomy to avoid injury and devascularization. The penetrance of ICG up to 10 mm allows for visualization of the CHD and CBD without dissecting out the structures (Fig. 12.1). This has potential as a major adjunct in this operation for pediatric patients, especially those with an anticipated difficult cholecystectomy such as patients with obesity or prolonged symptoms.

There have been multiple case series in the literature regarding the utility of ICG-FC in laparoscopic cholecystectomies in pediatric patients. In 2019, a case series demonstrated successful use of ICG-FC in five pediatric patients [9]. Another case series in 2019 of ICG-FC in 15 laparoscopic cholecystectomies is compared to 200 cases at the same center where ICG-FC was not utilized [10]. The analysis demonstrated shorter operative time and no complications in the ICG-FC group. There were four complications and two bile duct injuries in the non-ICG-FC group. In this series, ICG was given 18 h pre-op which minimized liver interference. A 2020 series compared 31 laparoscopic cholecystectomies using ICG-FC with 68 cases without the use of ICG-FC [11]. In this series, ICG was injected intraoperatively which led to a high amount of liver interference. However, analysis still demonstrated shorter operative times, lower costs, and no complications associated with ICG-FC in these patients. Another series in 2020 demonstrated successful use in 12 cases, and a final series in 2021 demonstrated use in 13 cases [12, 13]. Larger studies of prospective randomized trials are needed to determine ICG-FC impact on CBD injuries in pediatric laparoscopic cholecystectomy.

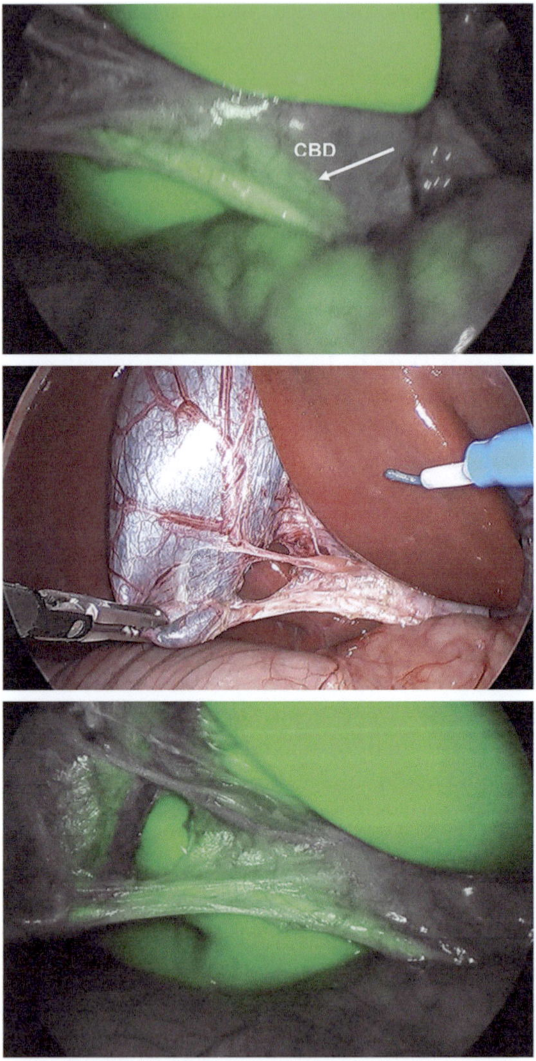

Fig. 12.1 Laparoscopic ICG view of the common bile duct and the cystic duct (arrow) reassuring the surgeon of the intraoperative biliary anatomy during laparoscopic cholecystectomy (top image). The critical view of safety was achieved (middle image) and the bile duct anatomy again confirmed by ICG-cholangiogram (bottom picture)

Kasai Portoenterostomy

An exciting potential use for ICG-FC in the pediatric population is patients undergoing Kasai portoenterostomy (KPE) for biliary atresia (BA). This operation requires extensive dissection of the fibrous cone at the porta hepatis. For a successful biliary drainage into the enteric system, it is important to ensure patency of the bile duct at the level of transection of the porta hepatis as well as ensuring that exposed micro bile ducts are not inadvertently closed during anastomosis. ICG-FC can serve as an adjunct to ensure patency at the level of transection and can even identify hilar micro bile ductules. Use of ICG in an operation for BA does demonstrate background liver fluorescence as ICG is not normally excreted as in patients with a normal biliary tract (Fig. 12.2). In BA cases, ICG application can be useful to aid the laparoscopic or open cholangiogram (Fig. 12.3), for complete dissection of the fibrous cone of the porta hepatis, and possibly as a predictor of postoperative drainage if bile accumulates in a Gelfoam patch during preparation of the Roux limb (Fig. 12.2).

The use of ICG-FC in KPE was demonstrated in two case series. The first in 2015 involved five pediatric patients undergoing KPE in whom ICG-FC was utilized after injection 24 h pre-op [14]. Serum and feces bilirubin were measured to ensure adequate drainage of bile into the enteric system on postoperative day 3. This demonstrated higher post-op normalization of bilirubin in the ICG-FC group compared to 35 patients without ICG use. A second case series in 2019 again demonstrated successful use of ICG-FC in ten patients undergoing KPE [15]. Data should continue to be collected with long-term follow-up in order to determine long-term patency of KPE using ICG-FC and impact on progression to revision or transplantation.

Hepatic Resection

Hepatic resection for hepatoblastoma (HB) is an important use of ICG-FC as aggressive surgical resection of the primary tumor and metastases improves survival [16]. ICG-FC has been utilized in

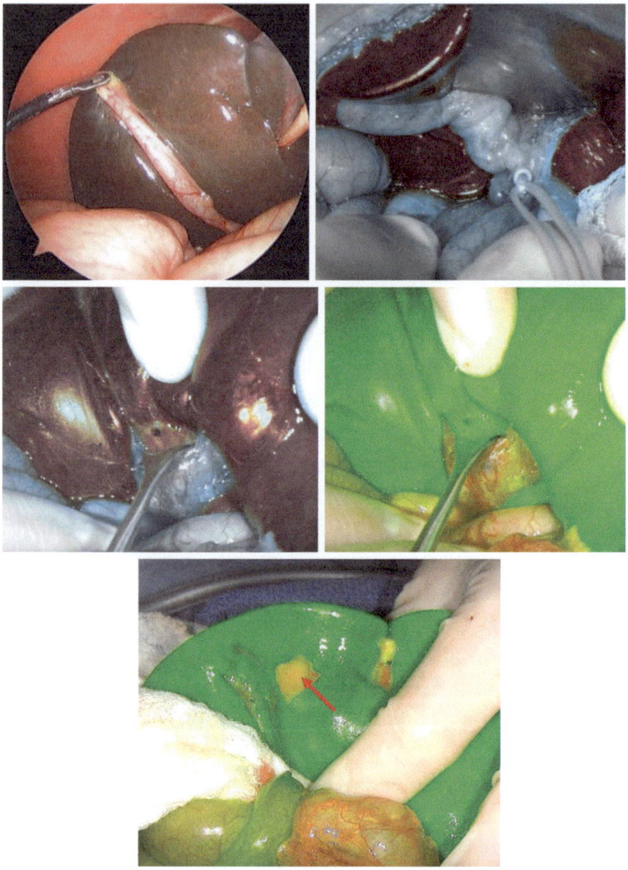

Fig. 12.2 Infant with biliary atresia. Laparoscopic view of the small and empty gallbladder and the liver (upper left). Color-segmented fluorescence (CSF) mode where any extrahepatic bile would appear red, similar to the liver, no bile outside of the liver, vessel loop around common bile duct (upper right). CSF mode (left) and overlay mode (right) of the cleanly dissected liver surface in the area of the fibrous cone; the portal vein is retracted (middle). The lower image shows a Gelfoam piece (arrow), which was left in the port hepatic, while the jejuno-jejunostomy of the Roux limb was fashioned. Note the missing fluorescence in the Gelfoam. The predictive value of this finding remains unclear

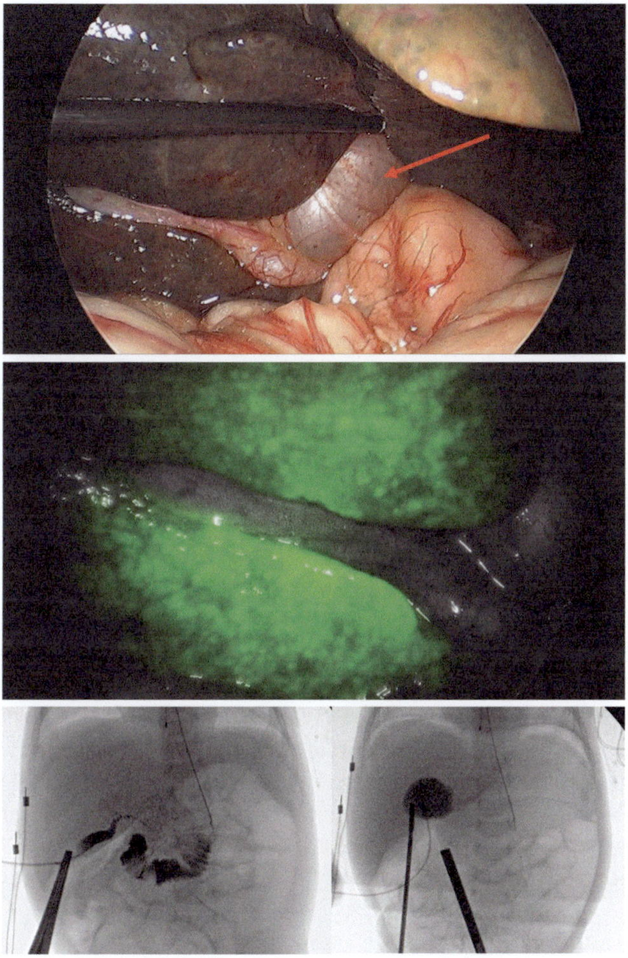

Fig. 12.3 Laparoscopic view of an infant with cystic biliary atresia thought to be a choledochal cyst on prenatal ultrasounds. Note the cirrhotic liver, the small and empty gallbladder, and the cyst in the porta hepatis (top). No fluorescence could be seen in the gallbladder or the porta hepatic cyst, virtually excluding the diagnosis of choledochal cyst (middle). A formal laparoscopic cholangiogram showed a patent bile system from the gallbladder to the duodenum but did not contrast the common hepatic duct or the intrahepatic bile system (bottom left). A laparoscopic cholangiogram into the sorta hepatic cyst showed an isolated cyst not connected the the bile system (bottom right). An open Kasai procedure, which was successful to achieve bile drainage

adult patients with hepatocellular carcinoma (HCC) with successful results. In 2009, a study demonstrated that ICG is particularly useful for liver tumors as ICG is not excreted normally from HCC as with normal liver parenchyma leading to retained ICG in the tumor for days following IV administration [16]. This novel discovery demonstrates the special utility of ICG in improving R0 resection of primary and metastatic liver tumors. After successful use in HCC in adult patients, use was extended to assess utility in HB for pediatric liver resections. In 2015, a cases series of three pediatric patients with HB demonstrated successful use of ICG in detecting viable recurrent and metastatic disease [17]. Two 2019 case series of 13 operations in one and ten operations in another demonstrated successful use of ICG in hepatic resections for HB [18, 19]. In a 2021 series, 29 patients had 25 liver resections with 13 specimens positive for HB on pathology [20]. Twelve of 13 were ICG-avid yielding a sensitivity of 92%. Ten lesions were ICG-avid with no evidence of HB yielding on specificity of 17%. This demonstrates the high level of false positivity utilizing ICG for detection of malignant tissue in the liver. Most false positives were due to liver inflammation or steatosis. Two other series in 2021 demonstrated efficacy of ICG-FC in resection of HB in 19 and 11 hepatic resections [21, 22]. ICG-FC has been utilized to resect several hepatoblastoma tumors with a high sensitivity and low specificity. This demonstrates that surgeons should be aware of the possibility of false positivity when utilizing this technology. ICG-FC is safe and sensitive in hepatic resection for HB. Larger prospective trials with long-term follow-up are needed to determine impact of ICG-FC on early recurrence and overall survival.

Intestinal Resection and Anastomosis

The serum protein-bound nature of ICG lends itself to fluorescence angiography (ICG-FA) which can serve a useful adjunct for assessing intestinal viability in the operating room. ICG is administered IV and assessed with NIR fluorescence in real time. Surgeons often rely on gross visual assessment of color and bleeding edges in addition to palpable mesenteric pulse to predict blood flow to intestinal segments that may be resected or used for anastomosis. ICG-FA can serve as an intraoperative tool to improve the accuracy in the prediction of bowel viability and preventing anastomotic stricture or dehiscence (Fig. 12.4).

In pediatric patients, the previous experience with ICG-FA in the literature is extremely limited but is promising for future use. Potential uses of ICG-FA in pediatric patients include malrotation with midgut volvulus, necrotizing enterocolitis, inflammatory bowel disease (IBD), Hirschsprung's disease (HD), cloaca, and anorectal malformations. The existing literature includes a single case report of one pediatric patient with small bowel volvulus requiring small bowel resection [23]. In this case, ICG-FA was concerning for malperfusion despite a normal gross appearance. The patient developed a late stricture requiring reoperation. In 2014, a swine model of mesenteric ischemia demonstrated utility of ICG-FA [24]. This was followed by a case series the same year of 24 adult patients who underwent colorectal surgery for a variety of pathologies (diverticular disease, colorectal cancer, and IBD) [25]. There were zero anastomotic leaks in this study after satisfactory analysis with intraoperative ICG-FA. The only study evaluating ICG-FA in pediatric colorectal surgery is a 2020 case

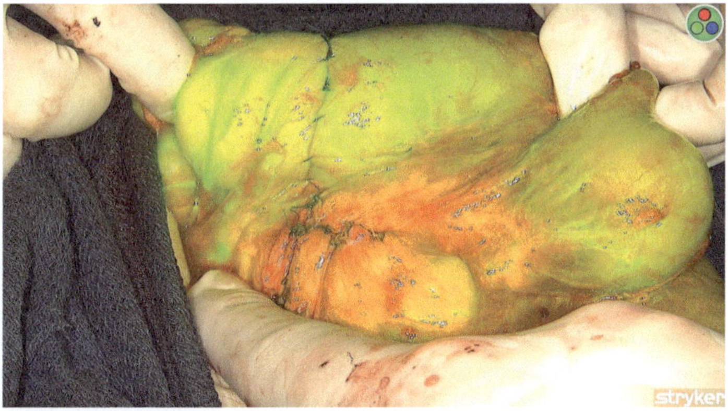

Fig. 12.4 Overlay mode of SPY Portable Handheld Imaging System, a handheld solution for perfusion assessment of a handsewn colonic end-to-end anastomosis after bowel resection

series including 13 patients to assess viability of tissue used for vaginal reconstruction or for bowel anastomosis [26]. Thirteen patients underwent operation for HD, nine patients with cloaca, and one patient with an anorectal malformation. The use of ICG-FA changed the operative plan in four patients and led to a decrease in leak rate from 7.4% to 3.5%.

There is great potential for ICG-guided surgery to improve outcomes for pediatric surgeons in colorectal surgery, esophageal surgery, necrotizing enterocolitis, volvulus, and tennis intestinal anastomoses but the data is only evolving at this time.

Pediatric Urology Clinical Applications

FGS has also played a valuable role in pediatric urology with applications in ureteral identification, partial and complete nephrectomies, deroofing of renal cysts, and varicocelectomy. FGS is believed to make these procedures faster and safer with continued improvement over time as the application of ICG expands.

Intraoperative Ureteral Identification

Intraoperative identification of the ureter can be challenging in complex pediatric surgery procedures such as pelvic or retroperitoneal masses and cysts, complex colorectal surgery, redo operations, or obesity. Ureteral identification can be more challenging during laparoscopic surgery. ICG offers real-time identification of ureter during surgery especially for laparoscopic or robotic cases. Intraureteral ICG has been administered for evaluation and identification of the ureters. In adults, this has been used in the setting of urothelial carcinoma and robotic sacrocolpopexy [27]. Similarly, an intraureteric ICG administration has been performed in pediatric patients undergoing a partial nephrectomy [28]. Additionally, ICG is extensively used to assess vasculature after administration via a peripheral IV. Thus, ICG can be valuable at the time of ureteral reconstruction by allowing the identification of diseased areas of the ureter, which would be marked by significant devascularization [27].

Our own protocol at the Children's Hospital of Pittsburgh includes that the patient is placed in the lithotomy position. A pediatric urologist or surgeon performs cystoscopy and places a 5 Fr open-tip ureteral catheter under fluoroscopy guidance. The tip is placed before or at the level of the renal pelvis. ICG is injected (2.5 mg/mL; 2 mL per ureter) and catheter clamped for the duration of the operation. Fluorescence-guided detection of the ureter using ICG is safe and ready for use and there is no systemic exposure. The disadvantage is that a ureteral catheter needs to be placed at the start of the procedure. ICG allows to "flip the switch to see the ureter" at any time during the procedure (Fig. 12.5).

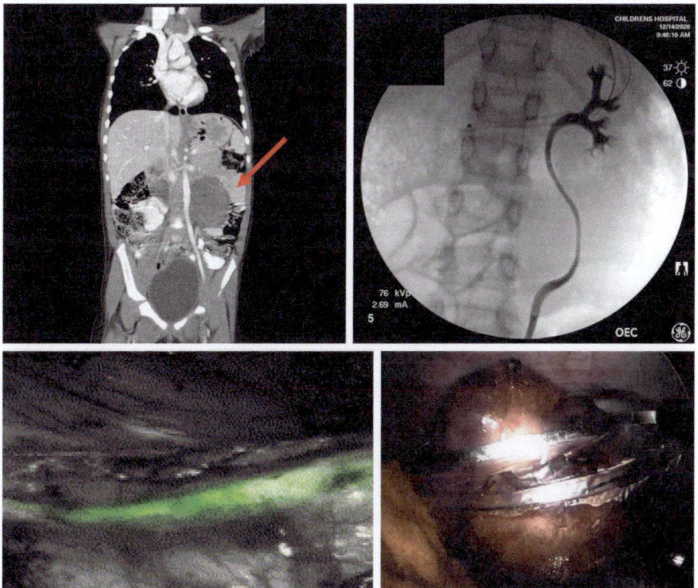

Fig. 12.5 A 6-year-old girl with large left retroperitoneal mass displacing the ureter. A ureteral catheter was placed and ICG injected. The ureter could be easily identified during the laparoscopic removal of the mass and spared

Partial Nephrectomies

A wide array of literature is published regarding the benefits of using FGS in pediatric and adult partial nephrectomies. ICG is often considered a valuable tool when challenging vascular anatomy is encountered. Diana et al. performed a sizeable multi-institutional study evaluating robot-assisted partial nephrectomies in adults after administering ICG, allowing for the evaluation of kidney perfusion intraoperatively. Their group evaluated 318 patients between 2010 and 2016 (with a median age of 61). This group performed partial nephrectomies for tumors with an average size of 30 mm, administering 2–4 mL of 2.5 mg/mL solution of ICG before or after renal artery clamping. They noted that the peak fluorescence occurred 2 min after injection. They performed a logistic regression analysis and found that ICG use independently predicted achieving the trifecta (warm ischemia time <25 min, no positive surgical margins, and absence of Clavien-Dindo > two complications) [28].

Similar success has been seen extensively in the realm of pediatric surgery. Because ICG allows for faster identification of intraoperative landmarks, it facilitates accurate dissection and resection, resulting in shorter operating times. Over four years, Esposito et al. performed a laparoscopic partial nephrectomy on 22 patients with a median age of 3.9 years for a nonfunctioning moiety of a duplex kidney. They prepared ICG to a concentration of 2.5 mg/mL and administered it via peripheral IV to identify the vasculature or ureteral catheter to delineate the ureter. Structures of interest became apparent within 30–60 s of the ICG injection. They administered the ICG in three phases: first, to identify ureter pre-op; second, to identify the vasculature; and lastly, to identify the avascular kidney after ligation. Overall, they found that ICG near-infrared laparoscopic partial nephrectomy led to shorter operative times [29]. In the same way, a separate group has used ICG to evaluate the vascular anatomy intraoperatively during a robot-assisted laparoscopic heminephrectomy. Herz et al. evaluated and operated on six patients with a median age of 4.75, diagnosed with an obstructed duplex ectopic ureter, duplex ureterocele, or duplex kidney. Interestingly, in certain patients, they found that segmental arterial mapping was more informative than a preoperative 3D CTA. Importantly, they noted avoidance of a critical complication by applying this system. They administered 0.5–1 mL of ICG (concentration of 2.5 mg/mL) and then waited 30–60 s, and then they activated the near-infrared fluorescence system [30]. Abdelhafeez et al. used ICG (administering a dose of 1.5 mg/kg the day before surgery) in eight pediatric patients with a median age of three years (seven had Wilms tumor and one had epithelioid angiomyolipoma). They routinely found that the normal kidney had higher uptake (fluorescence) compared to the kidney tumor, making the differentiation of renal tumor from normal kidney both easier and safer [31].

ICG allows for safer surgery because it allows for clear visualization of the ureter, clearly displays the blood supply, and demarcates the tissues of interest, more precisely identifying the area of excision. Furthermore, ICG allows for identifying abnormal vascular anatomy and permits early detection of iatrogenic injury. Interestingly, despite making surgery faster and safer, Esposito et al. found FGS resulted in a comparable length of stay, analgesia, and time to initiating feeding [29].

Varicocele

A common intervention that employs the use of FGS is varicocele repair. Esposito et al. evaluated lymphography with ICG (1 mg of ICG injected directly into the left testicle with the fluorescence of the lymphatics becoming apparent after 20–30 s). They evaluated 25 patients with an average age of 13.7, whom all had symptomatic high-degree varicoceles associated with testicular hypotrophy [32]. In a separate cohort, the same group performed a Palomo varicocelectomy in 30 boys with an average age of 16.7. Again, the lymphatic vessels demonstrated fluorescence and were accordingly spared [33]. In both cohorts, there was no conversion to open surgery, and at the time of follow-up, there was neither recurrence of the varicocele nor evidence of a postoperative hydrocele. They also evaluated their postoperative complications using ICG compared to isosulfan blue based on their previously published data, and they found that complications were lower in the ICG group. However, they were not statistically significant [34].

Cyst Deroofing

Comparably, there is great utility to using ICG in renal cyst deroofing. Fluorescence highlights the normal renal parenchyma within seconds, while the avascular cyst remains nonfluorescent. Because of excellent visualization, significant bleeding or damage was prevented, especially to the renal parenchyma [35]. Furthermore, the postoperative complication rate was lower and statistically different when evaluating renal cyst deroofing with ICG to no ICG [34].

Pediatric Thoracic Surgery Clinical Applications

ICG is also a valuable tool when performing thoracic surgery, allowing for the performance of a segmentectomy or wedge resection over a lobectomy or a more extensive resection. Sekine et al. evaluated the utilization of ICG for thoracoscopic segmentectomy in ten patients with a mean age of 72.8 with early lung cancer. To isolate pulmonary segments, ICG was injected directly into the implicated bronchioles. The target segments of the lung were then identified using the ICG fluorescence, obviating the intersegmental lines and planes. This is especially valuable in patients with emphysema, who may have anatomy with distorted segmental planes because of emphysematous changes. The segments were removed with either a stapler or electric cautery. They report that ICG did not shorten OR time or result in decreased blood loss [36]. Another group has also used ICG to evaluate the feasibility of using FGS to treat lung cancer. Tarumi et al. performed VATS segmentectomy with ICG to identify segmental fissures for lung cancer. However, unlike the previous group who had administered ICG directly into the bronchi, Tarumi et al. administered a dose of 3 mg/kg of ICG via peripheral IV after ligating the dominant pulmonary arteries. They noted fluorescence within minutes and marked the visceral pleura with electrocautery. This allowed them to maintain an excellent surgical view and identify the intersegmental line without re-inflating the lung [37].

FGS may hold a significant benefit in treating congenital pulmonary lesions. Shirota et al. evaluated and treated a group of pediatric patients with lung cysts. The authors used a thoracoscopic approach to treat congenital lung cysts, employing ICG (administering one to five IV 0.01 to 0.02 mg/kg injections) to perform a segmentectomy or partial lung resection instead of a traditional lobectomy [38]. The ICG allowed them to visualize blood flow easily. This would be a valuable tool for treating small lesions across multiple lobes.

Another group applied FGS in the setting of a thoracoscopic lobectomy to treat two patients with a mean age of 15.5 months, one with a congenital cystic adenomatoid malformation and the other with pulmonary extra-lobar sequestration. ICG (0.25 mg/mL/kg IV intraoperatively) was used to identify a plane between the cystic malformation and normal long parenchyma to elucidate the resection margins [12]. The same group also applied the utility of FGS in the setting of a thoracoscopic lymph node biopsy. Specifically, this was used in one six-year-old boy suspected of lymphoma with a noted malignant 2 cm hilar lymph node. ICG (0.5 mg/mL/kg intraparenchymal lung injection) facilitated identification and subsequent removal of the pathological lymph node [12].

Lung Metastasis

In the realm of pediatric surgery, hepatoblastoma frequently metastasizes to the lungs. Cho et al. evaluated 22 cases of hepatoblastoma; six of these patients had lung metastasis at the time of surgery, and two of these patients underwent thoracic surgery using ICG. ICG allowed for easy identification of the pulmonary lesions, given the lack of ICG uptake in normal lung tissue [21]. Yamamichi et al. evaluated a smaller cohort of three patients with hepatoblastoma: one with a primary tumor, another with a recurrent tumor, and a third with a metastatic lesion to the lung. All patients were evaluated with ICG (administered 0.5 mg/kg IV three to four days before the operation). In the patient with lung metastases, they were able to identify multiple metastatic lesions by positive fluorescence, and all were completely resected. These fluorescence-positive lesions were found to be consistent with hepatoblastoma tumor cells. They were able to resect a total of 24 nodules. Unfortunately, the patient subsequently developed recurrent lung metastases two months later and died of recurrent tumors [17]. Yoshida et al. used ICG (0.5 mg/kg the day prior to surgery) for lung metastasectomy of hepatoblastoma. In 16 patients (age range between 4 months and 11 years), they performed 61 ICG-assisted pulmonary metastasectomies (obtaining a total of 373 specimens). With ICG, their sensitivity was 92.6%, specificity 2.9%, PPV 71.4%, and NPV 13%. They noted they had 100 ICG-positive specimens histologically negative for tumor, noting changes consistent with regression of a metastatic tumor and non-specific changes of fibrosis and hemorrhage, representing ICG labeling of pulmonary tissue with abnormal blood flow [39].

Chylothorax

ICG can also be a valuable tool for evaluating the lymphatic system. Thus, it may have additional value in evaluating patients with chylothoraces. Shibasaki et al. used ICG lymphography to evaluate lymphatic dysfunction in patients with congenital chylothoraces, evaluating ten neonates with a median age of 29.5 days after birth and median gestation age of 35.5 weeks. They administered subcutaneous ICG (0.25 mg in the second interdigit regions of the hands and the first interdigit space of the feet). They then evaluated the trunk and extremities using an infrared camera. This allowed them to determine normal lymphatic flow from abnormal or pathological lymphatic flow, grading the lymphatic dysplasia as mild, moderate, severe, or lymphatic hypoplasia. Images and videos were obtained immediately, 3–6 h after, and 24 h after ICG [40]. Another group shared their experience using ICG to evaluate a six-month-old patient with Noonan syndrome. They used ICG to evaluate lymphatic flow after the patient developed bilateral chylothoraces after cardiac surgery. They administered 0.05 mL intradermally of 0.25 mg/mL of ICG to each dorsal foot, waited 1 h, administered a dose to each hand, and waited for 20 min. They noted diffuse uptake into the lymphatics of bilateral lower extremity lymphatics and inguinal lymph nodes. However, no meaningful fluorescence was appreciated in the upper extremities. They believe the impaired visualization of abnormal drainage pattern may have been secondary to the known lymphatic aberrations in patients with Noonan syndrome. More specifically, they believe they could not use this system to determine the site of leakage in the thoracic duct because of congenital lymphatic abnormalities or high cardiovascular pressures [41]. However, ICG may still hold value in evaluating patients with normal lymphatic anatomy or those patients with localized aberrant lymphatic anatomy.

Chylothoraces may occur not only after cardiac surgery but also after pediatric thoracic surgery. Postoperative chylothorax after esophageal atresia/tracheoesophageal fistula surgical repair is a severe complication. Another group used ICG and near-infrared fluorescence imaging to identify and ligate sites of chylous leakage. They performed ICG-NIR in ten patients (seven patients had their thoracic duct evaluated at the initial operation, and three patients were taken back to OR after conservative management failed to treat chylothorax) after awaiting 1 h after inter-toe ICG injection (0.025 mg of ICG). Using this system, they were able to identify the thoracic duct or the site of lymphatic leakage in each patient, and they appropriately sutured or ligated the area of concern [42]. Overall, despite the potential benefits, given the small numbers in pediatric cases, it is difficult to strongly recommend FGS for thoracic surgery at present. Additional ongoing research may change this in the future.

Pediatric Liver Transplant Surgery

Hepatic necrosis is a feared complication of liver transplant surgery. However, hepatic necrosis may also result in patients undergoing surgery for gastric adenocarcinoma. Lee, J.H., et al.

identified 31 patients with aberrant left hepatic arteries undergoing resection for gastric adenocarcinoma. The aberrant artery was identified in 19% preoperatively; the remainder of cases were found intraoperatively. They were able to appropriately preserve the aberrant left hepatic artery in cases where there was inadequate flow based on the fluorescence, thus preventing hepatic necrosis [43].

As discussed elsewhere, ICG cholangiography is a valuable tool when performing hepatobiliary surgery. Mizuno, S., et al. evaluated 108 patients who underwent a living donor liver transplantation. They reported that only 18 of the 108 underwent ICG cholangiography (0.025 mg/mL directly into the bile duct through a transcystic tube), and bile leakage occurred in 5.6% of the recipients, strictures occurred in 13.9% of the recipients, and 2.7% of the donors developed a biliary leak. However, the 18 that underwent ICG cholangiography did not develop any biliary complications in donors or recipients [44].

Quintero, J., et al. evaluated the use of ICG in the setting of liver failure. Pediatric acute liver failure is uncommon but results in death or the need for a liver transplant in 25–50% of cases. Indocyanine green plasma disappearance rate (ICG-PDR) may be used to predict the degree of liver damage. ICG-PDR was obtained upon admission when ALF was diagnosed, and it was repeated every 24 h until ALF resolution, liver transplant, or death. A lower ICG-PDR score translated to significant irreversible liver damage. The sensitivity was 92.3% and specificity was 97.1%, which are higher than King's College and Clichy's criteria. Additionally, PPV was 92.3%, and NPV was 97% [45].

In liver transplantation, patency of the hepatic artery, portal vein, and bile duct is important. Panaro, F., et al. used ICG fluorescence to evaluate the degree of perfusion in six liver transplantation procedures. Specifically, they aimed to evaluate the graft bile duct perfusion to determine the most appropriate area of duct transection prior to creating the anastomosis. They intravenously administered ICG (0.5 mg/kg) after liver transplant and revascularizing the organ. In 47 s, they were able to identify and differentiate the vascularized portion from the non-vascularized portion of the graft bile duct, which allowed them to determine where to transect the duct and create the appropriate anastomosis. They noted anomalies in two of their six patients regarding the vascularization of the bile duct, requiring them to resect the bile duct. By 12-month follow-up, none of the patients had any biliary complications [46]. Portal vein thrombosis is another severe complication that may lead to graft failure. Portal vein thrombosis is a severe complication after liver transplantation. Kawaguchi, Y., et al. report the case of a 60-year-old female who underwent a living donor liver transplant and immediately underwent ICG (0.93 mg) fluorescence imaging, which demonstrated inadequate perfusion of segment 4. Subsequent ultrasound demonstrated a thrombus in the portal vein of segment 4, which they were able to be removed successfully [47].

Thus, ICG has a broad range of uses in the setting of liver transplant in addition to the evaluation of hepatic artery, portal vein, and bile ducts intraoperatively. ICG may be used for preoperative evaluation of potential surgical candidates as a dynamic study as opposed to other scoring systems as well as for the preoperative evaluation of graft, allowing surgeons to exclude grafts that may be high risk or ineffective. Intraoperatively, it may play an additional role in liver mapping, cholangiography, tumor visualization, and partial liver graft evaluation. Additionally, it may allow for early identification of thrombosis, kinking, or changes in flow that would potentially prevent serious complications. Postoperatively, it may help predict early morbidity and mortality and it may also be used to assess graft function and regeneration [48, 49].

Pediatric Surgical Oncology Applications

Fluorescence-guided surgery has been used with increasing frequency for various applications in pediatric surgical oncology. ICG fluorescence can facilitate tumor identification, oncologic resection, margin delineation, and metastasectomy. Furthermore, as ICG has been documented to detect lesions as small as

0.062 mm, ICG fluorescence may allow for detection of lesions that might otherwise have been missed by preoperative imaging or intraoperative inspection or palpation [50].

Primary Hepatic Tumor Resection

One of the more established applications of ICG fluorescence in pediatric surgical oncology is resection of primary hepatic tumors in children specifically hepatoblastoma and hepatocellular carcinoma [22, 51, 52].

Intravenous injection of ICG 0.5 mg/kg is recommended 72 to 96 h prior to hepatic tumor resection [51, 53]. Hepatic tumors are more cholestatic and have a decreased ability to excrete ICG relative to normal liver parenchyma. This 72- to 96-h delay allows for optimal visualization of the hepatic tumor with decreased background noise [18]. However, if patients are unable to receive their ICG injection that far in advance, a lower dose of ICG can be administered closer to the time of their operation (e.g., 0.2–0.3 mg/kg of ICG 24–48 h before surgery), although there may still be a poor signal-to-noise ratio even with the lower dosing [22]. Similarly, patients with underlying liver disease, including liver cirrhosis as seen in biliary atresia, may retain ICG longer, contributing to increased background noise if ICG is administered too soon before an operation [54].

There are multiple reports documenting the successful use of ICG for resection of hepatoblastoma. ICG demonstrates excellent sensitivity for detecting hepatoblastoma tumors, particularly masses within 10 mm of the liver surface [19, 20]. In a case series of 11 patients undergoing hepatic resection with ICG guidance, ICG was 100% sensitive in identifying malignant lesions with high sensitivity across various histologic types (fetal hepatoblastoma, 100%; embryonal hepatoblastoma, 100%; mixed fetal-embryonal hepatoblastoma, 83%). However, specificity was low: seven of 16 lesions were ICG positive despite not demonstrating viable tumor on surgical pathology [6]. In addition, ICG may identify remote satellite lesions within the liver that may be too small for detection on preoperative cross-sectional imaging or intraoperatively by palpation [22]. ICG also demonstrates effectiveness for relapsed hepatoblastoma, including patients who previously underwent liver transplantation for management of hepatoblastoma and subsequently presented with relapse in the liver graft [55].

The high sensitivity and seamless integration into robotic or laparoscopic cameras make ICG a useful adjunct during both open and laparoscopic resections in children. It is particularly useful for laparoscopic-assisted oncologic resections, during which palpation of the liver surface is less feasible [52].

ICG can also be used to evaluate hepatic perfusion and delineate boundaries between liver segments during hepatectomy. Terasawa et al. developed a technique that would allow for assessment of the boundaries of tumor-bearing hepatic segments, both to determine a line of transection and to evaluate the perfusion of the preserved hepatic parenchyma [56]. After transecting the hepatic parenchyma and clamping the portal pedicle of the tumor-bearing hepatic segments, 1.25 mg of ICG is administered intravenously. This creates a visual line of demarcation between non-fluorescing tumor-bearing hepatic segments that are to be resected and surrounding fluorescing hepatic parenchyma to be preserved.

Non-hepatic Primary Tumor Resection

Until recently, most reports of fluorescent-guided resection of non-hepatic primary tumors were limited to case reports and series of adult patients. However, recent series have demonstrated the successful utilization of ICG as an adjunct during oncologic resection of non-hepatic tumors in children. Furthermore, prospective trials assessing the feasibility of ICG-mediated near-infrared imaging for resection and identification of margins in pediatric neoplasms are currently underway.

Esposito et al. utilized ICG for laparoscopic excision of abdominal lymphoma and robot-assisted resection of ovarian tumors in pediatric patients [12]. ICG was administered intravenously at a dosage of 0.5 mg/mL/kg for three patients with lymphoma. ICG allowed for assessment of the vascularization of the lymphoma tumor, helped define the level of resection in cases requiring mesenteric division, and was used to detect lymph nodes for biopsy or resection. Of the five patients with ovarian tumors, three were mature teratomas and two were seromucinous cystadenoma on pathology. Patients received an intravenous administration of ICG at a dosage of 0.5 mg/mL/kg. Within 20–30 s of injection, ICG allowed for delineation between the hypofluorescent ovarian tumor and normal salpinx and ovarian parenchyma. It also allowed for verification of perfusion to the salpinx and uterus following tumor resection.

In a large series of pediatric patients, Abdelhafeez et al. achieved fluorescence in 46 out of 52 tumors: nine osteosarcomas, six neuroblastomas, six non-rhabdomyosarcoma soft tissue sarcomas, five rhabdomyosarcomas, three Ewing sarcomas, two germ cell tumors, one chondroblastoma, one solid pseudopapillary neoplasm of the pancreas, one lymphoma, and one myoepithelial carcinoma of the chest wall (in addition to nine hepatoblastomas and two hepatocellular carcinomas) [51]. The majority of patients received 1.5 mg/kg of ICG intravenously over 15 min the day prior to surgery. Near-infrared imaging demonstrated an 88% sensitivity and 77% specificity rate for identifying tumors. Eighty-eight percent of malignant tumors demonstrated fluorescence versus 23% of benign lesions. ICG was unable to identify two primary adrenocortical tumors included in this series.

Background noise from ICG uptake of surrounding organs is a common concern in fluorescence-guided surgery. Abdelhafeez et al. reported that background noise was observed in 57% of procedures, including 100% of trunk and extremity resections, 68% of abdominal operations, and 40% of thoracic cases [51]. Of note, although background noise from adjacent organs was noted in all open abdominal and thoracic operations, it was only seen in 45% and 15% of minimally invasive abdominal and thoracic resections, respectively. This suggests that optimization of ambient light contamination may be a strategy for mitigating the effects of background noise during ICG-guided resections.

Future investigations are warranted for several areas pertaining to fluorescent-guided pediatric surgical oncology, including methods for mitigating background noise, evaluation of the efficacy of ICG-guided surgery for organ-sparing operations in cases such as bilateral Wilms tumors, optimizing identification of neuroblastoma and sarcoma metastases, and margin delineation in local control operations for neuroblastoma and sarcomas.

Pulmonary Metastasectomy for Primary Hepatic Tumors

Because ICG does not typically collect in normal lung tissue and metastatic lesions are commonly found in the periphery of the lung, ICG fluorescence allows for detection of very small, nonpalpable pulmonary metastases secondary to hepatic malignancies [21]. ICG is concentrated in hepatocytes and metastases from hepatic tumors, making it a beneficial adjunct for metastasectomy procedures [53]. The use of ICG for pulmonary metastasectomy via thoracotomy or thoracoscopy has been documented for both hepatoblastoma and hepatocellular carcinomas in pediatric patients [17]. It can detect pulmonary lesions as small as 0.062 mm in diameter [50]. A dose of 0.5 mg/kg of ICG administered approximately 24 h prior to surgery is generally recommended [57].

ICG is particularly helpful for thoracoscopic identification of metastatic lesions, where palpation is less feasible and the decrease in ambient light minimizes background noise compared to open resections [53]. Single lung ventilation with collapse of the affected lung should be utilized when medically feasible to enhance detection of lesions with ICG [21]. Given that ICG has less optimal penetration for lesions more than 10 mm below the surface of the lung, a secondary localization technique should be considered for deeper lesions [19]. To optimize detection of nodules, contrast mode, which demonstrates ICG signal over a dark background, can be used initially [53]. This is followed by overlay mode, which demonstrates ICG signal over the white light image of the lung, to guide wedge resection (Fig. 12.6).

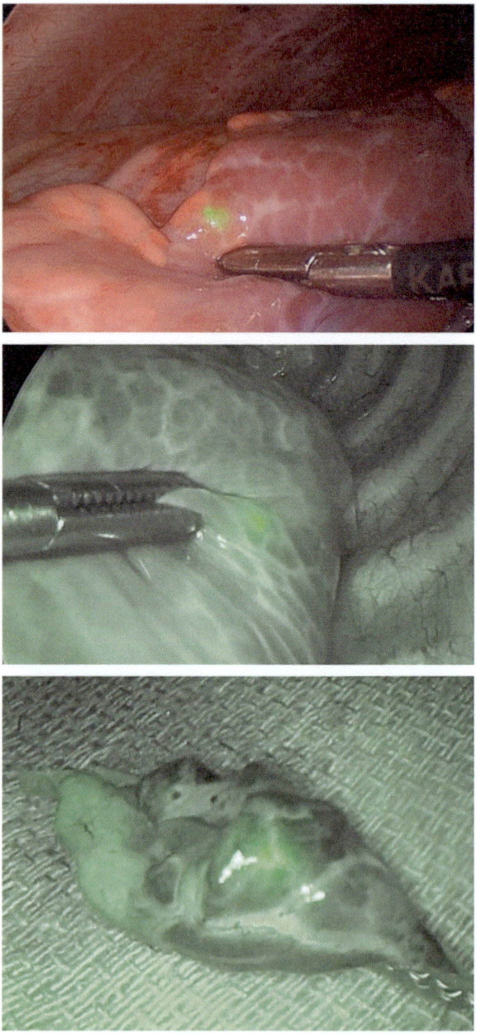

Fig. 12.6 A 2-year-old girl with PRETEXT III metastatic hepatoblastoma to the lung s/p cycle 3 chemotherapy and 3 left and 2 right pulmonary nodules. Therapeutic goal was to reach eligibility for liver transplant. Lung mets were easily identified with ICG and thoracoscopic SPY technology and removed with clear margins by wedge resection (lower picture). Note that ICG has to be given at 0.5 mg/kg 24 h in advance to the procedure. SPY technology allows thoracoscopic detection and parenchymal-sparing complete resection (Images courtesy of Drs. Densmore and Mowrer, Children's Hospital of Wisconsin)

Pulmonary Metastasectomy for Non-hepatic Tumors

ICG is also being increasingly used for pulmonary and pleural metastasectomy via thoracotomy or thoracoscopy for pediatric tumors of non-hepatic primary. Its use has been documented for pulmonary metastases secondary to nephroblastoma, neuroblastoma, chondroblastoma, and numerous sarcomas, including osteosarcoma, Ewing sarcoma, non-rhabdomyosarcoma soft tissue sarcoma, and rhabdomyosarcoma [57]. The surgical principles are similar to those for pulmonary metastasectomy for hepatic primary tumors.

In comparison to metastases secondary to hepatic primary tumors, metastases of non-hepatic primary tumors may require higher doses of ICG for optimal fluorescence (e.g., 3–4 mg/kg). ICG dosages up to 5 mg/kg administered approximately 24 h prior to surgery have been reported [58]. Although this is higher than the dosage currently approved by the US Food and Drug Administration (FDA), adverse events related to ICG administration are rare [5]. A higher concentration of ICG can be used (i.e., 5 mg/mL instead of 2.5 mg/mL) to decrease the volume of ICG injected [53].

In a series of 52 adult patients with a history of sarcoma who underwent pulmonary metastasectomy, additional lesions were detected with ICG in 59% of patients in the fluorescence-guided surgery cohort versus 25% of patients in the historical control cohort for whom additional lesions were detected with visual and tactile feedback alone ($p < 0.05$). Patients in the fluorescence-guided surgery group also had significantly improved median progression-free survival and longer time to recurrence in the lung compared to historical controls [58].

Further investigation is warranted to evaluate the effect of treatment necrosis and decreased tumor viability on ICG sensitivity of pulmonary nodules. However, ICG is a promising adjunct for pulmonary metastasectomy.

Lymph Node Identification and Sentinel Lymph Node Biopsy

Sentinel lymph node biopsy (SLNB) is an important technique for staging and regional lymph node assessment of malignancy (Figs. 12.7 and 12.8). Although well established for many types of

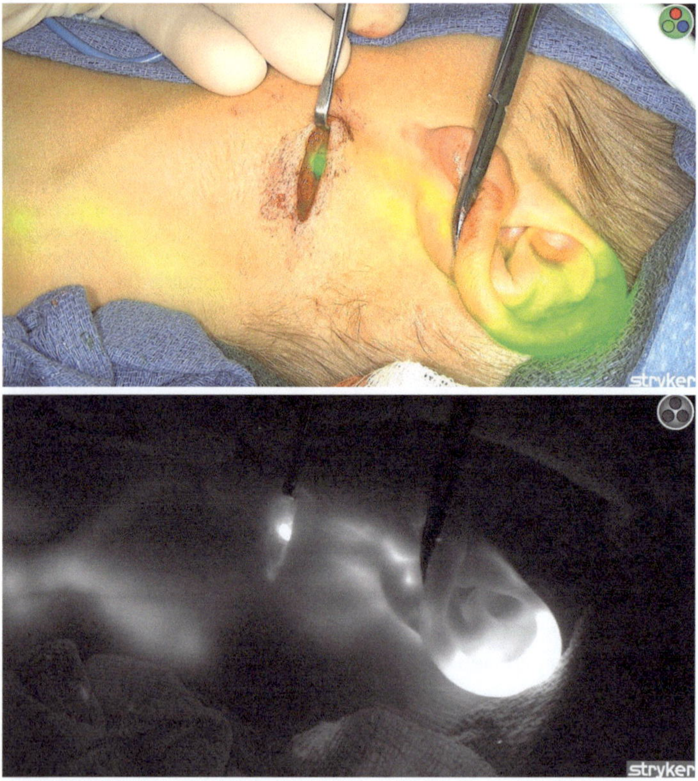

Fig. 12.7 ICG lymphangiography for sentinel lymph node biopsy for melanoma of the left ear using the SPY Portable Handheld Imaging System. The upper image shows the overlay mode and the lower image the SPY fluorescence mode. ICG is injected into the lesion on the upper ear. Note clear visibility of the lymph vessels leading to the sentinel node of the lesion (Images courtesy of Dr. Marcus Malek, UPMC Children's Hospital of Pittsburgh)

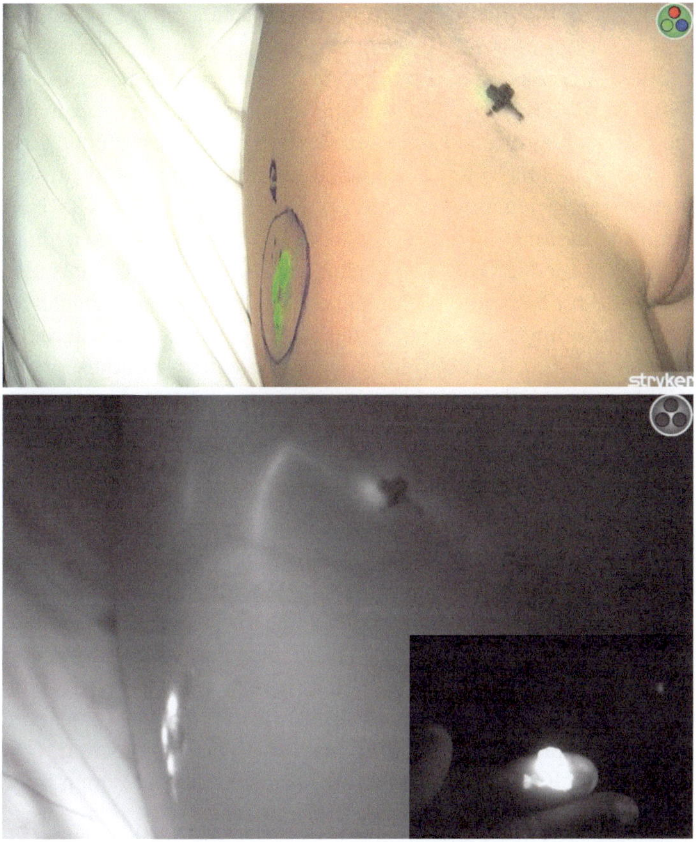

Fig. 12.8 ICG lymphangiography for sentinel lymph node biopsy for melanoma of the right upper thigh using the SPY Portable Handheld Imaging System. The upper image shows the overlay mode and the lower image the SPY fluorescence mode. ICG is injected into the lesion on the upper thigh. Note clear visibility of the lymph vessels leading to the sentinel node of the lesion. The right lower image shows the fluorescence of the resected sentinel lymph node (Images courtesy of Dr. Marcus Malek, UPMC Children's Hospital of Pittsburgh)

adult cancer, the role for SLNB in pediatric cancers is less defined [59]. SLNB is currently used in pediatric cases of melanoma and various sarcomas, including rhabdomyosarcoma and certain soft tissue sarcomas [59]. Technetium lymphoscintigraphy remains the gold standard for SLNB, with blue dyes such as lymphazurin or methylene blue often used in conjunction for visual identification of sentinel nodes. Valente et al. found that ICG with NIR fluorescence imaging was safe and performed similarly to technetium 99 m for SLNB in breast cancer patients [60]. ICG has also been used for SLNB and lymph node harvest in other adult cancer types, including melanoma, gynecologic cancers, and colorectal cancers [61–63]. It is currently unknown whether fluorescent or ICG lymphoscintigraphy is noninferior for SLNB or lymph node identification in pediatric patients. However, it can be used an adjunct for lymph node identification [12].

In pediatric patients, reports of ICG use for lymph node identification and SLNB have been more limited. Esposito et al. utilized ICG to detect a thoracic hilar lymph node for biopsy for suspected lymphoma [14]. A 0.5 mg/mL/kg of ICG was injected into the lung parenchyma intraoperatively to assist with lymph node identification [12]. In a series of pediatric patients with paratesticular rhabdomyosarcoma, Mansfield et al. injected 10 mg of ICG into the spermatic cord under either direct visualization or ultrasound guidance to facilitate retroperitoneal lymph node dissection [64]. Injection of ICG into the spermatic cord led to iliac lymph node avidity using near-infrared spectroscopy, with sequential spread along the ipsilateral para-aortic or para-caval lymph node chain. Recently, a case report described the use of ICG to increase lymph node harvest during laparoscopic Wilms nephroureterectomy [65]. Despite International Society of Pediatric Oncology (SIOP) and Children's Oncology Group (COG) protocols requesting more than six lymph nodes during Wilms nephroureterectomy, the median number of nodes obtained during both open and minimally invasive resections is approximately four. In this case report, 2 mL of 2.5 mg/mL ICG was injected into the normal renal parenchyma near the tumor in 0.5 mL aliquots. Seven hilar, suprahilar, pre-aortic, and para-aortic nodes subsequently demonstrated fluorescence, including several that would have gone undetected without ICG. However, further investigation is warranted evaluating injection sites other than the renal parenchyma so as to prevent violation of COG guidelines and potential upstaging of the tumor.

ICG lymphoscintigraphy can also be used for tumors of the trunk and extremities. 4 mL of ICG can be injected subcutaneously at a concentration of 1.25 mg/mL in four quadrants around the tumor intraoperatively (1 mL per quadrant) [53]. In smaller children, ICG is frequently visible through the skin when using a near-infrared imaging device. Sentinel lymph nodes are best visualized using a contrast mode, whereas other modes, such as the color-segmented fluorescence mode, can be utilized for identification of regions with high fluorescence intensity.

Further study is needed to evaluate the sensitivity and specificity of ICG lymphoscintigraphy for various cancer types in pediatric patients.

Pediatric Plastic Surgery Applications

There has been increasing utilization of ICG in pediatric plastic surgery for a variety of purposes, including assessment of flap perfusion, evaluation of lymphedema, and management of lymphatic malformations. Reconstruction of congenital anomalies has given way to the use of ICG for several operations unique to pediatric patients. For instance, Hinchcliff et al. described the use of intraoperative laser-assisted ICG angiography for a one-year-old with anterior plagiocephaly [66]. The patient underwent calvarial reconstruction for unilateral coronal synostosis, during which tension during closure was encountered. ICG was safely utilized to verify perfusion to the anterior and posterior flaps prior to closure. Tomioka et al. also utilized ICG to evaluate flap perfusion in a one-year-old who underwent web transplantation for syndactyly [67].

In a case series of 433 pediatric free tissue transfers, Upton et al. emphasized that technical considerations are more complex in pediatric transfers given technical factors such as patients' diminutive vessels, as well as challenges with postoperative immobilization [68]. Fried et al. described the use of ICG to verify perfusion of a free latissimus dorsi myocutaneous flap in a six-month-old for reconstruction of a temporal fossa defect after resection of a teratoma [69]. Intraoperative use of ICG in pediatric patients may mitigate the morbidity of flap failures or vascular complications requiring a return to the operating room for anastomotic revisions or flap repositioning [68]. Martins et al., in their case series of pediatric patients undergoing first-stage autologous total ear reconstruction, found that patients in the intraoperative laser-assisted ICG angiography treatment group were significantly less likely to undergo surgical revision in comparison to the non-ICG group [70].

ICG can also be used for real-time imaging of lymphatic anatomy and flow in the case of lymphedema or lymphatic malformations. ICG can detect lymphatic channels within one to two centimeters of the skin surface in the absence of fascia, muscle, or bone overlying the channels [33, 34]. Injection of ICG can aid in the visualization of lymphatic channels, valves, and flow, which can facilitate staging and management [71, 72]. Greives et al. injected 12.5 μg of ICG in 0.05 mL of saline into the dorsum of each hand and foot to evaluate lymphatic uptake in a 21-month-old with congenital lymphedema of the right hand and arm [73]. Imaging demonstrated normal lymphatic anatomy with decreased lymphatic contractile function of the right upper extremity relative to the unaffected extremities, which aided in determining appropriate management.

ICG can also facilitate identification, resection, and classification of lymphatic malformations. Shirota et al. used ICG to aid complete resection of a lymphatic malformation in the abdominal wall of a 15-year-old male [74]. The patient had failed management with sclerotherapy three times and MRI alone had failed to adequately determine the extent of the tumor. Kato et al. similarly used ICG lymphography to identify lymphatic malformations originating throughout the body in 20 pediatric patients ages 11 months to 10 years [75]. They identified four classic flow patterns: (1) strong detectable inflow, (2) multiple small observable inflows, (3) superficial lymph flow over a lesion, and (4) flow around a lymphatic malformation without connection to the lesion. By identifying lymphatic inflow using ICG lymphography, surgical resection or bypass using lymphatic venous anastomosis can be utilized for management of lymphatic malformations [75].

Pediatric Trauma Surgery Applications

The use of ICG in pediatric trauma surgery has been relatively limited despite numerous possible applications. Han et al. used ICG angiography to determine skin tissue viability in 19 pediatric patients after acute trauma [76]. ICG dosages up to 0.5 mg/kg were used for each patient. In 78.9% of cases, there was discordance between clinician assessment of viability and ICG angiography. All intraoperative decisions (e.g., primary skin-sparing repair vs. resection with or without skin graft or flap reconstruction) were made based on ICG results with 94.7% of cases demonstrating recovery without any evidence of postoperative necrosis. ICG may provide objective data to physicians determining skin and soft tissue viability in pediatric patients after acute traumatic injury. This technique has similarly been used in adult patients after degloving injuries to evaluate for tissue viability [77, 78].

Bauerly et al. further described the use of serial fluorescence microangiography to evaluate for progressive tissue ischemia in a 5-year-old secondary to acute pedal compartment syndrome after a crush injury [79]. The authors concluded that serial microangiography allows for evaluation of tissue ischemia and response to therapy (e.g., hyperbaric therapy). It also provides objective data when determining level of amputation, if indicated. This data can be especially valuable in young pediatric patients with challenging clinical diagnoses, such as compartment syndrome, who may not be as readily able to explain their symptoms or to follow commands.

Fluorescent technology may also be a useful adjunct in the management of burn wounds. Pediatric burn patients have a higher incidence of burn wound infection compared to adults [80]. Up to 75% of mortality in burn patients after initial resuscitation is due to infection [81]. In their case series of ten pediatric burn patients with 15 wounds, Farhan and Jeffery concluded that the MolecuLight i:X, a handheld noncontact fluorescence imaging device, could detect significant bacterial burden, subclinical bacterial colonization, and infection in pediatric burn wounds both instantly and reliably [82]. This technology could mitigate delays in care associated with wound biopsy and cultures.4.

Although there are reports of the use of fluorescence-guided surgery in other aspects of adult trauma, such as evaluating bowel perfusion after abdominal trauma or as a neuromonitoring tool in traumatic brain injury patients, the pediatric data is currently more limited [83, 84].

Pediatric Cardiac Surgery Applications

Many pediatric patients born with congenital heart defects require complex surgical reconstructions with intricate reconstruction of the coronary vasculature. Reconstruction of this atypical coronary anatomy is made increasingly complicated by the typical need for a staged approach that can allow for scarring of the epicardial anatomy between operations [85]. Fluorescence-guided surgery has allowed for reliable, noninvasive, and real-time intraoperative evaluation of the coronary anatomy.

There are reports of fluorescence-guided surgery being used in neonates as young as 2 days of life as adjuncts in cardiac surgery for a variety of congenital heart defects [86]. The successful utilization of ICG has been documented for numerous purposes, including evaluation of coronary anatomy and arterial anastomoses, assessment of shunt patency after reconstruction, assessment of reconstruction after pulmonary arterioplasty, evaluation of the aortic arch and arch anastomoses, and assessment of myocardial perfusion [87, 88]. ICG has also demonstrated utility in localizing the thoracic duct, for identifying abnormal lymphatic anatomy, and for the localization and management of iatrogenic abnormal lymphatic drainage or postoperative chylothorax. Said et al., in their case series of 15 patients, found that ICG techniques were most useful for assessing myocardial perfusion, for localizing epicardial coronary arteries (particularly in staged operations), and for evaluating the patency of systemic-to-pulmonary arterial shunts [86]. With regard to specific procedures, Kogon et al., in their case series of 30 patients, found that ICG fluorescence imaging demonstrated best image adequacy for Blalock-Taussig shunts (100%), coarctation repairs (86%), and coronary reimplantations (66%), versus hemi-Fontan or Fontan (40%) repairs and pulmonary artery reconstructions (33%) [88].

Evaluation of deeper structures with ICG, such as pulmonary arterial branches, may be more difficult in the absence of additional techniques to aid with exposure. Furthermore, although outflow from synthetic conduits can be assessed with ICG, synthetic grafts (e.g., expanded polytetrafluoroethylene [PTFE]) may demonstrate poor penetration of the dye [86, 88].

ICG fluorescence is a valuable adjunct in pediatric cardiac surgery. It allows for safe and reliable real-time localization of complex variant coronary anatomy, assessment of reconstructed shunts and vascular anastomoses, and evaluation of myocardial perfusion. This valuable data, in turn, allows surgeons to assess and refine their operations, to revise or perform any additional procedures, and to ensure improved outcomes before ever leaving the operating room.

Pediatric Neurosurgery Applications

ICG fluorescence has proven to be a useful adjunct for numerous applications in pediatric neurosurgery. One of the most valuable uses of ICG videoangiography (ICG-VA) has been for intraoperative evaluation of blood flow during microsurgical clipping of intracranial aneurysms [89, 90]. While clipping aneurysms, neurosurgeons aim to completely occlude the aneurysm without leaving any neck residuals [91]. However, they must also strive to maintain the patency and flow of any normal parent, branching, or perforating vessels near the lesion [92]. Wali et al. described the use of exoscopic 3D high-definition ICG-VA while clipping a 12 × 13 × 7 mm aneurysm arising from the M1/M2 junction in an 11-year-old with Alagille syndrome [91]. ICG was used to evaluate cerebral flow dynamics and middle cerebral artery outflow prior to clip placement. Furthermore, it demonstrated complete occlusion of the aneurysm without neck remnant after clip placement. Similarly, Nossek et al. utilized ICG for a 17-year-old patient with an enlarging mycotic aneurysm whose parent vessel supplied the motor cortex distal to the aneurysm [90]. ICG demonstrated collateral retrograde filling of the distal parent vessel that intraoperatively informed and guided the surgeon's plan for safe trapping and resection of the aneurysm. Traditionally, postoperative evaluation of neck residuals or unexpected vessel occlusion after microneurosurgical clipping has been evaluated with postoperative angiography and possible need for reoperation [92]. ICG-VA provides intraoperative real-time evaluation of aneurysm occlusion, neck remnants, and adjacent normal vessel patency, as well as possible clip revision, prior to leaving the operating room.

ICG-VA has also been utilized during surgical revascularization and assessment of patients with moyamoya disease. Moyamoya disease is an uncommon, chronic cerebrovascular disease characterized by progressive occlusion of the supraclinoid internal carotid arteries resulting in formation of fine "moyamoya" collateral vessels at the base of the brain [93]. In children, this can manifest clinically as transient ischemic attacks or cerebral infarction [94]. Revascularization surgery, in the form of direct, indirect, or combined bypass, is a treatment option for patients with symptomatic moyamoya disease or asymptomatic moyamoya disease with impaired cerebral hemodynamics [95]. During revascularization, neurosurgeons often strive to preserve the middle meningeal artery (MMA) because it provides collateral flow through the dura matter and its anterior branch provides collateral flow to the anterior cerebral artery. However, the anterior branch is easily damaged during conventional frontotemporal craniotomy because it frequently runs through the bony tunnel in the lesser wing of the sphenoid bone. Tanabe et al. found that the MMA can frequently be visualized using ICG-VA in pediatric patients prior to craniotomy, which may increase the likelihood of its preservation. They found that visualization of the anterior branch with ICG is possible when the diameter of the MMA is greater than 1.3 mm and the sphenoid bone overlying it is less than 3 mm in thickness. Hori et al. and Ambekar et al. further utilized ICG to evaluate for patency of the anterior branch of the MMA, as well as to evaluate blood flow through a bypass, including superior temporal artery to middle cerebral artery anastomoses [93, 96]. Uchino et al. calculated the blood flow index using ICG intensity-time curves to assess for changes in cerebral perfusion after direct bypass [97]. Uchino et al. and Horie et al. report changes in ICG-VA, as well as differences between adult and pediatric populations, that may aid in predicting postoperative cerebral hyperperfusion in select patient populations.

ICG is also a useful adjunct for the resection of tumors and complex vascular lesions. Ueba et al. used ICG and FLOW 800 to discriminate between arterialized draining veins and feeding arteries during resection of a spinal hemangioblastoma in a 19-month-old [98]. The slope of the average signal intensity was steeper for feeding arteries than arterialized veins. This information reportedly guided surgeons with intraoperative planning and resection, delineating the lesion and minimizing trauma to the spinal cord. It also prevented inadvertent violation of the hemangioblastoma, which could have caused significant blood loss.

There are also reports of fluorescence-guided surgery for less established purposes in pediatric neurosurgery. For instance, Sanchez Fernandez et al. used combination of ICG and fluorescein during repeat surgical intervention for an 11-year-old status post craniotomy and evacuation of a subdural empyema with progressive cerebritis on MRI during the week after his initial surgery [99]. ICG and fluorescein demonstrated damage of cortical vascularization and avascularized tissue, respectively, that were subsequently excised with good clinical outcomes. Sugimoto et al. used ICG-VA to evaluate flow through a rare intracranial pial arteriovenous fistula in a three-year-old [100]. ICG-VA allowed for precise localization of two fistulous points between the M2 portion of the middle cerebral artery and a large varix, which were clipped with subsequent demonstration of normal flow.

ICG-VA is a useful, reliable, real-time adjunct for numerous procedures in pediatric neurosurgery, including clipping of aneurysms and arteriovenous malformations, surgical revascularization with subsequent assessment of anastomoses and changes in cerebral hemodynamics, and resection of neoplastic and vascular lesions.

Conclusions and Future Directions

Fluorescence-guided surgery (FGS) using ICG is an emerging technology in pediatric surgery. As hospitals are acquiring this new technology, there is great promise to improve outcomes for our patients. Predominant applications are in cancer surgery to facilitate complete resection or detecting metastasis in the lung, solid organs, or lymph nodes. ICG-guided sentinel node resection has the potential to replace other technologies already available today. ICG allows assessment of perfusion in a variety of procedures where tenuous anastomoses are fashioned such as in pull-through procedures for patients with Hirschsprung's disease or anorectal malformations, esophagectomies for esophageal atresia patients, or intestinal atresia or necrotizing enterocolitis. Benefits of applications for rare cases such as biliary atresia or choledochal cyst are being explored. Also for pediatric surgeons, ICG-guided cholangiograms should be the routine to increased safety during gallbladder surgery. Pediatric surgery as a surgical field with a particular wide spectrum harbors a multitude of potential applications for this new technology that can guide interventions. Large case series and randomized prospective trials are missing in the pediatric surgery world today in the more recent field of ICG-guided surgery. The pediatric surgery community needs to produce more robust data to define best practices and guidelines for the benefit of our small patients.

References

1. Alander JT, et al. A review of indocyanine green fluorescent imaging in surgery. Int J Biomed Imaging. 2012;2012:940585.

2. Le-Nguyen A, et al. The use of indocyanine green fluorescence angiography in pediatric surgery: a systematic review and narrative analysis. Front Pediatr. 2021;9:736242.
3. Garski TR, et al. Adverse reactions after administration of indocyanine green. JAMA. 1978;240(7):635.
4. Benya R, Quintana J, Brundage B. Adverse reactions to indocyanine green: a case report and a review of the literature. Catheter Cardiovasc Diagn. 1989;17(4):231–3.
5. Shafy SZ, et al. Fluorescence imaging using indocyanine green dye in the pediatric population. J Pediatr Pharmacol Ther. 2020;25(4):309–13.
6. Chu W, et al. Anaphylactic shock after intravenous administration of indocyanine green during robotic partial nephrectomy. Urol Case Rep. 2017;12:37–8.
7. Lee T, et al. Anaphylactic shock after intravenous fluorescein administration for intraoperative cystoscopy. Obstet Gynecol. 2018;131(4):727–9.
8. Raval MV, Lautz TB, Browne M. Bile duct injuries during pediatric laparoscopic cholecystectomy: a national perspective. J Laparoendosc Adv Surg Tech A. 2011;21(2):113–8.
9. Guillén G, et al. Pilot experience with indocyanine green navigation in pediatric surgery. Cir Pediatr. 2019;32(3):121–7.
10. Esposito C, et al. Twenty-five year experience with laparoscopic cholecystectomy in the pediatric population-from 10 mm clips to indocyanine green fluorescence technology: long-term results and technical considerations. J Laparoendosc Adv Surg Tech A. 2019;29(9):1185–91.
11. Calabro KA, Harmon CM, Vali K. Fluorescent cholangiography in laparoscopic cholecystectomy and the use in pediatric patients. J Laparoendosc Adv Surg Tech A. 2020;30(5):586–9.
12. Esposito C, et al. Image-guided pediatric surgery using indocyanine green (ICG) fluorescence in laparoscopic and robotic surgery. Front Pediatr. 2020;8:314.
13. Esposito C, et al. Indocyanine green (ICG) fluorescent cholangiography during laparoscopic cholecystectomy using RUBINA™ technology: preliminary experience in two pediatric surgery centers. Surg Endosc. 2021;35(11):6366–73.
14. Hirayama Y, et al. Near-infrared fluorescence cholangiography with indocyanine green for biliary atresia. Real-time imaging during the Kasai procedure: a pilot study. Pediatr Surg Int. 2015;31(12):1177–82.
15. Yanagi Y, et al. The outcome of real-time evaluation of biliary flow using near-infrared fluorescence cholangiography with Indocyanine green in biliary atresia surgery. J Pediatr Surg. 2019;54(12):2574–8.
16. Gotoh K, et al. A novel image-guided surgery of hepatocellular carcinoma by indocyanine green fluorescence imaging navigation. J Surg Oncol. 2009;100(1):75–9.

17. Yamamichi T, et al. Clinical application of indocyanine green (ICG) fluorescent imaging of hepatoblastoma. J Pediatr Surg. 2015;50(5):833–6.
18. Yamada Y, et al. Fluorescence-guided surgery for hepatoblastoma with indocyanine green. Cancers (Basel). 2019;11(8):1215.
19. Souzaki R, et al. Navigation surgery using indocyanine green fluorescent imaging for hepatoblastoma patients. Pediatr Surg Int. 2019;35(5):551–7.
20. Lake CM, et al. Indocyanine green is a sensitive adjunct in the identification and surgical management of local and metastatic hepatoblastoma. Cancer Med. 2021;10(13):4322–43.
21. Cho YJ, et al. The advantages of indocyanine green fluorescence imaging in detecting and treating pediatric hepatoblastoma: a preliminary experience. Front Pediatr. 2021;9:635394.
22. Whitlock RS, et al. Pathologic correlation with near infrared-indocyanine green guided surgery for pediatric liver cancer. J Pediatr Surg. 2022;57(4):700–10.
23. Iinuma Y, et al. Intraoperative near-infrared indocyanine green fluorescence angiography (NIR-ICG AG) can predict delayed small bowel stricture after ischemic intestinal injury: report of a case. J Pediatr Surg. 2013;48(5):1123–8.
24. Diana M, et al. Enhanced-reality video fluorescence: a real-time assessment of intestinal viability. Ann Surg. 2014;259(4):700–7.
25. Ris F, et al. Near-infrared (NIR) perfusion angiography in minimally invasive colorectal surgery. Surg Endosc. 2014;28(7):2221–6.
26. Rentea RM, et al. Preliminary use of indocyanine green fluorescence angiography and value in predicting the vascular supply of tissues needed to perform cloacal, anorectal malformation, and hirschsprung reconstructions. Eur J Pediatr Surg. 2020;30(6):505–11.
27. Pathak RA, Hemal AK. Intraoperative ICG-fluorescence imaging for robotic-assisted urologic surgery: current status and review of literature. Int Urol Nephrol. 2019;51(5):765–71.
28. Diana P, et al. The role of intraoperative indocyanine green in robot-assisted partial nephrectomy: results from a large, multi-institutional series. Eur Urol. 2020;78(5):743–9.
29. Esposito C, et al. Technical standardization of ICG near-infrared fluorescence (NIRF) laparoscopic partial nephrectomy for duplex kidney in pediatric patients. World J Urol. 2021;39(11):4167–73.
30. Herz D, et al. Segmental arterial mapping during pediatric robot-assisted laparoscopic heminephrectomy: a descriptive series. J Pediatr Urol. 2016;12(4):266.e1–6.
31. Abdelhafeez AH, et al. Indocyanine green-guided nephron-sparing surgery for pediatric renal tumors. J Pediatr Surg. 2021;57:174.

32. Esposito C, et al. Indocyanine green fluorescence lymphography: a new technique to perform lymphatic sparing laparoscopic palomo varicocelectomy in children. J Laparoendosc Adv Surg Tech A. 2019;29(4):564–7.
33. Esposito C, et al. Clinical application and technical standardization of indocyanine green (ICG) fluorescence imaging in pediatric minimally invasive surgery. Pediatr Surg Int. 2019;35(10):1043–50.
34. Esposito C, et al. Near-infrared fluorescence imaging using indocyanine green (ICG): emerging applications in pediatric urology. J Pediatr Urol. 2020;16(5):700–7.
35. Esposito C, et al. Laparoscopic or robotic deroofing guided by indocyanine green fluorescence and perirenal fat tissue wadding technique of pediatric simple renal cysts. J Laparoendosc Adv Surg Tech A. 2020;30(4):471–6.
36. Sekine Y, et al. A simple and effective technique for identification of intersegmental planes by infrared thoracoscopy after transbronchial injection of indocyanine green. J Thorac Cardiovasc Surg. 2012;143(6):1330–5.
37. Tarumi S, et al. Clinical trial of video-assisted thoracoscopic segmentectomy using infrared thoracoscopy with indocyanine green. Eur J Cardiothorac Surg. 2014;46(1):112–5.
38. Shirota C, et al. Thoracoscopic surgery for congenital lung cysts: an attempt to limit pulmonary resection in cases of lesions involving multiple lobes. Pediatr Surg Int. 2021;37(2):213–21.
39. Yoshida M, et al. Clinicopathological study of surgery for pulmonary metastases of hepatoblastoma with indocyanine green fluorescent imaging. Pediatr Blood Cancer. 2022;69(7):e29488.
40. Shibasaki J, et al. Evaluation of lymphatic dysplasia in patients with congenital pleural effusion and ascites using indocyanine green lymphography. J Pediatr. 2014;164(5):1116–1120.e1.
41. Pham KT, et al. Multimodality lymphatic imaging of postoperative chylothorax in an infant with Noonan syndrome: a case report. Eur J Med Res. 2020;25(1):55.
42. Shirotsuki R, et al. Novel thoracoscopic navigation surgery for neonatal chylothorax using indocyanine-green fluorescent lymphography. J Pediatr Surg. 2018;53(6):1246–9.
43. Lee JH, et al. Real-time identification of aberrant left hepatic arterial territories using near-infrared fluorescence with indocyanine green during gastrectomy for gastric cancer. Surg Endosc. 2021;35(5):2389–97.
44. Mizuno S, et al. Biliary complications in 108 consecutive recipients with duct-to-duct biliary reconstruction in living-donor liver transplantation. Transplant Proc. 2014;46(3):850–5.

45. Quintero J, et al. Indocyanine green plasma disappearance rate: a new tool for the classification of paediatric patients with acute liver failure. Liver Int. 2014;34(5):689–94.
46. Panaro F, et al. Indocyanine green fluorescence angiography during liver and pancreas transplantation: a tool to integrate perfusion statement's evaluation. Hepatobiliary Surg Nutr. 2018;7(3):161–6.
47. Kawaguchi Y, et al. Evaluation of hepatic perfusion in the liver graft using fluorescence imaging with indocyanine green. Int J Surg Case Rep. 2015;14:149–51.
48. Majlesara A, et al. Indocyanine green fluorescence imaging in hepatobiliary surgery. Photodiagn Photodyn Ther. 2017;17:208–15.
49. Dai B, et al. Advantages of using indocyanine green in liver transplantation: a narrative review. Ann Transl Med. 2022;10(2):110.
50. Kitagawa N, et al. Navigation using indocyanine green fluorescence imaging for hepatoblastoma pulmonary metastases surgery. Pediatr Surg Int. 2015;31(4):407–11.
51. Abdelhafeez A, et al. Indocyanine green-guided pediatric tumor resection: approach, utility, and challenges. Front Pediatr. 2021;9:689612.
52. Chung PHY, Chok KSH, Wong KKY. Indocyanine green fluorescence-assisted laparoscopic hepatectomy for hepatocellular carcinoma in a pre-adolescent girl: a case report. Hong Kong Med J. 2020;26(4):342–4.
53. Goldstein SD, et al. Evolving applications of fluorescence guided surgery in pediatric surgical oncology: a practical guide for surgeons. J Pediatr Surg. 2021;56(2):215–23.
54. Lau CT, Au DM, Wong KKY. Application of indocyanine green in pediatric surgery. Pediatr Surg Int. 2019;35(10):1035–41.
55. Takahashi N, et al. Living donor liver re-transplantation for recurrent hepatoblastoma in the liver graft following complete eradication of peritoneal metastases under Indocyanine green fluorescence imaging. Cancers (Basel). 2019;11(5):730.
56. Terasawa M, et al. Applications of fusion-fluorescence imaging using indocyanine green in laparoscopic hepatectomy. Surg Endosc. 2017;31(12):5111–8.
57. Yamamichi T, et al. Computed tomography-guided marking using a dye-staining method for preoperative localization of tiny pulmonary lesions in children. Pediatr Surg Int. 2021;37(9):1265–72.
58. Azari F, et al. Impact of intraoperative molecular imaging after fluorescent-guided pulmonary metastasectomy for sarcoma. J Am Coll Surg. 2022;234(5):748–58.
59. Sadeghi R, et al. Sentinel lymph node biopsy in pediatric Wilms tumor. J Pediatr Surg. 2022;57:1518.
60. Valente SA, et al. Near infrared fluorescent lymph node mapping with indocyanine green in breast cancer patients: a prospective trial. J Am Coll Surg. 2019;228(4):672–8.

61. Frumovitz M, et al. Near-infrared fluorescence for detection of sentinel lymph nodes in women with cervical and uterine cancers (FILM): a randomised, phase 3, multicentre, non-inferiority trial. Lancet Oncol. 2018;19(10):1394–403.
62. Cahill RA, et al. Near-infrared (NIR) laparoscopy for intraoperative lymphatic road-mapping and sentinel node identification during definitive surgical resection of early-stage colorectal neoplasia. Surg Endosc. 2012;26(1):197–204.
63. Bluemel C, et al. EANM practice guidelines for lymphoscintigraphy and sentinel lymph node biopsy in melanoma. Eur J Nucl Med Mol Imaging. 2015;42(11):1750–66.
64. Mansfield SA, et al. Alternative approaches to retroperitoneal lymph node dissection for paratesticular rhabdomyosarcoma. J Pediatr Surg. 2020;55(12):2677–81.
65. Pachl MJ. Fluorescent guided lymph node harvest in laparoscopic Wilms nephroureterectomy. Urology. 2021;158:189–92.
66. Hinchcliff KM, Yao A, Taub PJ. Laser-assisted indocyanine green imaging to assess perfusion of scalp closure in an infant. J Craniofac Surg. 2013;24(6):2004–6.
67. Tomioka YK, et al. Foot web space transfer for congenital syndactyly. Plast Reconstr Surg Glob Open. 2020;8(12):e3292.
68. Upton J, Guo L. Pediatric free tissue transfer: a 29-year experience with 433 transfers. Plast Reconstr Surg. 2008;121(5):1725–37.
69. Fried FW, et al. Free latissimus dorsi myocutaneous flap in a 6-month-old child for reconstruction of a temporal fossa defect after Teratoma resection. Ann Plast Surg. 2019;82(1):62–3.
70. Martins DB, et al. Intraoperative indocyanine green laser angiography in pediatric autologous ear reconstruction. Plast Reconstr Surg Glob Open. 2016;4(5):e709.
71. Narushima M, et al. Indocyanine green lymphography findings in limb lymphedema. J Reconstr Microsurg. 2016;32(1):72–9.
72. Cheng MH, Liu TT. Lymphedema microsurgery improved outcomes of pediatric primary extremity lymphedema. Microsurgery. 2020;40(7):766–75.
73. Greives MR, et al. Near-infrared fluorescence lymphatic imaging of a toddler with congenital lymphedema. Pediatrics. 2017;139(4):e20154456.
74. Shirota C, et al. New navigation surgery for resection of lymphatic malformations using Indocyanine green fluorescence imaging. Am J Case Rep. 2017;18:529–31.
75. Kato M, et al. Flow pattern classification in lymphatic malformations by indocyanine green lymphography. Plast Reconstr Surg. 2019;143(3):558e–64e.
76. Han T, et al. The role of ICG angiography in decision making about skin-sparing in pediatric acute trauma. Front Pediatr. 2022;10:851270.

77. Ferguson S, Turker T. Delayed perfusion evaluation in extremity trauma. J Clin Orthop Trauma. 2021;23:101655.
78. Pruimboom T, et al. Potential of near-infrared fluorescence image-guided debridement in trauma surgery. Case Reports Plast Surg Hand Surg. 2018;5(1):41–4.
79. Bauerly NA, et al. Utilization of fluorescence microangiography in pediatric acute compartment syndrome: a case report. J Foot Ankle Surg. 2020;59(1):201–5.
80. Jeschke MG, et al. Morbidity and survival probability in burn patients in modern burn care. Crit Care Med. 2015;43(4):808–15.
81. Ansermino M, Hemsley C. Intensive care management and control of infection. BMJ. 2004;329(7459):220–3.
82. Farhan N, Jeffery S. Utility of MolecuLight i:X for managing bacterial burden in pediatric burns. J Burn Care Res. 2020;41(2):328–38.
83. Afifi I, et al. The use of Indocyanine green fluorescent in patients with abdominal trauma for better intraoperative decision-making and less bowel anastomosis leak: case series. J Surg Case Rep. 2021;2021(6):rjab235.
84. Forcione M, et al. Cerebral perfusion and blood-brain barrier assessment in brain trauma using contrast-enhanced near-infrared spectroscopy with indocyanine green: a review. J Cereb Blood Flow Metab. 2020;40(8):1586–98.
85. Pourmoghadam KK, et al. Avoiding coronary injury in congenital heart surgery by laser-assisted indocyanine green dye imaging. World J Pediatr Congenit Heart Surg. 2014;5(2):326–9.
86. Said SM, Marey G, Hiremath G. Intraoperative fluorescence with indocyanine green in congenital cardiac surgery: potential applications of a novel technology. JTCVS Tech. 2021;8:144–55.
87. Vogt PR, Bauer EP, Graves K. Novadaq spy intraoperative imaging system--current status. Thorac Cardiovasc Surg. 2003;51(1):49–51.
88. Kogon B, et al. The role of intraoperative indocyanine green fluorescence angiography in pediatric cardiac surgery. Ann Thorac Surg. 2009;88(2):632–6.
89. Kim DL, Cohen-Gadol AA. Indocyanine-green videoangiogram to assess collateral circulation before arterial sacrifice for management of complex vascular and neoplastic lesions: technical note. World Neurosurg. 2013;79(2):404.e1–6.
90. Nossek E, Setton A, Chalif DJ. Trapping and resection of cortical MCA mycotic aneurysm in eloquent area. Acta Neurochir. 2018;160(3):579–82.
91. Wali AR, et al. First-in-human clinical experience using high-definition exoscope with intraoperative indocyanine green for clip reconstruction of unruptured large pediatric aneurysm. World Neurosurg. 2021;151:52.

92. Dashti R, et al. Microscope-integrated near-infrared indocyanine green videoangiography during surgery of intracranial aneurysms: the Helsinki experience. Surg Neurol. 2009;71(5):543–50. discussion 550
93. Hori S, et al. Surgical anatomy and preservation of the middle meningeal artery during bypass surgery for moyamoya disease. Acta Neurochir. 2015;157(1):29–36.
94. Horie N, et al. Indocyanine green videoangiography for assessment of postoperative hyperperfusion in moyamoya disease. Acta Neurochir. 2014;156(5):919–26.
95. Tanabe N, et al. Indocyanine green visualization of middle meningeal artery before craniotomy during surgical revascularization for moyamoya disease. Acta Neurochir. 2017;159(3):567–75.
96. Ambekar S, et al. Intraoperative assessment of STA-MCA bypass patency using near-infrared indocyanine green video-angiography: a preliminary study. Neurol India. 2012;60(6):604–7.
97. Uchino H, et al. Intraoperative assessment of cortical perfusion by indocyanine green videoangiography in surgical revascularization for moyamoya disease. Acta Neurochir. 2014;156(9):1753–60.
98. Ueba T, et al. Efficacy of indocyanine green videography and real-time evaluation by FLOW 800 in the resection of a spinal cord hemangioblastoma in a child: case report. J Neurosurg Pediatr. 2012;9(4):428–31.
99. Sánchez Fernández C, et al. Combined microsurgical fluorescence for optimizing resection in refractory empyema and cerebritis. Childs Nerv Syst. 2020;36(9):1835–41.
100. Sugimoto T, et al. Effectiveness of intraoperative indocyanine green videoangiography in direct surgical treatment of pediatric intracranial pial arteriovenous fistula. J Neurosurg Pediatr. 2015;15(1):55–9.

Use of Fluorescence Guidance in Neurosurgery

13

Brendan Jones and Maxwell Almenoff

Introduction

Indocyanine green (ICG) has become well-established as an adjunct in multiple surgical fields as it augments reality to allow for accurate identification of anatomic structures and assessment of blood flow [1]. Due to the binding of indocyanine to plasma proteins, it is maintained in the vasculature and has become recognized as versatile tool in vascular neurosurgery. Assuring the integrity of tissue perfusion is the most important principle in neurovascular surgery [2]. The first described use of fluorescent visualization of cerebral blood vessels in neurovascular surgery was in 1967 by Feindel et al. [3], and in 1994, Wrobel et al. [4] described a case of ICG angiography in aneurysm surgery. However, it wasn't until 2003 when Raabe et al. [5] used microscope-integrated indocyanine green (M-ICG) angiography to assess vessel patency that neurosurgery as a field began to

B. Jones (✉)
Department of General Surgery, West Virginia University School of Medicine, Morgantown, WV, USA

M. Almenoff
Department of Cardiovascular and Thoracic Surgery, Vascular Surgery, West Virginia University Heart and Vascular Institute, Morgantown, WV, USA

N. Szoka et al. (eds.), *The SAGES Manual of Fluorescence-Guided Surgery*, https://doi.org/10.1007/978-3-031-40685-0_13

widely investigate and adopt the technique [6]. Prior to this time, intraoperative digital subtraction arteriography (DSA) was required for assessment of cerebral blow flow [5]. Raabe et al. [5] demonstrated that ICG angiography was a simple method to provide real-time information on multiple phases of blood flow down to vessels less than 0.5 mm in diameter, thus opening the door to a multitude of neurosurgical applications (Fig. 13.1). The use of indocyanine has since broadened to other areas within neurosurgery with the four main uses being neurovascular, endoscopic endonasal approaches, ventricular surgery, and neurooncological procedures; this chapter will focus on the neurovascular uses of indocyanine green. Within neurovascular procedures ICG is commonly used for assessing aneurysm morphology and perforator vessel preservation. The ability to identify the obliteration or patency of vessels is also pertinent in arteriovenous malformations and dural fistula surgery.

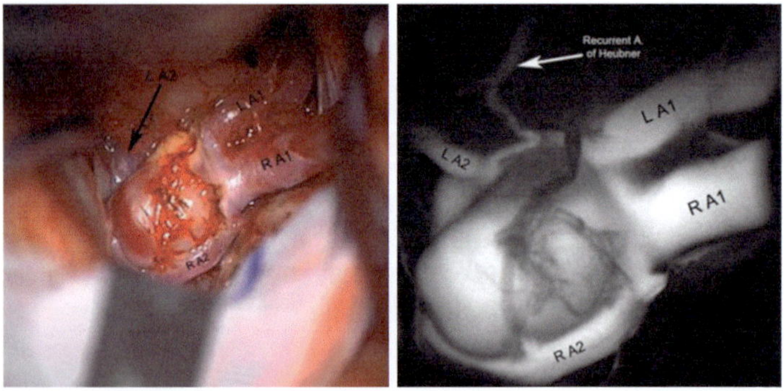

Fig. 13.1 For the exposed operative field (*left*), ICG videoangiography (*right*) provides a real-time assessment of the flow through both large and small (recurrent artery of Heubner) vessels. *LA1* left A1 segment of the ACA, *LA2* left A2 segment of the ACA, *RA1* right A1 segment of the ACA, *RA2* right A2 segment of the ACA [7]

The use of ICG angiography has been fairly easy to integrate into the field of neurosurgery, largely due to the prevalence of microscopic surgery. Multiple companies have equipped their microscopes with near infrared sensitive digital cameras capable of viewing the ICG diffusion within the cerebral vessels [6]. With integration of ICG angiography into the operative microscope, simplicity and speed are improved.

ICG Use in Aneurysm Repair

Aneurysm treatment depends on complete exclusion of the aneurysm sac and patency of the supplying arteries. While alternative treatments such as coiling and stenting have made advances, microsurgical clipping should still be considered the durable and definitive treatment for intracranial aneurysms [8]. Sindou et al. [9] found that incomplete clipping accounts for up to 4–8% of all clipping cases [6]. If imaging is only completed postoperatively, the findings may result in repeat surgery, and studies suggest a 2–8% rate of residual aneurysm filling and a 4–12% rate of parent or branching artery occlusion on postoperative angiography [2]. Prior to ICG, neurosurgeons had several intraoperative methods to assess aneurysm blood flow such as contact Doppler ultrasonography, blood flowmetry, and the gold standard of contrast-enhanced (digital subtraction) angiography (DSA). Starting with the case series by Raabe et al. in 2003, ICG angiography has been studied in aneurysm clipping. ICG offers an easy, rapid, and minimally invasive method of allowing evaluation of complete aneurysm exclusion, neck remnant, and blood flow in parent and perforating arteries (Fig. 13.2). Many of the studies since Raabe et al. [5] have compared ICG to Doppler ultrasonography or DSA to assess anatomy pre- and post-clipping, clip positioning, presence of aneurysm residuals, and patency of normal vessels. It is recommended that the surgeon use an objective intraoperative technique rather than relying on visual assessment alone [6].

ICG, while not without its limitations, does offer benefit over some of the existing methods of flow detection. DSA, which has been shown to have a significant impact on 7–34% of cases when

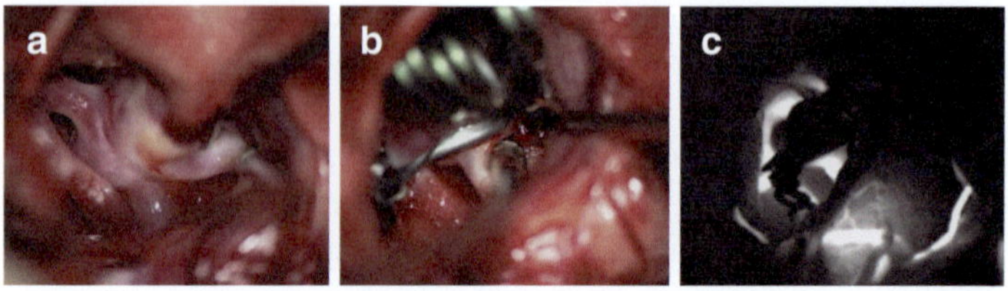

Fig. 13.2 Middle cerebral artery aneurysm with the neck dissected and clear view of the parent vessel and its two branches (**a**), after retraction showing the neck of the clipped MCA aneurysm (**b**), and intraoperative ICG videoangiography showing the patency of the branches of the MCA and complete exclusion of the aneurysm from the circulation (**c**) [10]

used intraoperatively, is expensive, requires additional specially trained staff, and has a complication rate of 0.4–3.5% [7]. A minimum of 20 min is typically needed to set up and perform intraoperative DSA, a length of time that may exceed the ischemic limit of cerebral tissue in certain cases. Clip adjustment after DSA is associated with a 33% rate of stroke. Doppler ultrasonography exhibits good correlation with postoperative angiography and is inexpensive and noninvasive and does not add significant time to the case, but interpretation of signals is subjective, and such factors as the angle of insonation, thickness of the vessel wall, and investigation point may affect the outcome of the assessment [2, 6].

Aneurysm clipping is often completed with two doses of ICG; one dose being administered prior to clipping and the second to confirm the position of the clip and exclusion of the aneurysm. With an up to 42-min visualization window, no additional doses are needed in the pre-clipping step, and the patency of parent and surrounding perforating arteries can be easily assessed. However, a second dose is typically required for post-clipping evaluation due to "trapping" of the ICG in the aneurysm which could simulate incomplete clipping [11]. Eliava et al. [6] demonstrated in their series that it takes approximately 10 min to complete aneurysm clipping after ICG administration. The use of ICG also allowed the surgeon to quickly recognize stenosis or incomplete exclusion and reposition the clip accordingly. Vessels less than

1 mm in diameter are well assessed with the operating microscope and ICG allowing for the accurate assessment of perforating arteries [2]. These small perforating arteries may be below the level of detection for DSA, and Oliveira et al. [12] showed a 1.6% rate of clip adjustments based on ICG detection of compromised flow through perforating arteries.

Despite a greater than 90% correlation with intra/postoperative DSA, ICG angiography cannot completely remove all risk of improperly placed clips [2]. Eliava et al. [6] described a case where postoperative selective angiography revealed a remnant aneurysmal neck that was unable to be evaluated intraoperatively due to inability to directly view the area because of the location. Several other studies have demonstrated a small rate of unexpected neck residuals and close vessel occlusion at a rate of 4–6% [7, 8, 13]. In the series of 15 patients, one patient also had mild stenosis of the internal carotid artery that was only noted on control angiography and not on ICG angiography. Studies have demonstrated clip repositioning rates of 2–38% with the use of ICG; part of this variation is due to the lack of standardization of ICG technique, potential limited experience, and varied patient groups. ICG angiography was noted to be crucial to case success in three cases where blood flow, not visible by Doppler ultrasonography, was visible by ICG angiography. A comparison of intraoperative DSA to ICG, with 100 patients in each group, by Hardesty et al. [14] demonstrated no reliable difference in the risk of postoperative ischemia (4% vs 3%), unexpected aneurysm filling (4% vs 2%), or parent vessel compromise (2% vs 2%).

ICG is not without its drawbacks. Mainly, the fluorescence can only be traced within the limits of visibility; important structures may be easily obscured by vessel branches, a clip, or the aneurysm itself. A comparison of contrast-enhanced angiography and ICG by Washington et al. [7] did not favor ICG. In this study, the conclusion of 14.3% of cases was discordant, largely due to the fact that only visible vessels were assessed by ICG. Within the seven cases of discordance from this study, five of the cases underwent clip adjustment leading to complete aneurysm occlusion or restoration of patency in branch vessels. No specific aneurysm characteristics were more likely to contribute to discordance on multivariate analysis, but there was a trend toward anterior communicating artery location leading to discordance on univariate analysis. This finding aligns with the findings of Gruber et al. [15] and Dashti et al. [13] that deep-seated aneurysms are poorly imaged with ICG. Similarly, Roessler et al. [16] demonstrated a 9.1% identification rate with selective angiography of small (<2 mm) neck aneurysm remnants and a residual 6 mm aneurysm following ICG. These findings suggest that DSA may still serve a vital role in complex aneurysms where hidden parts of the parent, branching, and perforating vessels and undissected portions of the aneurysm dome are difficult to directly visualize with ICG (Fig. 13.3). ICG can also be affected by calcified or atherosclerotic vessels and thrombosis within the aneurysm. However, intraoperative DSA also has its limitations with a reported 7.9% residual aneurysm and 4.8% rate of distal arterial branch occlusion detected on postoperative DSA. Despite the aforementioned finding, the study of 295 patients by Roessler et al. [16] is one of the largest to date and also demonstrated a 9% repositioning rate and a 4.5% rate of incomplete clipping after ICG administration, findings that may not have been detected with Doppler or flowmetry.

The use of ICG has advanced beyond microscope integrated use, and in 2013 the first described use of endoscopic-ICG (E-ICG) use for neurovascular use was reported by Bruneau et al. [18]. Aneurysm clipping was performed on an unruptured anterior communicating artery aneurysm using a similar two bolus protocol and a 0° NIR-optimized endoscope. The E-ICG provided high-resolution, panoramic views with additional information on the aneurysm exclusion and parent and perforating artery patency that would be potentially obscured without an angled camera. In 2014, Mielke et al. [19] published a series of 26 patients with ruptured and non-ruptured aneurysms comparing M-ICG and E-ICG. The series showed that in 11 of 26 patients, E-ICG added information by increasing fluorescence time, offering different viewing angles and enlarged views of the vessels and aneurysms. An additional series by Yoshioka and Kinouchi [20] and Cho et al. [21] demonstrated successful use of E-ICG in aneurysm clipping.

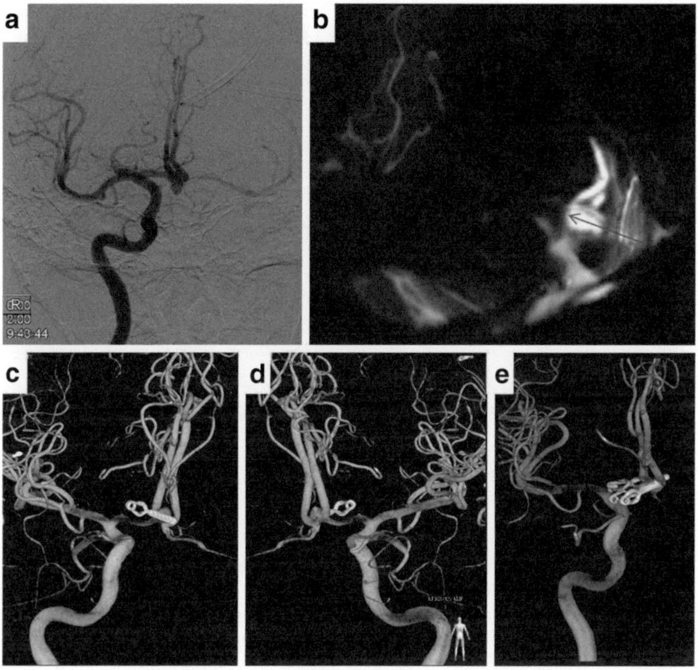

Fig. 13.3 (**a**) Preoperative anteroposterior angiography with right internal carotid injection in a patient with an anterior communicating artery aneurysm. (**b**) Indocyanine green videoangiography after clipping. There is no evidence of residual aneurysm. The direction of the arrow denotes the direction of the clip. Postoperative anteroposterior angiography (**c**, **d**) showed residual aneurysm. The patient underwent reclipping, and angiography (**e**) after reclipping showed complete obliteration of the aneurysm [17]

Cho et al. [21] specifically selected ICA-PCoA and ICA-AChA aneurysms due to the higher incidence of incomplete clipping and branch compromise (Fig. 13.4). With the use of endoscopic ICG, all necessary anatomic information and assessment of the clipping was possible despite limited microscopic views. The main advantage of endoscopy is enhanced visualization, better magnification, and dynamic vision which improves the ability to view less accessible regions, particularly posterior to the clip and beyond the direct view of the microscope. Critical to the success

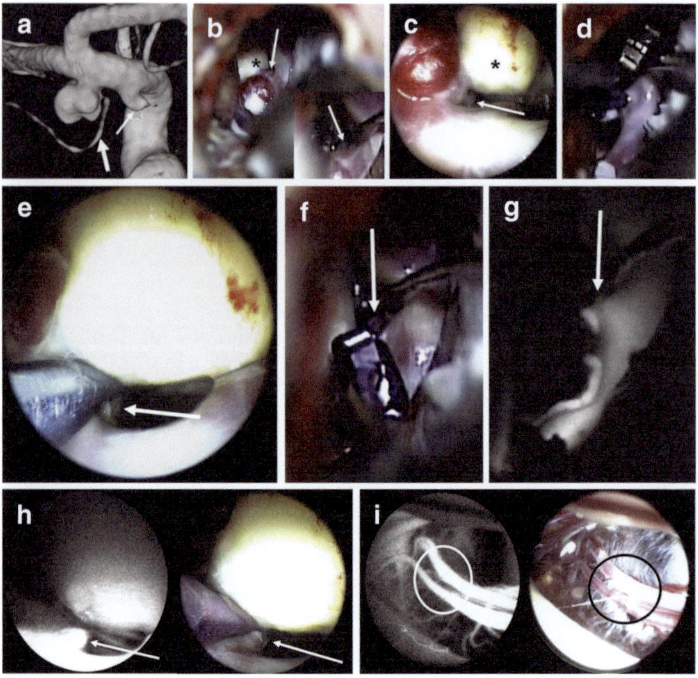

Fig. 13.4 A 59-year-old man with an unruptured left internal carotid artery (ICA) anterior choroidal artery (AChA) aneurysm measuring approximately 7 mm (case 8). (**a**) The AChA (thick arrow) and PCoA (thin arrow) were observed on medioposterior view of three-dimensional reconstructed left ICA angiography. (**b**, **c**) The orifice of the AChA (arrows) at the aneurysm neck was identified with the microscope (**b**) (with a magnifying view at the right lower side) and endoscope (**c**), with a hard atherosclerotic anterior aneurysm wall (asterisks). (**d**, **e**) After clipping, the orifice of the AChA was not visualized with the microscope (**d**); however, it was shown to be compromised by the standard clip (arrow) with the endoscope (**e**). (**f**, **g**) A miniclip was instead applied, and the orifice of the AChA (arrows) was shown on microscopic indocyanine green angiography with no indocyanine green filling within the sac. (**h**, **i**) Dual-channel endoscopic indocyanine green angiography of fluorescent (left panels) and visible color light (right panels) imaging also visualized the intact orifice (arrows in **h**) and trunk proper (circles in **i**) of the AChA [21]

of E-ICG procedures is the maintenance of a clear surgical field. Without a clear field, visual perception may be distorted and "false" vascular structures visualized.

Compared with other forms of vascular assessment, ICG angiography is approximately ten times more expensive than Doppler ultrasonography and four times more expensive than flowmetry. ICG is considered a cost-effective replacement to intraoperative DSA. Studies comparing the cost of ICG and other standard flow assessments are lacking with Nishiyama et al. [22] being one of the few to look at per-patient cost of intraoperative imaging.

Washington et al. [7] note that a combination of ICG and DSA may be the most effective for maximizing the safety and efficacy of aneurysm surgery. Care should be taken when relying on ICG for aneurysms where the field of view is limited or there are complex flow dynamics.

ICG Use in Arteriovenous Malformation

The goal of surgical intervention of arteriovenous malformations (AVM) is the removal of the AVM nidus and complete excision. Microsurgical resection is the only treatment option that immediately eliminates the risk of hemorrhage from the AVM and any remaining residual nidus with a high chance of re-rupture. DSA can be used intraoperatively for assessment of AVMs, but it comes with increased operating time and expense. The DSA images are not integrated into the microscopic view like ICG and must be interpreted separately, diverting the surgeon's attention away from the operative field.

ICG can help distinguish vessels in physiological and pathological states; with arterialized veins emitting fluorescence in the late arterial phase. Using ICG can help the surgeon identify AVM arteries and veins early and plan operative steps. Deep-seated AVMs are somewhat troublesome for ICG as the location is not amenable to direct visualization; in these cases DSA is the gold standard, but ICG can be a helpful adjunct.

ICG Use in Extracranial-Intracranial Bypass

ICG has always had a leading role in bypass surgery, and use with neurovascular bypass was incorporated after the benefit was demonstrated in coronary artery bypass. Extracranial-intracranial bypass plays an important role in management of complex intracranial aneurysms, moyamoya disease, and cerebral ischemia. Early bypass graft occlusion and bypass failure are the main obstacles of EC-IC bypass surgery, which leads to cerebral ischemia and resulting morbidity. Intraoperative assessment of bypass graft function can reduce complications, but techniques such as Doppler ultrasonography and thermal artery imaging are limited in respect to image quality and spatial resolution, thus limiting the ability to detect flow in perforating arteries. DSA is the gold standard but is associated with limitations as mentioned previously. Historically, the immediate postoperative bypass patency rate has been cited between 89% and 96%. Multiple factors contribute to the patency of the graft including graft and donor vessel diameter, atherosclerotic changes in the donor vessel, cerebral blood flow demand, and flow direction within the bypass [23]. ICG has been reliably shown to detect stenosis and nonfunctioning bypasses and can help judge flow and anatomic relationships at the anastomotic site. Woitzik et al. [24] demonstrated a patency rate of EC-IC bypass of 100% after introducing the usage of ICG; prior to ICG the patency rate was less than 90%. The use of ICG localized the site of failure to the anastomosis and allowed for surgical revision and restored flow in six cases reported by Woitzik et al. [24].

While ICG can rapidly allow identification of parent and recipient arteries, further advancement in the quantitative and qualitative evaluation of blood flow is underway. Awano et al. [25] measured ICG perfusion area to assess hemodynamic changes following superficial temporal artery (STA) and middle cerebral artery (MCA) bypass surgery in moyamoya disease and non-moyamoya ischemic stroke. The group showed a significant increase in cortical oxygen saturation in the moyamoya disease cohort thought to be attributable to the increase of blood flow demand and pressure gradient between the STA and recipient vessels [26]. Januszewski et al. [23] attempted to classify the type of flow through bypass grafts to predict early graft failure and need for intraoperative revision. The group characterized flow through the graft into three types: type I being robust and anterograde (early arterial phase), type II being delayed anterograde flow (usually corresponding to capillary or venous phase), and type III being delayed anterograde flow without continuity to the bypass site or no flow at all. This classification makes use of the three phases of ICG distribution: arterial, capillary, and combined arteriovenous due to the recirculation of dye. On postoperative imaging, four occluded grafts (11%) were found in the series, all of which were type II or III. Based on these findings, Januszewski recommended revision of most type II flow grafts as failure is not likely to be related to competitive flow. ICG was found to be accurate and comparable to DSA in this series.

Discussion of Hyperperfusion After STA-MCA

ICG can also be of use in detecting patients who may be at risk for cerebral hyperperfusion. Two studies performed by Horie et al. [27] and Uchino et al. [28] examined ICG intensity-time curves and semiquantitative analysis of ICG-video angiography (ICG-VA), respectively. This can be applied in both patients with moyamoya disease and atherosclerotic disease. A blood flow index, calculated on the basis of the ICG intensity-time curve, with an increase of greater than threefold, may be predictive of the occurrence of hyperperfusion. Additionally, ICG-VA and analysis with specialized software may allow for recognition of flow parameters and hemodynamic changes that may be indicative of transient neurologic event complications, but to date no evidence has shown a correlation with improved patient outcomes.

Intraoperative Vessel Identification

Intraoperative vessel identification can also be performed with ICG-VA in aneurysm bypass and indirect bypass. While preoperatively there are multiple modalities to assist in selection of an appropriate donor vessel for EC-IC bypass, ICG can be used intraoperatively for mapping and preparation of the donor vessel. ICG-VA has also been used for selective targeting of the most suitable recipient artery, and this has been well-described in the treatment of complex MCA aneurysm. As a terminal branch of the MCA (M4) is preferred as a recipient vessel in this case, ICG-VA can detect the direction of flow and delayed or reversed filling time of M4 branches during arterial phase and other vascular structures during the capillary and venous phases. A primary and secondary identification protocol has been described by Esposito et al. [29, 30] in which delayed filling of superficial M4 branches during either phase demarcates the supplied cortical area and any artery within this area can be selected as the recipient. The secondary identification consists of a provocative temporary occlusion. ICG-VA can then be repeated after anastomosis to rule out residual filling of the aneurysm. A "flash fluorescence" technique has also been described by Lawton (Fig. 13.5). This technique helps identify an adequate recipient artery through occlusion of the afferent artery and subsequent flash fluorescence with ICG of efferent arteries after removal of the clip. This method can reduce unnecessary sylvian fissure dissection and allows for anastomosis to be performed on the cortical surface without brain retraction. Transdural ICG-VA use in STA-MCA bypass has helped in delineation of superficial vessel anatomy and allowed for tailoring of the dural incision and prevention of vessel damage during dural opening and microsurgical dissection.

There is also a report by Yokoyama et al. [31] of E-ICG use in the treatment of recurrent skull base tumors. ICA angiography was performed after identification of a possible branch feeding the tumor; this information was used as the basis for deciding whether to deliver intra-arterial chemotherapy [11].

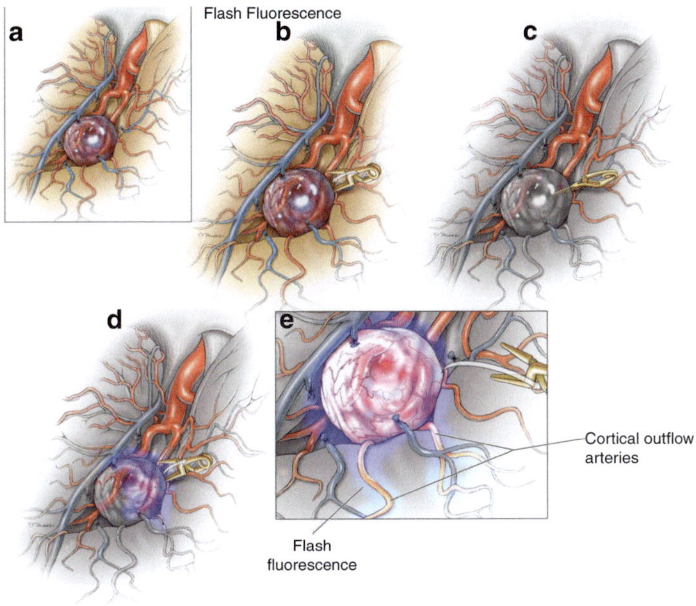

Fig. 13.5 Use of flash fluorescence technique to identify the efferent arteries of the aneurysm using ICG-VA. (**a**) Identification of candidate bypass recipient arteries among the surface M4 branches is difficult but could be improved using the following steps. (**b**) Temporary clip occlusion of the aneurysm inflow (afferent arteries) proximal to the aneurysm. (**c**) ICG-VA demonstrating initial fluorescence in uninvolved arterial branches. (**d**) Removal of temporary clip for aneurysm reperfusion. (**e**) Fluorescence seen in the efferent arteries to identify the most suitable recipient on the cortical surface for the bypass [26]

Standard ICG Dosing

The standard dose of ICG is 0.2–0.5 mg/kg [26]. Januszewski et al. [23] described a standard injection, through a peripheral vein, of 25 mg of ICG dissolved in 10 mL of water. Cavallo et al. [26] reported dissolving 25 mg in 5 mL of water and flushing immediately with 10 mL of normal saline. Redosing is suggested at 20 min to ensure adequate clearance of the tracer with the total cumulative dose not to exceed 5 mg/kg.

Conclusion

Over the past decade, the use of ICG angiography in neurosurgery has expanded. This technique has found use in multiple aspects of neurosurgery and offers additional tool in the surgeon's kit. Series in neurovascular bypass, aneurysm exclusion, and AVM have demonstrated the utility of ICG-VA. This technology may even help in the early recognition of postsurgical complications with the application of software that can analyze flow using ICG intensity. ICA-VA can be time-saving in some cases and simpler to interpret but is limited in its ability to view deeper vessels. This limitation has been somewhat overcome by the introduction of E-ICG. Additional studies are still needed to further determine when ICG is superior to other imaging methods.

References

1. Alius C, Tudor C, Badiu CD, Dascalu AM, Smarandache CG, Sabau AD, Tanasescu C, Balasescu SA, Serban D. Indocyanine green-enhanced colorectal surgery—between being superfluous and being a game-changer. Diagnostics. 2020;10:742.
2. Balamurugan S, Agrawal A, Kato Y, Sano H. Intra operative indocyanine green video-angiography in cerebrovascular surgery: an overview with review of literature. Asian J Neurosurg. 2011;6(2):88–93.
3. Feindel W, Yamamoto YL, Hodge CP. Intracarotid fluorescein angiography: a new method for examination of the epicerebral circulation in man. Can Med Assoc J. 1967;96:1–7.

4. Wrobel CJ, Meltzer H, Lamond R, Alksne JF. Intraoperative assessment of aneurysm clip placement by intravenous fluorescein angiography. Neurosurgery. 1994;35:970–3.
5. Raabe A, Beck J, Gerlach R, Zimmerman M, Seifert V. Near-infrared indocyanine green video angiography: a new method for intraoperative assessment of vascular flow. Neurosurgery. 2003;52(1):132–9.
6. Eliava SS, Shekhtman OD, Pilipenko YV, Okishev DN, Kheyreddin AS, Kisar'ev SA, Kaftanov AN. Intraoperative indocyanine green fluorescence angiography in brain aneurysm surgery. The first experience of the technique use and a literature review. Problems Neurosurg Named After N.N. Burdenko. 2015;1:28–36.
7. Washington CW, Zipfel GJ, Chicoine MR, Derdeyn CP, Rich KM, Moran CJ, Cross DT, Dacey RG Jr. Comparing indocyanine green videoangiography to the gold standard of intraoperative digital subtraction angiography used in aneurysm surgery. J Neurosurg. 2013;118:420–7.
8. Ozgiray E, Akture E, Patel N, Baggott C, Bozkurt M, Niemann D, Baskaya MK. How reliable and accurate is indocyanine green video angiography in the evaluation of aneurysm obliteration? Clin Neurol Neurosurg. 2013;115(7):870–8.
9. Sindou M, Acevedo JC, Turjman F. Aneurysmal remnants after microsurgical clipping: classification and results from a prospective angiographic study (in a consecutive series of 305 operated intracranial aneurysms). Acta Neurochir (Wien). 1998;140:1153–9.
10. Norat P, Soldozy S, Elsarrag M, Sokolowski J, Yagmurlu K, Park MS, Tvrdik P, Yashar M, Kalani S. Application of indocyanine green videoangiography in aneurysm surgery: evidence, techniques, practical tips. Front Surg. 2019;6:1–7.
11. Catapano G, Sgulo F, Laleva L, Columbano L, Dallan I, de Notaris M. Multimodal use of indocyanine green endoscopy in neurosurgery: a single-center experience and review of the literature. Neurosurg Rev. 2018;41:985–98.
12. de Oliveira JG, Beck J, Seifert V, Teixeira MJ, Raabe A. Assessment of flow in perforating arteries during intracranial aneurysm surgery using intraoperative near-infrared indocyanine green video videoangiography. Neurosurgery. 2007;61(3 Suppl):63–72.
13. Dashti R, Laakso A, Niemela M, Porras M, Hernesniemi J. Microscope integrated indocyanine green video-angiography in cerebrovascular surgery. Acta Neurochir Suppl. 2011;109:247–50.
14. Hardesty DA, Thind H, Zabramski JM, Spetzler RF, Nakaji P. Safety, efficacy, and cost of intraoperative indocyanine green angiography compared to intraoperative catheter angiography in cerebral aneurysm surgery. J Clin Neurosci. 2014;21(8):1377–82.
15. Gruber A, Dorfer C, Standhardt H, Bavinzski G, Knosp E. Prospective comparison of intraoperative vascular monitoring technologies during cerebral aneurysm surgery. Neurosurgery. 2011;68:657–73.

16. Roessler K, Krawagna M, Dorfler A, Buchfelder M, Ganslandt O. Essentials in intraoperative indocyanine green videoangiography assessment for intracranial aneurysm surgery: conclusions from 295 consecutively clipped aneurysms and review of the literature. Neurosurg Focus. 2014;36:1–7.
17. Sharma M, Ambekar S, Ahmed O, Nixon M, Sharma A, Nanda A, Guthikonda B. The utility and limitations of intraoperative near-infrared indocyanine green videoangiography in aneurysm surgery. World Neurosurg. 2014;82(5):607–13.
18. Bruneau M, Appelboom G, Rynkowski M, Van Cutsem N, Mine B, De Witte O. Endoscope-integrated ICG technology: first application during intracranial aneurysm surgery. Neurosurg Rev. 2013;36:77–84; discussion 84–5.
19. Mielke D, Malinova V, Rohde V. Comparison of intraoperative microscopic and endoscopic ICG angiography in aneurysm surgery. Neurosurgery. 2014;10(Suppl 3):418–25; discussion 425. https://doi.org/10.1227/NEU.0000000000000345.
20. Yoshioka H, Kinouchi H. The roles of endoscope in aneurysmal surgery. Neurol Med Chir (Tokyo). 2015;55:469–78. https://doi.org/10.2176/nmc.ra.2014-0428.
21. Cho W, Kim JE, Kang H, Ha EJ, Jung M, Lee C, Shin I, Kang U. Dual-channel endoscopic indocyanine green fluorescence angiography for clipping of cerebral aneurysms. World Neurosurg. 2017;100:316–24.
22. Nishiyama Y, Kinouchi H, Senbokuya N, Kato T, Kanemaru K, Yoshioka H, et al. Endoscopic indocyanine green video angiography in aneurysm surgery: an innovative method for intraoperative assessment of blood flow in vasculature hidden from microscopic view. J Neurosurg. 2012;117:302–8.
23. Januszewski J, Beecher JS, Chalif DJ, Dehdasjti AR. Flow-based evaluation of cerebral revascularization using near-infrared indocyanine green videoangiography. Neurosurg Focus. 2014;36:1–8.
24. Woitzik J, Horn P, Vajkoczy P, Schmiedek P. Intraoperative control of extracranial-intracranial bypass patency by nearinfrared indocyanine green videoangiography. J Neurosurg. 2005;102:692–8.
25. Awano T, Sakatani K, Yokose N, Kondo Y, Igarashi T, Hoshino T, et al. Intraoperative EC-IC bypass blood flow assessment with indocyanine green angiography in moyamoya and non-moyamoya ischemic stroke. World Neurosurg. 2010;73:668–74.
26. Cavallo C, Gandhi S, Zhao X, Belykh E, Valli D, Nakaji P, Preul MC, Lawton MT. Applications of microscope-integrated indocyanine green videoangiography in cerebral revascularization procedures. Front Surg. 2019;6:1–10.
27. Horie N, Fukuda Y, Izumo T, Hayashi K, Suyama K, Nagata I. Indocyanine green videoangiography for assessment of postoperative hyperperfusion

in moyamoya disease. Acta Neurochir. 2014;156:919–26. https://doi.org/10.1007/s00701-014-2054-4.
28. Uchino H, Kuroda S, Hirata K, Shiga T, Houkin K, Tamaki N. Predictors and clinical features of postoperative hyperperfusion after surgical revascularization for moyamoya disease: a serial single photon emission CT/positron emission tomography study. Stroke. 2012;43:2610–6. https://doi.org/10.1161/strokeaha.112.654723.
29. Esposito G, Dias S, Burkhardt JK, Bozinov O, Regli L. Role of indocyanine green videoangiography in identification of donor and recipient arteries in cerebral bypass surgery. Acta Neurochir Suppl. 2018;129:85–9. https://doi.org/10.1007/978-3-319-73739-3_12.
30. Esposito G, Regli L. Selective Targeted cerebral revascularization via microscope integrated indocyanine green videoangiography technology. Acta Neurochir Suppl. 2014;119:59–64. https://doi.org/10.1007/978-3-319-02411-0_10.
31. Yokoyama J, Ishibashi K, Shiramizu H, Ohba S. Impact of endoscopic indocyanine green fluorescence imaging on superselective intra-arterial chemotherapy for recurrent cancer of the skull base. Anticancer Res. 2016;36:3419–24.

Use of Fluorescence Guidance in Cardiothoracic Surgery

14

Derek Muehrcke

Indications

The ability to accurately identify coronary artery anatomy and ensure patent bypass grafts is critical to surgical outcome during open heart surgery. Coronary artery bypass graft patency is the major predictor of long-term survival after coronary artery bypass grafting surgery [1]. Technical anastomotic problems are a major source of early graft closure [2, 3]. The ability to reliably assess the patency of coronary artery bypass grafts using intraoperative fluorescence imaging has been shown to improve short-term patient outcomes after coronary artery bypass grafting [4] and to reduce hospital cost of CABG [5, 6]. Several techniques have been used to assess intraoperative graft flow and patency. Most have had drawbacks limiting their use. These have been reviewed previously by Balacumaraswami and Taggert [7]. Electromagnetic

Supplementary Information The online version contains supplementary material available at https://doi.org/10.1007/978-3-031-40685-0_14.

D. Muehrcke (✉)
Cardiovascular and Thoracic Surgery at Flagler Hospital, Saint Augustine, FL, USA

N. Szoka et al. (eds.), *The SAGES Manual of Fluorescence-Guided Surgery*, https://doi.org/10.1007/978-3-031-40685-0_14

flowmetry, based on principles of electromagnetic induction, can quantitate blood flow accurately under experimental conditions where it assumes laminar flow. However, in the clinical setting, flow values fluctuate with movement and changing hematocrit, and consequently, its use has been short lived [8–10]. Continuous wave (CW) and pulsed wave (PW) Doppler velocity measurements have been used to assess intraoperative graft patency. Although, easy to use, continuous wave (CW) and pulsed wave (PW) Doppler velocity measurements are based on the principle of a change in Doppler velocity, detectors have no range resolution and PW Doppler systems were affected by the angle of insonation [10]. Epicardial ultrasound scanning [11] uses an epicardial probe, which provides satisfactory images of coronary stenosis and graft anastomoses but does not provide real-time angiographic images. Thermal coronary angiography, based on the creation of thermal images with an infrared camera, depends on the temperature difference between the myocardium and the coronary arteries generated with the use of cold or warm saline or cardioplegic injections. Although this provides images of graft function, resolution varies depending on temperature differences [12]. None of these techniques produce reliable or consistent results.

Intraoperative Techniques of Graft Patency Assessment

There are three currently used popular methods of measuring graft patency in CABG surgery. The best but most expensive method is coronary angiography. It does represent the gold standard to determine graft patency. Coronary angiography provides a clear multiplane visual assessment of all proximal and distal anastomoses. It is however invasive, expensive, and difficult to perform after heart surgery without having a cardiologist and cardiac catheterization lab available.

Transient time flowmetry (TTFM) and intraoperative fluorescence imaging (IFI) are currently the two most popular methods of assessing intraoperative coronary artery bypass graft patency.

Both are relatively inexpensive and easy to perform and can provide real-time intraoperative assessment of graft patency. Below we will discuss both of these techniques: their methodology, current experience, results, and limitations.

Transit-Time Flowmetry (TTFM)

Transit-time flowmetry (Medistim AS, Norway) is a technique based on the principle of transit-time ultrasound technology. It uses a perivascular flow probe, which consists of two ultrasonic transducers and a fixed acoustic reflector, which holds the graft perpendicular to the position of the transducers and the reflector. The transit time taken from the wave of ultrasound to travel from one transducer to another is derived by the flow meter and provides an accurate measure of flow volume [13].

Technique

The flow probes require the use of an ultrasound gel applied to the lumen of the flow probe. It is important to ensure the graft occupies at least 75% of the area within the probe to get an accurate reading (Fig. 14.1). The coupling agent (gel) improves ultrasound imaging. Results are quantitatively reported as mean graft flow and a flow waveform is generated. In addition to the flow waveform, the systems provide various calculated derivatives such as mean graft flow (MGF), pulsatile index (PI), and diastolic flow index (DFI).

Mean graft flow is expressed as mL/min which indicates the quantity of graft flow at the time of the measurement. Mean graft flow values above 40 mL/min indicate satisfactory flow, and values less than 5 mL/min are considered unsatisfactory, prompting revision [13]. When mean graft flow value between 5 mL/min and 40 mL are obtained, interpretation depends on certain derived values such as PI and DFI. PI is expressed as an absolute number of the value obtained by the dips between the maximum flow and the minimum flow divided by the mean flow. It gives an estimate

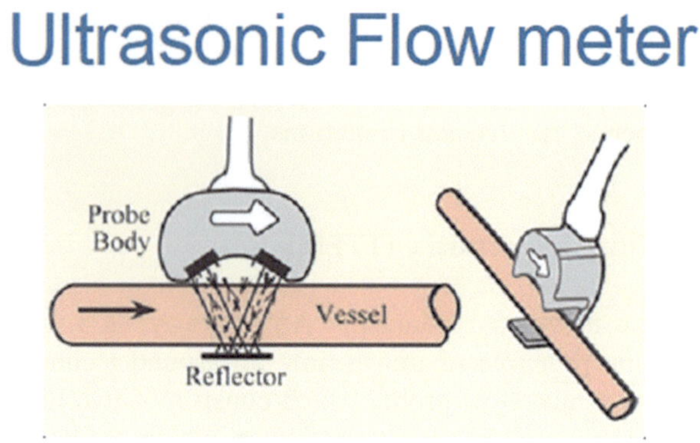

Fig. 14.1 TTFM flow probe with bypass graft inserted for reading of flow expressed as mL/min. The ultrasound flow meter measures the velocity of a fluid with ultrasound to calculate volume flow. Using ultrasound transducers, the flow meter can measure the average velocity along the path of an emitted beam of ultrasound, by averaging the difference in measured transit time between the pulses of ultrasound propagating into and against the direction of flow

of the resistance to graft flow. Generally, a PI value of more than 5 is considered to indicate unsatisfactory graft flow [14] and revision should be considered; however, PI alone cannot be used to determine graft revision. DFI is expressed with the percentage of total graft flow which occurs during diastole. A predominant diastolic flow in the graft with a DFI that is more than 50 is considered normal, similar to the native coronary blood flow [15]. A DFI less than 50 is cause for concern. Unfortunately, there are no images of graft flow produced using this technique to help validate visually marginal or concerning derived values.

Current Experience and Results

Several groups have reported the clinical usefulness of TTFM to assess graft patency.

D'Ancona et al. reported the need to revise 37 of 1147 graft (3%) in 33 of 409 off-pump coronary artery bypass grafts (8%).

They emphasize the reliance on correct analysis of TTFM flow patterns to correct the abnormalities, since interpretation of the derived values is variable and may be inconclusive [16].

Likewise, Taggert's group [17] has used TTFM in over 100 patients, and it was found to be useful in confirming graft patency in the majority of patients with good mean graft flow values. Using both TTFM and intraoperative fluorescence imaging (IFI) modalities in the same patient, they found that in the majority of grafts, both TTFM and IFI reliably confirmed graft patency. However, in 3.8% of grafts (10% of patients) with low mean graft flow situations, where TTFM indicated the need to revise the grafts, IFI confirmed satisfactory visual antegrade flow. Because the flow through the grafts could be visualized, no revisions were performed. Taggert expressed concerns that TTFM may overestimate the need for graft revision.

TTFM has been used in the assessment of graft patency with a greater degree of accuracy compared with other flow measurement modalities, such as electromagnetic flowmetry, which varies with movement and hematocrit and Doppler flowmeters, which vary with the angle of insonation [18, 19]. It has correctly identified occluded grafts when other tests suggested a patent graft. This includes situations where a pulse was felt in an occluded graft (as a tactile pulse can be felt in occluded grafts which can be misinterpreted as "flow"). TTFM can detect graft occlusion even when the ECG remains normal and echocardiography identifies normal wall motion. Jakobsen noted that only one of the five cases with TTFM documented graft occlusion was the graft impairment reflected in abnormal ECG findings [20]. Walpoth and colleagues describe two cases in which TTFM detected graft occlusion despite adequate perfusion of the graft assessed by the surgeon's fingers, which was corrected on the operating room table [21].

TTFM unfortunately does not always reliably predict graft or anastomotic stenosis as reported by several groups. Hirotani and colleagues evaluated TTFM measurements in a series of 291 in situ internal mammary artery grafts and 190 saphenous vein grafts in 171 patients. They compared the intraoperative measurements with postoperative coronary angiogram performed before hospital discharge [19]. They found that mean graft flow, as measured by TTFM failed to predict stenosis or partially occluded grafts on postoperative angiograms. Jakobsen and Kjaergard reported 1.8% graft revision rate in a series of 280 CABG patients [20].

Limitations

In the majority of patients with good MGF (>40 mL/min), TTFM reliably indicates graft patency. However, in low mean graft flow situations, interpretation of PI and DFI values is arbitrary, and there is considerable uncertainty regarding adequacy of graft patency. Transit-time flow measurement is a very easy device to use; however, it does not show a visual image of the graft. When the graft is subjected to spasm, or the stenosis of the native coronary artery is not very severe, flow measurement data may not be diagnostic.

Intraoperative Fluorescent Imaging (IFI) System

Principle

SPY intraoperative fluorescence imaging received FDA 510(K) clearance in 2005 as a system to assess graft patency after CABG surgery. The IFI system SPY™ (STRYKER corporation, Kalamazoo MI) depends on the fluorescent properties of indocyanine green (ICG) dye. ICG rapidly binds to the plasma proteins when injected intravenously and is therefore confined to the intravascular compartment. Indocyanine green is excreted unchanged by the liver with a half-life of 3–5 min; thus, there is no potential for nephrotoxic effects for those patients with compromised renal function. The dye also has an excellent safety profile. The incident of allergic reactions to ICG is approximately 1 in 40,000, and it has been reported mainly in patients with an allergy to iodine [22]. The risk of allergic reactions is strongly dose dependent, being greatest with a dose in excess of 0.5 mg/kg weight. A lower density laser with a total output of 2.7 w spread over an area of

7.5 cm × 7.5 cm at a distance of 30 cm has a depth of penetration of about 1–2 mm to avoid thermal damage. ICG fluoresces when illuminated with a laser light of 806 nm and emits light at the longer wavelength at 830 nm. The imaging camera head is a charged couple device video camera and is positioned over the exposed heart, and the laser is activated before the first pass of a bolus of ICG through the field of view. Images of the coronary arteries and bypass grafts are acquired at a rate of 30 frames/s and may be viewed in real time. The near-infrared light can maximally penetrate 1–2 mm of soft tissue. The fluorescence sequentially shows illumination of the graft or coronary artery lumen, a blush of the epicardium occurs as the dye passes through the microcirculation, and, finally, washout occurs as the dye enters the coronary veins.

The ICG dye transmission time is dependent on various factors including the systemic arterial pressure, competitive native coronary blood flow on the severity of native proximal coronary stenosis, distal coronary vascular resistance, and conduit diameter. The proximal target coronary artery snaring with a silastic sling facilitates anastomotic visualization and largely eliminates competitive flow [16]. Skeletonized internal thoracic artery (ITA) and radial artery (RA) conduit provider better visualization than pedicle ones. The appearance of fluorescent images, as the dye passes through the bypass graft, confirms graft patency.

Technique

There are three different techniques we use to visualize CABG grafts and one technique we use to identify epicardial coronary arteries during redo bypass surgery or for intramyocardial vessel identification. We typically perform coronary artery bypass grafting using the cardiopulmonary bypass machine with the heart arrested. We feel this technique allows us to bypass more vessels, improves long-term graft patency, and improves long-term survival than off-pump bypass techniques. However, the techniques can easily be used with off-pump bypass grafting, with special attention to not allowing air down the grafts being assessed.

A direct handheld injection of ICG down individual vein grafts is used to assess each vein graft distal anastomosis and to assess perfusion of the heart (Video 14.1). The important internal thoracic artery to left anterior descending artery bypass graft is assessed by injection ICG dye into the heart-lung machine. Imaging of each graft takes only 2–3 min (Video 14.2). Typically, we perform our vein graft anastomoses first followed by the IMA to LAD anastomosis. Each distal vein graft anastomosis can be tested by injecting 10 ccs of contrast down the vein graft (or free arterial graft) through a syringe. The concentration of the ICG used has decreased with the newer SPY-PHI handheld cameras as they have improved penetration. The concentration we use is made up by placing 0.3 ccs (0.375 mg) of ICG (concentration 2.5 mg/mL) into 500 ccs of normal saline (final concentration 0.00075 mg/mL). Thirty-five ccs of this solution is mixed with 10 ccs of heparinized blood mixed with nitroglycerine (0.38 mg) for direct injection down the vein grafts or free internal thoracic artery grafts. Ten ccs of the final mixture is injected down the vein graft as images are acquired, and then the graft is flushed with heparinized blood as a washout. Care must be taken not inject air down the grafts, especially when performing off-pump bypass grafting. The images develop instantaneously in real time. We specifically look for tactile flow resistance through the vein graft, and the ICG contrast image through the anastomosis, and the epicardial artery. The tactile response of how hard or easy it is to inject the solution gives feedback as to the flow in the bypassed vessel. The rate of hand-injected flow is determined by several factors including the diameter of the vein, the size of the anastomosis, the size of the epicardial artery grafted, and the resistance in the vascular bed distal to the anastomosis. Moreover, we look for the three phases of fluorescence. The first is the arterial phase, where the vein graft, anastomosis, and artery are illuminated. The second phase is where the myocardium is illuminated, and the third phase is the venous phase when the veins on the heart are imaged.

An injection of the ICG into the heart-lung machine is used to assess IMA to coronary artery flow when the cross clamp is on, as the in situ graft is the only source of blood flow to the heart with the cross clamp on (Video 14.2). Flow through the in situ IMA graft is evaluated by injecting 0.8 cc of undiluted ICG dye (1.0 mg) into the heart-lung machine. Imaging will take 10–15 s to occur. There should be a brisk transition from the IMA graft into the left anterior descending coronary artery.

At the end of the procedure after performing the proximal anastomoses, all proximal anastomoses are assessed simultaneously by injecting 0.3 ccs of undiluted ICG (0.375 mg) into the central line (Video 14.3). This is followed by a 10-cc flush of normal saline. Visualization of the proximal anastomoses will take 10–15 s to appear as the dye works its way through the heart to the aorta. Revisions are based on the findings of the gross blood flow images. The images are then recorded on computer hard drive as well as a copy of selected screenshots which are placed into the patient's chart. Repeat ICG injections can be administered at short intervals (after 2 or 3 min after the dye washes out) and still generate excellent image quality. Any extravasated dye from a leak at the anastomosis may obscure images.

The determination of a left anterior descending toe left anterior descending artery occlusion can be identified easily intraoperatively (Video 14.4). If there is no flow, then the graft can be revised immediately to insure a patent graft (Video 14.5). In a similar fashion, an occluded proximal bypass vein graft can de identified (Video 14.6). These grafts can also be revised immediately to ensure open grafts at the end of the procedure (Video 14.7).

Peals and Pitfalls of Bypass Graft Imaging

The most important concern with intraoperative imagine using ICG is the concentration of the dye. We have significantly decreased the concentration of the dye solution with the more powerful handheld SPY-PHI camera. Using a too concentrated dye solution washes out the images and details such as kinks and narrowing and even twists in an anastomosis can be obscured. A too dilute solution will fail to identify epicardial vessels under scar tissue in redo bypass surgery and may not allow an intramyocardial epicardial vessel to be seen. Moreover, too dilute of a dye solution not show graft narrowing.

When performing a root injection of 30–60-cc ICG dye directly into the root through the anti-grade cardioplegia needle to evaluate for epicardial vessels obscured by overlying scan tissue in redo procedures (Video 14.8), care must be taken not to introduce are into the root when doing this. When the heart is arrested, the dye will not be washed out, as no flush out is used, so the operator has much more time to find the images. The difficulty occurs when one has to mark the location of the illuminated vessel while visualizing on a camera screen, not looking at the heart. One technique we have found helpful is to use a sterile felt marking pen and touch dots along the illuminated vessel which can easily be seen on the camera screen. The surgeon then has to just connect the dots with a scalpel to find the subtended epicardial vessel. We have found attempting to draw a straight line over the obscured epicardial vessel while looking at the camera screen is very difficult and leads to errors in finding the surface vessels. Similar to operating using a video-assisted thoracoscope (VATS) screen, one's movements are opposite to the images viewed. As such there is learning curve. When looking for buried intramyocardial vessels, the new SPYPHI scope appears to have deeper tissue penetration and allow finding obscured vessel easier. We have no experience using a more concentrated solution to see if even deeper penetration of the images occurs facilitating identification of intramyocardial vessels.

Another pitfall of the intraoperative assessment of bypass grafts is when extravasation occurs out of a leaky distal anastomosis, as the contrast is not washed away. The dye can stain the epicardial surface and obscure some images as the fluorescent dye remains. Usually this is not a problem as the flow through the anastomosis is easily seen on subsequent injections.

One interesting area of ongoing study is the possibility to assess the presence of competitive flow through the important IMA to LAD anastomosis if one calculates the pixel intensity to the anterior wall using qualification hardware. With the cross clamp off, serial central line injections of ICG with the IMA occluded using a soft vascular clap first and then subsequently with the IMA not occluded are used to generate pixel intensity grafts. The difference represents the flow to the anterior wall of the heart provided by the IMA graft (Fig. 14.2). The additional flow to the anterior wall from the IMA blood supply can be quantitated by subtracting these two values. Obviously, separate images are recorded for each injection and compared. The lack of increased flow may be a sign of competitive flow due to a non-physiologic proximal coronary artery stenosis. The importance to competitive blood flow is unknown. The next areas of research will include attempting to quantitate blood flow to the myocardium. It is important to realize that the intensity of the surface pixels may not reflect the heterogenous blood flow which occurs deeper

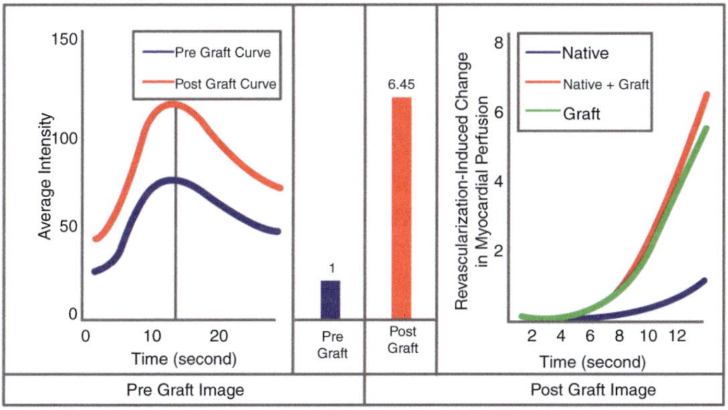

Fig. 14.2 Pixel intensity measurements approximate myocardial blood flow using the SPY Q analysis program. Measurements are made with the cross-clamp off. In the left panel, the blue represents anterior wall pixel intensity (blood flow), to the native myocardium (pre-grafting; IMA occluded). The red line represents the average pixel intensity after grafting with the IMA (post-grafting; IMA graft open). If the native flow is normalized to a value of 1 (middle panel), then the increased flow with the new IMA graft is quantitated to 6.45 times the blood flow. The right panel shows myocardial perfusion of the native vessel (blue), the improved flow with a new IMA graft (red), and the flow added to the anterior wall (green) [30]. Reproduced with rights: Mitsuo Kusano. IICG Fluorescent Imaging and navigation Surgery. Springer. Chap. 6 Takahashi, M, Masuda M, Miyajima K, et al. Innovative SPY Intra-operative Imaging and Validation Technologies for Coronary Artery Bypass Grafting Surgery. Figure 14.3, 2016

in the myocardium and endocardial surfaces. This will always be a limitation to blood flow analysis using this technique. Not to mention the very un-physiologic state being studied with an arrested heart in diastole. To truly asses changes in myocardial blood flow before and after bypass grafting, the heart must be assessed not only under similar work conditions, but all layers of the myocardium need to be assessed, which is not feasible during bypass grafting surgery.

Validation Studies

Takahashi and associates [23] were one of the first authors to compare IFI with TTFM in off-pump cases in Japan. Each patient served as their own control. They demonstrated high-quality IFI images in 290 grafts of 72 off-pump CABG cases (mean of 4.0 grafts per patient). Four anastomoses (1.4%), including 2 proximal and 2 distal, were revised because of defects detected by SPY images. In one case (Fig. 14.3), the SPY system revealed no blood flow in a radial sequential graft, although transit-time flow meter measurements taken on the sequential portion of the bypass graft showed a diastolic dominant pattern with intermediate flow of 24 mL/min. SPY images revealed the proximal portion of the radial artery graft, between the aorta and the obtuse marginal artery, to be non-patent, allowing them to revise the graft while the patient was still on the operating table. After revision, slide B on the right demonstrates IFI imaging showing both the aorta to obtuse marginal 1 graft and the sequential obtuse marginal 1 to obtuse marginal 2 graft the be patent. The TTFM flow increased from 22 mL/min top 55 mL/min in the sequential portion of the graft. The authors concluded that using the SPY system, technical failures could be completely resolved during surgery. They stated that the use of the SPY system for intraoperative graft validation during off-pump CABG may become the gold standard for surgical management in the near future. Importantly, Takahashi was able to demonstrate a significant flaw in TTFM analysis, that is, the inability to visually assess the bypass grafts. He demonstrated

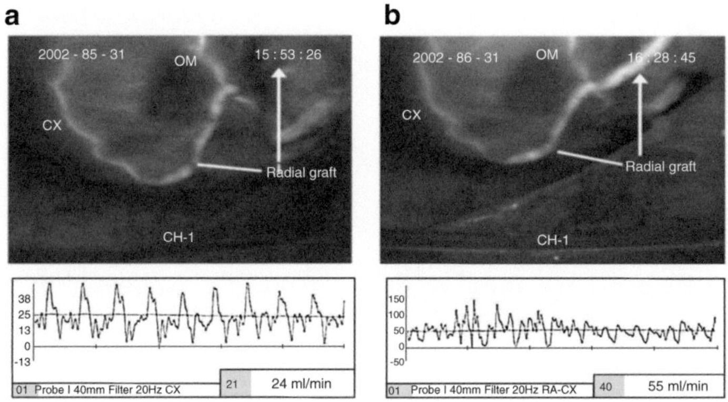

Fig. 14.3 Slide A represents the IFI images of a radial sequential graft from the circumflex obtuse marginal 1 to the circumflex obtuse marginal 2. By IFI the free radial graft from the aorta to the obtuse marginal 1 is occluded; however, the flow measured on the sequential obtuse marginal 1 to obtuse marginal 2 reveals a flow of 24 mL/min. After revision, slide B on IFI imaging shows both the aorta to obtuse marginal 1 graft and the sequential obtuse marginal 1 to obtuse marginal 2 graft the be patent. The TTFM flow increased from 22 mL/min to 55 mL/min [31]. (Reproduced with permission: Takahashi, Msao, Ishikawa, Toshihiro. SPY: an innovative intra-operative imaging system to evaluate graft patency during off-pump coronary artery bypass grafting. Interactive CardioVascular and Thoracic Surgery 3 (2004) 479–483)

two cases where sequential grafts were used wherein TTFM was unable to identify graft closure correctly.

In another patient depicted in Fig. 14.4, an in situ internal mammary artery has been used as a sequential graft between the diagonal and the left anterior descending (LAD) artery. Intraoperative fluorescence imaging reveals that the sequential portion between the diagonal and the LAD artery is occluded despite the TTFM flow measuring a flow of 22 mL/min, when measured in the IMA to diagonal graft. The images on the right were taken after the graft was revised in the operating room. It demonstrates excellent flow through both anastomoses of the sequential diagonal to LAD graft. The TTFM flow was unchanged (22 mL/min) after revision. In both cases presented, the TTFM was not helpful in detecting a significant intraoperative graft occlusion because of a lack of visual assessment of the graft.

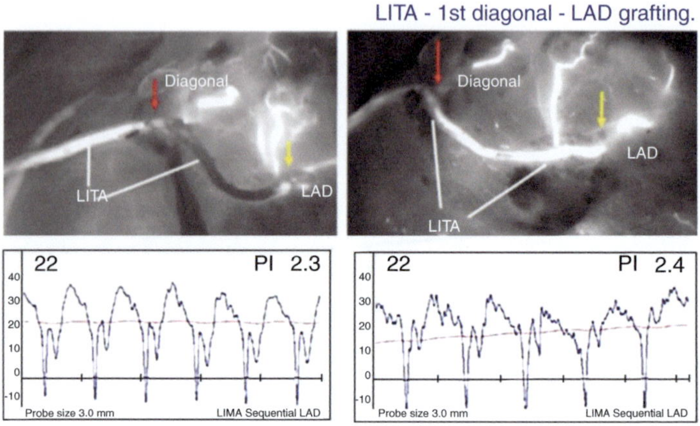

Fig. 14.4 Sequential IMA to diagonal and LAD graft. On the left the diagonal to LAD sequential graft is occluded by IFI; however, TTFM measured a flow of 22 mL/min. After revision IFI shows the entire sequential graft to be patent; however, there was no change in the TTFM flow of 22 mL/min [31]. (Reproduced with permission: Takahashi, Msao, Ishikawa, Toshihiro. SPY: an innovative intra-operative imaging system to evaluate graft patency during off-pump coronary artery bypass grafting. Interactive CardioVascular and Thoracic Surgery 3 (2004) 479–483)

Desai and colleagues [24] also noted that early CABG failures may be corrected if identified intraoperatively. These researchers like Takahashi compared the diagnostic accuracy of transit-time ultrasound flow measurement and ICG fluorescent-dye graft angiography. Both imaging studies were performed in each patient, as they acted as their own control. Virtually all cases were performed with cardioplegic arrest on the cardiopulmonary bypass machine. Patients undergoing isolated CABG with no contraindications for postoperative angiography were enrolled in the study. Patients were randomly assigned to be evaluated with either ICG angiography (ICG) and then transit-time ultrasonic flow measurement or transit-time flow then ICG angiography. Interestingly, all patients underwent X-ray angiography on postoperative day 4. The primary end-point of the trial was to determine the sensitivity and specificity of the two techniques versus standard X-ray angiography to detect graft occlusion or greater than 50% stenosis in the graft or peri-anastomotic area. A total of 106 patients were enrolled, and X-ray angiography was performed in 46 patients. In total, 139 grafts were reviewed with all 3 techniques and 12 grafts (8.2%) were demonstrated to have greater than 50% stenosis or occlusion by the reference standard. The sensitivity and specificity of ICG to detect greater than 50% stenosis or occlusion was 83.3% and 100%, respectively. The sensitivity and specificity of transit-time ultrasonic flow measurement to detect greater than 50% stenosis or occlusion was 25% and 98.4%, respectively. The p value for the overall comparison of sensitivity and specificity between ICG and transit-time flow ultrasonography was 0.011. The difference between sensitivity for ICG and transit-time flow measurement was 58% with a 95% confidence interval (CI) of 30% to 86%, $p = 0.023$. The authors concluded that ICG provided a better diagnostic method of detecting clinically significant graft errors than did transit-time ultrasound flow measurement. They also had patients who had marginal TTFM graft flows (5–40 mL/min) but had occluded grafts when visualized using ICG.

In a separate study, Wasada and associates [25] evaluated the intraoperative fluorescence imaging (IFI) system in the real-time assessment of graft patency during off-pump CABG. Patients undergoing off-pump CABG received IFI analysis, intraoperative transit time flowmetry, and postoperative X-ray angiography. A total of 507 grafts in 137 patients underwent analysis. Of all the IFI analyses, 379 (75%) grafts were visualized clearly up to the distal anastomosis. With regard to anastomosis location, anterior location was associated with a higher percentage of fully analyzable images (90%). More than 80% of images were analyzable, irrespective of graft type; six grafts with acceptable transit-time flowmetry results were diagnosed with graft failure by IFI, which required on-site graft revision. All revised grafts' patency was confirmed by postoperative X-ray angiography. Conversely, 21 grafts with unsatisfactory transit-time flowmetry results demonstrated acceptable patency with IFI. Graft revision was considered unnecessary in these grafts, and 20 grafts (95%) were patent by postoperative X-ray angiography. Compared with slow washout, fast washout was associated with a higher preoperative ejection fraction, use of internal mammary artery grafts, and anterior anastomosis location. The authors concluded that the IFI system enabled on-site assessment of graft patency, providing both morphologic and functional information. They concluded that this technique may help reduce procedure-related, early graft failures in off-pump bypass patients.

Interpretation

Several researchers have attempted to quantitate myocardial perfusion or graft flow using IFI. None have been able to quantitate myocardial blood flow reliably using the pixel intensity measurements which are used in assessing graft patency. It is important to understand that as a result of the low energy used in the laser to obtain images using IFI, only 2 mm of the myocardial surface can be imaged. Therefore, any quantitative analysis presumes that myocardial blood flow is universal through the entire thickness of the ventricular wall. This obviously may be not true and represents a potential inaccuracy of this methodology. Nonetheless, Detter et al. [26] have shown that myocardial blood flow is reduced in a step-like fashion with greater degrees of coronary stenosis. Moreover, Yamamato [27] has shown a similar association looking at the flow in the vessel itself, not the myocardium. Both attempted to assess myocardial flow by measuring peak pixel intensity and time to peak pixel intensity.

Detter et al. [26] attempted to quantify the blood supply to the heart by measuring the maximum pixel intensity of the myocardium and time to maximum intensity during the myocardial phase of IFI imaging. They evaluated the ability of IFI to quantitatively assess the effect of coronary stenosis of variable severity on myocardial perfusion using two separate methods. They compared the effect of variable coronary artery stenosis in vivo (coronary stenosis of 25%, 50%, 75%, and 100% flow restriction) using IFI compared to the gold standard assessment using the fluorescent microsphere method. Using open-chest pigs, graded stenosis and total occlusion of the left anterior descending coronary artery were created. They showed that increasing graded stenosis and total vessel occlusion reduced normalized background-subtracted peak fluorescence intensity and the slope of fluorescence intensity significantly. Moreover, background-subtracted peak fluorescence intensity and slope of fluorescence intensity (analyzed by ICG) demonstrated good linear correlation with fluorescent microsphere-derived myocardial blood flow. These quantitative assessments of myocardial blood flow using IFI are mostly used to show an increase or no change in myocardial blood flow following bypass grafting (Figs. 14.5 and 14.6). They concluded that the impairment of myocardial perfusion in response to increased coronary stenosis severity and total vessel occlusion can be quantitatively assessed by ICG and correlates well with results obtained by fluorescent microsphere assessment.

Ferguson et al. have also reported that the change in fluorescence intensity is a direct indicator of the change in the myocardial perfusion using perfusion pixel analysis [28]. Using this methodology his group has used IFI to assess competitive flow after bypass grafting. He has shown that when there is no increase in myocardial perfusion after grafting, the native vessel stenosis is likely not physiologically significant despite how tight the native vessel stenosis appeared visually. This may help reduce the incidence of early graft closure by better understanding which types grafts are more prone to competitive flow after they are constructed. Looking at 167 bypass patients with 359 grafts (53% arterial), all grafts were widely patent by IFI, and 24% of the arterial and 22% of the saphenous vein grafts showed no regional myocardial perfusion change in response to bypass grafting, consistent with competitive flow. In 165 in situ internal mammary grafts to the left anterior descending artery (>70% visual stenosis on preoperative angiogram), 40 had no change in regional myocardial perfusion, and 32 of the 40 had competitive flow imaged. They concluded that an important number of angiographic patient bypass grafts demonstrated no change in regional myocardial perfusion suggesting anatomical, but nonfunctional stenosis in the target vessel epicardial coronary arteries. In in situ arterial grafts imaged, competitive flow was associated with nonfunctional stenosis in the target vessel epicardial coronary artery. During the

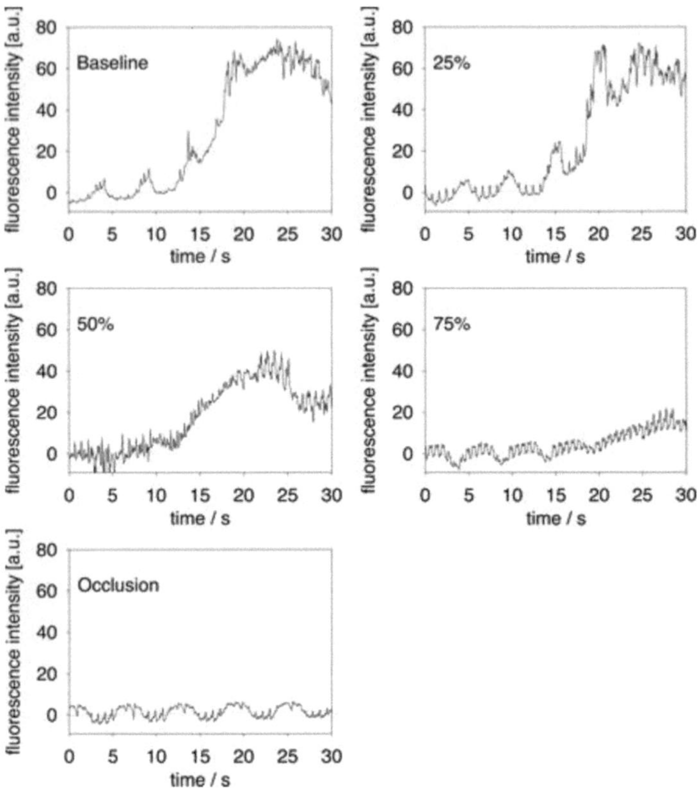

Fig. 14.5 Time-intensity curves of the left ventricular anterior wall analyzed by slope of fluorescence intensity (SFI) in a representative experiment at baseline and four graded coronary stenosis (25%, 50%, 75%, and 100% flow restriction). a.u. equals arbitrary units. One can see the diminished intensity of the fluorescence with increasing degrees of vessel stenosis. (Reproduced with permission: Detter C, Wipper S, Russ D, If and A, Burdorf L, Thein E, et al. Fluorescent cardiac imaging: a novel intraoperative method for quantitative assessment of myocardial perfusion during graded coronary artery stenosis. Circulation. 2007;116 (9):1007–14)

discussion of this paper [29], it was pointed out that the surgeon only finds out that graft has competitive flow after the graft has been performed, thereby limiting the usefulness of the technique.

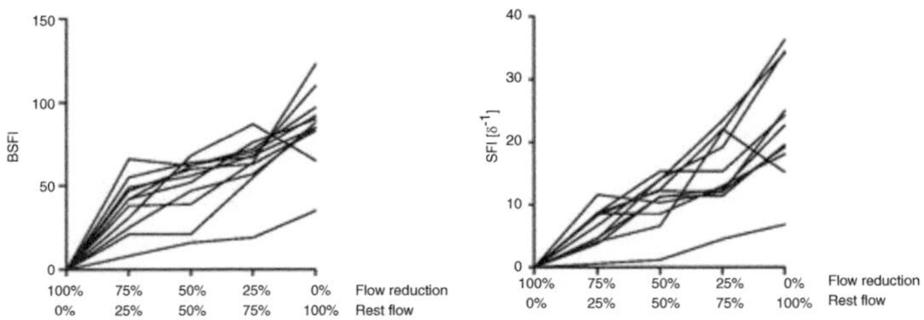

Fig. 14.6 Background-subtracted peak fluorescence intensity (BSFI) (left) and slope of fluorescence intensity (SFI) (right) obtained at baseline and four graded coronary stenosis (25%, 50%, 75%, and 100% flow restriction) in 11 animals (Reproduced with permission: Detter C, Wipper S, Russ D, If and A, Burdorf L, Thein E, et al. Fluorescent cardiac imaging: a novel intraoperative method for quantitative assessment of myocardial perfusion during graded coronary artery stenosis. Circulation. 2007;116 (9):1007–14)

Moreover, as the IFI in this study was not performed under stress, the physiologic importance of the epicardial stenosis may have been underestimated. Moreover, Sabik [29] pointed out that there is likely a benefit to bypassing coronary arteries without significant fraction flow reserve numbers as 80% of the grafts remain patient at a year, and the long-term effect is likely beneficial to the patient as their disease is likely to progress.

While some authors have found IFI helpful in evaluating stenosis at the anastomosis [24, 30], direct assessment of the severity of vessel stenosis by IFI can be limited. While the previously mentioned studies have illustrated that the extent of changes in ICG fluorescence intensity of the myocardial wall is useful, the human myocardium is often covered with an epicardial fat pad that limits ICG fluorescence imaging and therefore making analysis often times inaccurate.

Therefore, Yamamoto et al. [31], using an ex vivo model, studied the effect of vessel stenosis on the maximum intensity and time to maximum intensity in the vessels only, not the myocardium. During near-infrared (NIR) angiography, the fluorescence intensity was calculated during pre- and post-stenosis in an artificial ex vivo circuit, using NIR angiography. They measured the time to maximum fluorescence intensity and the absolute maximum intensity. They found that severe stenosis (greater than 75%) attenuated the increase in ICG fluorescence intensity in the vessel but not the time to maximum fluorescence. The conventional visual qualitative NIR angiographic assessment may produce a false result, due to the human eye not being able to perceive a difference in the intensity of the fluorescence. The anastomoses may appear normal as the flow rate (time to peak intensity) is not affected by greater degrees of stenosis. The surgeon is likely to see flow through the anastomosis but not perceive a diminished intensity of the fluorescent dye. The estimation is made worse by the fact that the time to maximal intensity if one looks at the flow through the vessel only is the same whether there is a tight stenosis at the anastomosis or not. This technique cannot detect small differences over time [32]. Since arterial stenosis attenuates increases in ICG fluorescence intensity through vessels, quantitative analysis using NIR angiography could predict vessel stenosis. This quantitative assessment may provide a more precise evaluation of vessel stenosis or graft complications, as this ex vivo study was able to detect vessel stenosis exceeding 75%.

Clinical Results

The ability to reliably assess the patency of coronary artery bypass grafts using intraoperative fluorescence imaging has been shown to improve short-term patient outcomes after coronary artery bypass grafting [4] and to reduce hospital cost of CABG [5, 6].

SPY imaging has been the topic of a substantial body of evidence supporting its use in CABG surgery. In 2009, cardiac surgeon researchers presented results from 350 patients undergoing CABG including SPY imaging enrolled in the VICTORIA Multicenter Registry. VICTORIA data showed that the complication rates, including reoperation and long length of stay, were 50% lower than expected compared to similar patients enrolled in the Society of Thoracic Surgeon's (STS) national cardiac database. The STS database is one of the longest-standing and largest existing medical datasets that exist today [4].

The Centers for Medicare and Medicaid independently studied cost data in 2008 and 2009 and concluded that the use of SPY in CABG resulted in average cost reductions of $2000–4000 per patient (Table 14.1). In today's healthcare environment, cost savings resulting from reductions in complications are critical to achieving the goals of healthcare reform. Moreover, an improvement in graft patency will likely lead to a reduced readmission rate and hospital reimbursement penalties. This represented a 10% decrease in cost for the average CABG patient after the cost of the procedure was included (CMS 2009) (Table 14.2). Similar results were reported by the Sentara Heart Hospital [6].

A Sentara Heart Hospital independent study of more than 700 patients undergoing CABG demonstrated that total costs of CABG were 4.2% lower and average length of stay was 6–16% lower in 358 patients where the CABG procedure included SPY imaging versus the 225 cases performed without SPY.

Table 14.1 Results of a study performed by the Centers for Medicaid and Medicare service to determine the cost saving associated with the use of SPY angiography

MS-DRG	Number of cases	Average length of stay	Average cost
Bypass + CATH + MCC with SPY	88	9.82	$29,258
Bypass + CATH+ MCC without SPY	10,224	11.14	$33,886
Other cardiac procedures + MCC with SPY	159	6.3	$22,342
CABG with CATH with SPY	60	12.82	$38,842
CABG with CATH without SPY	17,393	13.55	$41,207
CABG w/o CATH with SPY	69	8.75	$25,308
CABG w/o CATH without SPY	26,934	8.7	$29,334

On average patients having IFI during CABG surgery realized 10% hospital cost savings (12). These savings occurred after taking into consideration the cost of performing the angiography

Table 14.2 CMS data evaluating cost of intraoperative fluorescent-guided imaging during coronary artery bypass grafting (CMS data)

SPY CMS Confirms Cost Impact of SPY in CABG

MS-DRG	# of Cases	Average Length of Stay	Average Cost*
Bypass+ CATH + MCC Cases with SPY	88	9.82	$29,258
Bypass +CATH+MCC Cases without SPY	10,224	11.14	$33,886
Other cardiac Procedures+ MCC with SPY	159	6.3	$20,404
Other Cardiac Procedures + MCC without SPY	24,640	6.52	$22,342

MS-DRG	# of Cases	Average Length of Stay	Average Cost*
CABG w/o CATH Cases with SPY	60	12.82	$38,842
CABG w/o CATH Cases without SPY	17,393	13.65	$41,207
CABG w/o CATH- cases with SPY	69	8.75	$25,308
CABG w/o Cath Cases without SPY	26,934	8.7	$29,334

CMS confirmed that CABG with SPY resulted in an average cost savings of 10% for hospitals nationwide in all DRG' s, after already taking into account the cost of SPY

The above improved clinical results and cost reductions using IFI during CABG surgery have helped to make a strong case for the use of IFI in all CABG cases.

Pitfalls

This technology had several drawbacks. First, IFI does not provide an exact graft flow quantity measurement. Quantitative graft flow measurement software is currently being investigated but not accurate enough to be clinically useful. Second, the laser light source is of relatively low power to ensure safe clinical use. However, this limited the penetration of the light through tissue to about 2 mm. Thus, clear images could not be obtained when the coronary artery has a deep intramyocardial location or is covered by epicardial fat. The pedicled conduits with significant amounts of overlying tissue were also less well visualized. However, these investigators believed that full skeletonizing of the arterial conduits is a very useful and important technique for complete arterial revascularization of all the coronary vascular regions. The technique allows direct illumination of all bypass grafts (potentially difficult on the back of the heart). The entire graft often cannot be imaged in the same sequence by a single central injection. As a result of these drawbacks, Waseda et al. found that only 75% of the grafts were completely visualized [25]. While it appears IFI has an advantage over TTFM in sensitivity, it is also more cumbersome, time-consuming, and expensive.

The official position of The American College of Cardiology Foundation/American Heart Association guideline on "coronary artery bypass graft surgery" [33] is: "Over the past 20 years, the patency rate of all graft types has improved gradually, so that the present failure rate of LIMA grafts at 1 year is about 8% and of SVGs roughly 20%." Many patients being referred for CABG nowadays have far advanced CAD, which is often diffuse and exhibits poor vessel runoff. Technical issues at the time of surgery may influence graft patency, and intraoperative imaging may help to delineate technical from nontechnical issues. Because coronary angiography is rarely available intraoperatively, other techniques have been developed to assess graft integrity at this time, most often the transit-time flow and intraoperative fluorescence imaging. The transit-time flow is a quantitative volume-flow technique that cannot define the severity of graft stenosis or discriminate between the influence of the graft conduit and the coronary arteriolar bed on the mean graft flow. Intraoperative fluorescence imaging, which is based on the fluorescent properties of indocyanine green, provides a "semi-quantitative" assessment of graft patency with images that provide some details about the quality of coronary anastomoses. Although both methods are valuable in assessing graft patency, neither is sufficiently sensitive nor specific to allow identification of more subtle abnormalities. It is hoped that such imaging may help to reduce the occurrence of technical errors.

Pediatric Heart Surgery

One of the largest growth areas in the field of cardiac surgery using intraoperative fluorescent imaging is in the field of pediatric/congenital surgery. Kogon [34] described his group's experience using intraoperative indocyanine green fluorescent angiography in pediatric surgery. In the surgical reconstruction for congenital heart defects, vessel and anastomotic site patency is critical to success. Indocyanine green fluorescent angiography offers the potential for a reliable and rapid method of intraoperative assessment. They used intraoperative fluorescent imaging in the following repairs: coronary artery reimplantation, coarctation, palliative shunts, and pulmonary artery reconstructions to assess the utility of intraoperative fluorescent imaging.

Unlike angiography, intraoperative fluorescent imaging offers the potential for a reliable noninvasive, inexpensive, and rapid method of intraoperative assessment of vessel anastomotic patency. For congenital heart surgery, the current methodology of evaluating repairs intraoperatively is transesophageal echocardiography.

This modality is excellent for intracardiac lesions. There is frequently indirect to poor resolution of surrounding vasculature. The gold standard for vascular imaging is conventional angiography, which can be performed intraoperatively using mobile fluoroscopy unit. However, this is cumbersome and potentially nephrotoxic, often requires additional sites of vascular access, and has not been except the routine for congenital heart surgery. Certain congenital heart operations involve complicated blood vessel reconstructions and delicate anastomosis. Thrombosis, narrowing, and occlusion of vessels, particularly at the suture lines, often contribute to morbidity and mortality. Clearly, with these operations there is a particular risk for these problems, and conventional imaging techniques are suboptimal.

Coronary artery implantation is required for several congenital heart lesions/defects and is required during the arterial switch procedure for transposition of the great vessels, during repair of anomalous left coronary artery from the pulmonary artery, and during a Ross procedure or aortic root replacement. A widely patent coronary ostium without twisting or kinking of the proximal artery is critical to success, and problems can lead to myocardial ischemia and subsequent infarction.

Repair for coarctation of the aorta involves opening of a narrow area of the aorta to provide unobstructive flow from the aortic arch to the descending aorta. Residual ductal tissue or anastomotic problems can result in an aortic coarctation necessitating subsequent percutaneous or surgical intervention.

Placement of a palliative shunt is a common palliative operation for congenital heart disease and is typically used in patients with inadequate or ductal dependent pulmonary blood flow. This commonly takes the form of a systemic to pulmonary artery shunt (Blalock-Taussig shunt). Partial occlusion typically results in decreased peripheral oxygen saturations and hypoxemia. When children are shunt-dependent after surgery, relying on shunt patency for survival, occlusion may be life-threatening. In these cases, surgical or catheter-based intervention may be urgently required to restore patency.

Pulmonary artery reconstruction for stenosis can occur anywhere along the right ventricular outflow tract; in its most severe form, pulmonary atresia, the native branch and pulmonary branches can be severely hypoplastic or even discontinuous. Occasionally, major aortopulmonary collaterals contribute to pulmonary blood flow. In these indices combination of branch or distal pulmonary artery reconstruction and unifocalization of collaterals is often required. Either technically challenging operations, it would be extremely adventitious to detect potential problems with vessels and anastomotic patency prior to leaving the operating room, voiding the need for subsequent postoperative cardiac catheterization, cardiac-based intervention, or surgical reoperation, along with the associated morbidity and mortality.

This approach has limitations; reasons for unsuccessful imaging include a small incision and difficult exposure, overlying structures obscuring the view of the desired area, nonuniform dye column, over- or under-dosing of Indocyanine green dye, bleeding with resultant extravasation of dye, and minimal penetrance through polytetrafluoroethylene (Gore-Tex) (W. L. Gore &

Associates). Although some of these difficulties have been overcome by the increase in experience as the study progressed, others have not. For early successful repair such as the hemi-Fontan, Fontan, and pulmonary artery reconstructions, Kogon's group found the inability to obtain a uniform dye column at the side of interest, and overlying structures obscuring the view of the desired area will likely provide ongoing persistent obstacles to the cases. In the future, there may be situations in the intensive care unit where the technology would be advantageous. Often after complex reconstructions in neonates, the myocardium was edematous and cardiac function is marginal. The chest is left open intentionally to increase cardiac domain and allow for myocardial recovery. If these patients fail to progress their accent using critical condition to the cardiac catheterization, they have to evaluate the surgical repair. This could potentially be avoided with open chest bedside imaging in the intensive care unit.

Kogon's group also found adequate postoperative images obtained in 18 of 30 (60%) patients. Image adequacy was high as per Blalock-Taussig shunts (100%), coarctation repairs (86%), and coronary reimplantation (66%) and low for hemi-Fontan (0%), Fontan (40%), and pulmonary artery reconstructions (33%).

All adequate images showed vessel or anastomotic site patency, which corresponded to the subsequent postoperative echocardiograms and CT angiograms. They found that indocyanine green fluorescent imaging provided an additional intraoperative imaging modality. It potentially will reduce the need for subsequent postoperative interventions, along with the associated morbidity and mortality.

Unfortunately, the current method of evaluation of surgical repair intraoperatively is limited echocardiogram, either transesophageal or epicardial. Although this modality is excellent for some lesions, there is frequently indirect or poor resolution of anatomy in others. In addition, the results are often subject to misinterpretation due to operator dependency.

Another area in congenital heart surgery where intraoperative fluorescent imaging has used is for intraoperative coronary imaging prior to the procedure or planning purposes [35]. A clear understanding of the coronary anatomy is critical during congenital heart surgery, especially when a ventriculotomy is planned, as the right ventricular outflow tract reconstructions and biventricular repairs. Typically, major epicardial coronary arteries are easily identified during the first-time operations. However, for intraoperative and re-operative surgeries, epicardial adhesions can obscure coronary vessels making the identification challenging.

A clear understanding of the coronary anatomy is critical in congenital heart surgery, especially during procedures requiring direct coronary manipulation, such as arterial switch operations for transposition of the great vessels. Further understanding of the coronary anatomy and course is also important when repairing lesions such as tetralogy of Fallot, where abnormal coronary patterns can dictate operative strategy (i.e., transannular repair versus RV to PA conduit) and primary (non-redo) surgery; the epicardial vessels are easily identified by direct inspection and injury that could be avoided in cases requiring ventriculotomy. In the re-operative setting however, the ability to precisely delineate epicardial coronary artery anatomy is more limited. Epicardial adhesions can obscure the heart surface anatomy rendering the epicardial coronary vessels less obvious, therefore placing them at high risk for injury during the ventriculotomy. Preoperative imaging of the coronary arteries has traditionally been accomplished through several modalities including echocardiography, angiography, and the axial images with computer tomography and magnetic resonance imaging. All these can provide important anatomical information for preoperative planning; however, each has limitations in its ability to precisely define coronary anatomy. In redo right ventricular outflow tract (RVOT) reconstruction for tetralogy of Fallot and double-outlet right ventricle (DORV) and in complex biventricular repairs requiring intracardiac baffles and RV-PA conduits, the surgeon may be left questioning the exact location of epicardial vessels despite multiple preoperative imaging studies. In these cases, it is critical that the surgeon be able to precisely identify coronary arteries in order to avoid their injury when performing a ventriculotomy. To mitigate the risk of coronary artery injury, intraoperative fluorescent imaging can be used to obtain real-time coronary artery imaging for the operative planning.

Fein's group has described the application of intraoperative fluorescent imaging and congenital heart surgery to obtain real-time coronary artery visualization for operative planning in order to avoid coronary injury. They found the imaging to show the precise coronary anatomy, enabling identification of the optimal ventriculotomy site. Intraoperative fluorescent imaging is a safe and effective technique for characterizing coronary anatomy. This technique enhances procedural planning and helps to minimize the risk of coronary injury during preoperative congenital heart surgery. We have similarly used this technique to locate difficult to find intramyocardial vessels and obscured epicardial vessels in redo bypass surgery in adults [36].

Conclusions

Intraoperative fluorescent imaging is a helpful technique to visualize coronary artery anatomy when planning cardiac procedures, assessing postoperative congenital reconstructions, and to evaluate bypass grafts in real time. The technique has several drawbacks which are important to recognize; however, when used correctly, it is associated with improved clinical results and cost savings. Future research may allow more accurate myocardial blood flow quantification and recognize situations of competitive flow.

References

1. Desai ND, Miwa S. Kodama d, et al. improving the quality of coronary bypass surgery with intraoperative angiography: validation of a new technique. J Am Coll Cardiol. 2005;46:1521–5.
2. Puskas JD, Williams WH, Mahoney EM, et al. Off-pump vs conventional coronary artery bypass grafting: early and 1-year graft patency, cost, and quality-of-life outcomes: a randomized trial. JAMA. 2004;291:1841–9.
3. Khan NE, De SA, Mister R, et al. A randomized comparison of off-pump and on-pump multivessel coronary-artery bypass surgery. N Engl J Med. 2004;350:21–8.

4. Ferguson TB et al. Intra-operative angiography in CABG as a quality metric: the Victoria registry, poster presented at the American Heart Association meeting, November 2009.
5. Department of health and human Centers for Medicare & Medicaid Services 42 CFR Parts 412, 413, 415, and 489, [CMS-1406-P] RIN 0938-AP39, Medicare Program; Proposed Changes to the Hospital Inpatient Prospective Payment Systems for Acute Care Hospitals and Fiscal Year 2010 Rates and to the long-term care hospital prospective payment system and rate year 2010 rates, Sept 2009.
6. Data on File at Sentara Heart Hospital and NOVADAQ (Stryker, Kalamazoo Mich).
7. Balacumaraswami L, Taggert DP. Digital tools to facilitate intraoperative coronary artery bypass graft patency assessment. Semin Thorac Cardiovasc Surg. 2004;16:266–71.
8. Louagie YA, Haxhe JP, Buche M, et al. Intraoperative electromagnetic flowmeter measurements in coronary artery bypass grafts. Ann Thorac Surg. 1994;57:357–64.
9. Dennis J, Wyatt DG. Effects of hematocrit value upon electromagnetic flowmeter sensitivity. Circ Res. 1969;24:875–86.
10. Beard JD, Evans JM, Skidmore R, et al. A Doppler flowmeter for use in theatre. Ultrasound Med boil. 1986;12:883–9.
11. Haaverstad R, Vitale N, Williams RI, et al. Epicardial colour-Doppler scanning of coronary artery stenosis and graft anastomoses. Scand Cardiovasc J. 2002;36:95–9.
12. Falk V, Walther T, Philippi A, et al. Thermal coronary angiography for intraoperative patency control of arterial and saphenous vein coronary artery bypass grafts: results in 370 patients. J Card Surg. 1995;10:147–60.
13. D'Ancona G, Karamanoukian HL, Ricci M, et al. Graft revision after transient time flow measurements in off-pump coronary artery bypass grafting. Eur J Cardiothorac Surg. 2000;17:287–93.
14. Mindich BP, Rubinstein M, Urrutia CO, et al. Reduction of technical graft problems utilizing ultrasonic flow measurements. New York: NY Thorac Society; 2001.
15. D'Ancona G. Karamanoukian H, Ricci M. et al: myocardial revascularization on the beating heart after recent acute myocardial infarction. Heart Surg Forum. 2001;4:74–9.
16. D'Ancona G, Karamanoukian H, Ricci M, et al. Intraoperative graft patency verification in cardiac and vascular surgery. 1st ed. Armonk, NY: Futura Publishing Company; 2001.
17. Taggart DP, Choudhary B, Anastasiadis K, et al. Preliminary experience with a novel intraoperative fluorescence imaging technique to evaluate the patency of bypass grafts in total arterial revascularization. Ann Thorac Surg. 2003;75:870–3.

18. Canver CC, Dame NA. Ultrasonic assessment of internal thoracic artery graft flow in the revascularized heart. Ann Thorac Surg. 1994;58:135–8.
19. Hirotani T, Kameda T, Shirota S, et al. An evaluation of the intraoperative transit time measurements of coronary bypass flow. Eur J Cardio Thorac Surg. 2001;19:848–52.
20. Jakobsen HL, Kjergard HK. Severe impairment of graft flow without electrocardiographic changes during coronary artery bypass grafting. Scand Cardiovasc J. 1999;33:157–9.
21. Walpol BH, Bosshard A, Kipler B, et al. Failed coronary artery bypass anastomosis detected by intraoperative coronary flow measurement. Eur J Cardiothorac Surg. 1998;14:576–81.
22. Speich R, Saesseli B, Hoffman U, et al. Anaphylactic reaction after indocyanine-green administration. Ann Intern Med. 1988;109:345–6.
23. Takahashi M, Ishikawa T, Higashidani K, Katoh H. SPY: an innovative intra-operative imaging system to evaluate graft patency during off-pump coronary artery bypass grafting. Interact Cardiovasc Thorac Surg. 2004;3:479–83.
24. Desai ND, Miwa S, Kodaama D, et al. A randomized comparison of intra-operative Indocyanine green angiography and transit-time flow measurement to detect technical errors in coronary artery bypass grafts. J Thorac Cardiovasc Surg. 2006;132:585–94.
25. Wasada K, Ako J, Hasegawa T, et al. Intraoperative fluorescence imaging system for on-site assessment of off-pump coronary artery bypass graft. J Am Coll Cardiol Img. 2009;2:604–12.
26. Detter C, Wipper S, Russ D, Iffland A, Burdorf L, Thein E, et al. Fluorescent cardiac imaging: a novel intraoperative method for quantitative assessment of myocardial perfusion during graded coronary artery stenosis. Circulation. 2007;116(9):1007–14.
27. Yamamoto M, Orihashi K, Nishimori H, Wariishi S, Fukutomi T, Kondo N, et al. Indocyanine green angiography for intra-operative assessment in vascular surgery. Eur J Vasc Endovasc Surg. 2012;43(4):426–32.
28. Ferguson TB Jr, Chen C, Babb JD, et al. Fractional flow reserve-guided coronary artery bypass grafting: can intraoperative physiologic imaging guide decision making? J Thorac Cardiovasc Surg. 2013;146(4):824–35.
29. Sabik J. Discussion to: Ferguson TB Jr, Chen C, Babb JD, et al. fractional flow reserve-guided coronary artery bypass grafting: can intraoperative physiologic imaging guide decision making? J Thorac Cardiovasc Surg. 2013;146(4):824–35.
30. Yamamoto M, Sasaguri S, Sato T. Assessing intraoperative blood flow in cardiovascular surgery. Surg Today. 2011;41(11):1467–74.
31. Yamamoto M, Orihashi K, Nishimori H, Handa T, Kondo N, Fukutomi T, et al. Efficacy of intraoperative HyperEye medical system angiography for coronary artery bypass grafting. Surg Today. 2015;45(8):966–72.
32. Benson RC, Kues HA. Fluorescence properties of indocyanine green as related to angiography. Phys Med Biol. 1978;23(1):159–63.

33. Hills KD, Smith PK, Bittl JL, et al. 2100 ACCF/AHA Guidelines for coronary artery bypass graft surgery. A report of the American College of Cardiology Foundation/American Heart Association task force on practice guidelines. Developed in collaboration with the American Association for Thoracic Surgery. Society of Cardiovascular Anesthesiologist, and Society of Thoracic Surgeons. J Am Coll Cardiol. 2011;58(24):e123–210.
34. Kogon B, Fernandez J, Kanter K, et al. The role of intraoperative Indocyanine green fluorescence angiography in pediatric surgery. Ann Thorac Surg. 2009;88:632–6.
35. Feins EN, Si MS, Baird CW, Emani SM. Intraoperative coronary artery imaging for planning. Semin Thorac Cardiovasc Surg Pediatr Card Surg Annu. 2021;23(C):11–6.
36. Muehrcke DD, Shimp W, Casillas M. Intraoperative angiogrphy to find an intramyocardial artery. Clin Surg. 2021;6:3025.

Bibliography

PREVENT IV Investigators. Efficacy and safety of edifoligide, an E2F transcription factor decoy, for prevention of vein graft failure following coronary artery bypass graft surgery—PREVENT IV: a randomized controlled trial. JAMA. 2005;294:2446–54.

Taggart DP. Biochemical assessment of myocardial injury after cardiac surgery: effects of a platelet activating factor antagonist, bilateral internal thoracic artery grafts, and coronary endarterectomy. J Thorac Cardiovasc Surg. 2000;120:651–9.

Yusuf S, Zucker D, Peduzzi P, et al. Effect of coronary artery bypass graft surgery on survival: overview of 10-year results from randomized trials by the coronary artery bypass graft surgery trialists collaboration. Lancet. 1994;344:563.

Lytle B, Blackstone E, Loop F, et al. Two internal thoracic artery grafts are better than one. J Thorac Cardiovasc Surg. 1999;117:855.

Taggart DP, D'Amico R, Altman DG. Effect of arterial revascularization on survival: a systematic review of students comparing bilateral and single internal mammary arteries. Lancet. 2001;358:870–5.

Lytle BW, Loop FD, Taylor PC, et al. Vein graft disease: the clinical impact of stenosis in saphenous vein bypass grafts to coronary arteries. J Thorac Cardiovasc Surg. 1992;103(5):831–40. [PubMed: 1569763].

Halabi AR, Alexander JH, Shaw LK, et al. Relation of early saphenous vein graft failure to outcomes following coronary artery bypass surgery. Am J Cardiol. 2005;96:1254–9.

Use of Fluorescence Guidance in Urologic Surgery

15

David Zekan, Andrew Williams, Amr Elbakry, and Adam Luchey

Introduction

Anastomoses are a vital part of urologic surgery cases, used for urinary diversions, ureteral reimplantation, and other upper and lower urinary tract reconstruction. However, a considerable complication that can arise is anastomotic leak and stricture. While many factors have been implicated, a major cause of anastomotic leak and strictures is poor blood flow leading to tissue ischemia [1, 2]. The quality of organ perfusion is often only assessed by the surgeon's impression, taking into account the active bleeding margin, palpable pulsation, and lack of discoloration [3, 4], which, unfortunately, have low predictive value for risk of anastomotic leakage [5]. Recent advancements have led to a promising alternative: SPY fluorescence imaging. SPY-ELITE and its portable handheld model SPY-PHI are fluorescent imaging machines that are able to better assess blood flow in vessels and tissue when

D. Zekan (✉) · A. Elbakry · A. Luchey
West Virginia University Department of Urology, Morgantown, WV, USA
e-mail: dszekan@hsc.wvu.edu

A. Williams
West Virginia University School of Medicine, Morgantown, WV, USA

N. Szoka et al. (eds.), *The SAGES Manual of Fluorescence-Guided Surgery*, https://doi.org/10.1007/978-3-031-40685-0_15

used with near-infrared fluorescent dyes [1]. Such assessment of perfusion is widely applicable in urologic surgery, expanding uses far beyond just anastomotic analysis. The most commonly used immunofluorescent dye is indocyanine green (ICG), most commonly given intravenously (IV) and active for only 150–180 s before being excreted into the bile [6]. The IV dose of ICG has very low rates of adverse side effects with only 0.05% of patients having mild allergic reactions [7]. With the use of ICG and SPY, the recommended dose is 0.02 mg/kg body weight, but this can vary based on intended use as outlined below [8]. ICG is water soluble and binds almost exclusively to plasma proteins concentrating the fluorescence mostly to vasculature [4]. The fluorophore operates within the near-infrared spectrum, absorbing light in the 805 nm wavelength and emitting at 835 nm [4]. Most human tissue is relatively transparent at these wavelengths allowing for visualization depth of 10–20 mm, which is generally sufficient for use in urologic surgery [4]. The various camera recording options available on the SPY systems allow for detection of even small perfusion deficits within tissues and anastomoses while offering beautifully crisp images of the organs [4]. When ICG first became available, it was described as a "hammer looking for a nail," and its intended function was well-established in its ability to find and display perfusion; however, its clinical benefit and overall practicality were still underreported [6]. Recently, ICG and SPY technologies have been utilized in urologic surgery in an attempt to improve patient outcomes and streamline surgeries [6]. Here, we outline the various uses of ICG and SPY technologies in urologic cases and specific methods for replicability.

Ureteral Identification

Although a majority of its uses are intravenous, ICG injected retrograde into the ureters also provides promise for ureteral identification. This is crucial when working in conjunction with colorectal and gynecologic surgery, who traditionally rely on ureteral stent placement for ureteral identification and prevention of iatrogenic ureteral injuries. However, stenting vs. no stenting shows no difference in prevention of ureteral injury but aids in identification of an injury after it occurs. These injuries are increasing in incidence with use of laparoscopic and robotic technology to aid in pelvic surgeries [9]. Bilateral ureters are known to fluoresce green when injected intraluminally with methylene blue. However, studies vary with respect to reliability of fluorescence, reporting 50–91% visualization when viewed under NIRF (near-infrared fluorescence). The use of intraluminal ICG as described below (with injection through an open-ended ureteral catheter, nephrostomy tube, or both) boasts a 100% success rate for ureteral visualization in both colorectal and gynecologic surgery [9].

Ureteral Reconstruction

The use of ICG in upper tract reconstruction comes in two forms: intraluminal use of ICG to visualize ureters and areas of stricture and IV use to determine ureteral viability prior to reconstruction. Bjurlin et al. describe its IV use in robotic pyeloplasties, ureteral reimplants, ureterolysis, and ureteroureterostomies (UU) per the protocol outlined below. In all cases described (42 in total), they boast an overall 95.2% success rate with a 100% symptomatic (flank pain) and radiographic (hydroureteronephrosis) success rate in included cases aside from ureterolysis (71.4%), which is known to be less efficacious at baseline. Clavien grade 1–3 complications occurred in 14.3% of patients, including transient lower extremity weakness (one patient), enterotomy requiring small bowel resection (one patient), ureteral stone requiring nephrostomy tube (one patient), postoperative bleed requiring surgical exploration (one patient), and ureteral stent migration requiring repositioning (two patients) [10] (Fig. 15.1).

Lee et al. describe use of intraluminal ICG in UUs treating short ureteral strictures robotically in the hands of a single surgeon. Intraluminal injection was performed as described below, with injection above and below the level of stricture using a ureteral catheter, nephrostomy tube, or combination of the two. In a case series including seven patients with short mid-ureteral stric-

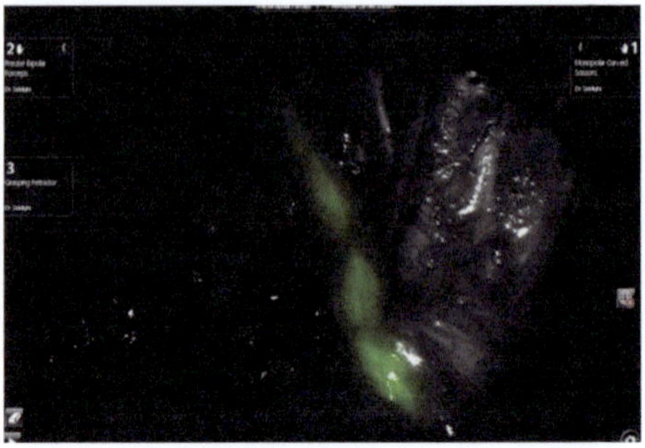

Fig. 15.1 Intraluminal injection of ICG for ureteral identification under NIRF [11]

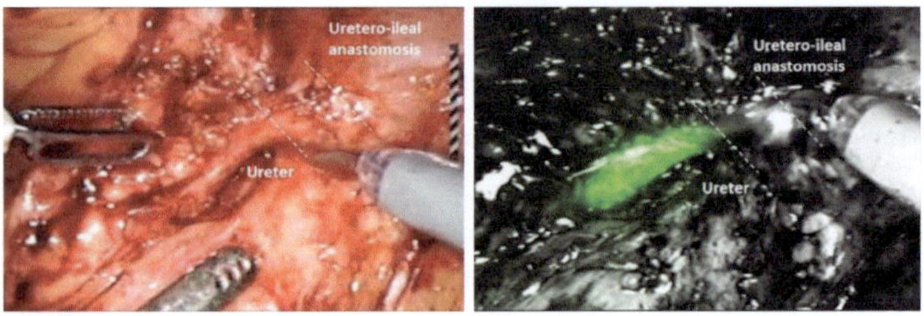

Fig. 15.2 Use of NIRF with IV ICG to differentiate diseased (ischemic) ureteral segment from healthy ureteral segment during robotic ureteral reimplantation for benign uretero-anastomotic stricture [13]

tures, they demonstrate the ability to delineate disease from healthy ureteral segments in all patients, with mean excision length of 1.6 ± 0.7 cm. A single patient with dense peri-hepatic adhesions experienced gallbladder laceration at the time of surgery, requiring robotic cholecystectomy, with no attributable complications to ICG administration. At follow-up (mean 5.9 ± 1.5 months), no patient had clinical or radiographic evidence of continued stricture [12]. Thus, both IV (Fig. 15.2) and intraluminal (Fig. 15.3) use of ICG during benign ureteral reconstruction is feasible, and its addition to the case presents minimal, if any, risk to the patient. Needed are long-term studies comparing outcomes (persistence and recurrence of stricture) between open, laparoscopic, and robotic techniques for benign reconstruction with and without the use of ICG.

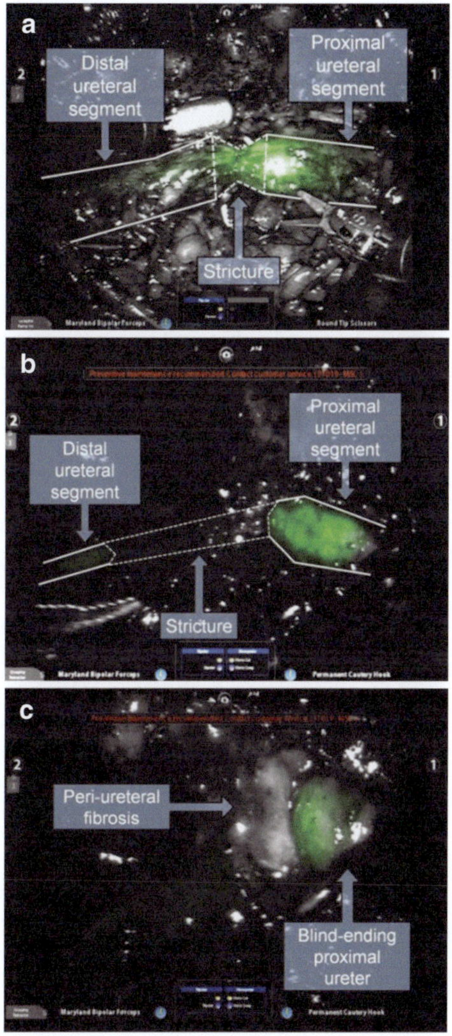

Fig. 15.3 Use of NIRF to differentiate diseased from healthy ureter during UU [12]

Partial Nephrectomy

The use of ICG and SPY angiography for upper tract pathology extends beyond just pyeloplasties and UUs, also aiding in partial nephrectomies. Partial nephrectomy offers superior functional outcomes compared to radical nephrectomy in small renal masses [14]. To minimize ischemia to healthy tissue, SPY angiography can be used to properly identify hilar vessels and tumor-specific vasculature to be clamped before resection [15]. Furthermore, tumors are often well demarcated on the SPY imaging, appearing hypofluorescent compared to surrounding parenchyma [15]. The use of ICG dye allows for better localization of malignant tissue for more precise resections [16]. Mitsui et al. utilized ICG dye and fluorescent imaging to visualize the tumor margins during surgery and validated these margins ex vivo. They found that even in complex cases, ICG allowed for easy discrimination between normal and cancerous tissues [16]. Their case series demonstrates 100% ex vivo differentiation within 60 min of ICG injection in 16 cases, with 14 of 16 tumors showing hypofluorescence in vivo. The remaining two were endophytic with overlying normal parenchyma. High and low fluorescence were both used to rule out residual tumor, which was confirmed on pathologic specimens [16]. Similarly, Angell et al. describe the ability to achieve differential fluorescence between renal tumors and surrounding normal parenchyma with a test dose of ICG and then re-dose at the time of tumor resection. Differential fluorescence was achieved in 65 of 70 tumors (82%), excluding tumors that could not be visualized as they were completely endophytic [17]. While the difference in tissue fluorescence between tumors and normal kidney parenchyma is easily discernable, tissue fluorescence of the tumor itself cannot adequately determine malignant and benign masses [18].

The use of fluorescent imaging also allows for better postoperative renal function when compared to conventional methods [14, 19]. Borofsky et al. utilized ICG dye to visualize renal vasculature during partial nephrectomy allowing them to more specifically cross-clamp distal vessels feeding the tumor ("zero ischemia" partial nephrectomy), rather than conventional cross-clamping of the main renal artery [14]. They demonstrated successful selective clamping in 27 of 34 patients (79.4%). While this method did lead to increased operating time, it also led to significantly better postoperative kidney function with a reduction in glomerular filtration rate (GFR) of only 1.8% compared to 14.9% reduction in the renal artery cross-clamp at a mean follow-up of about 13 days [14]. Shao et al. found similar significant results with 3-month postoperative GFR decrease of 16.7% in multiple feeder clamping compared to 26.2% decrease in GFR for renal artery clamping [19]. Fluorescent imaging also allows the surgeon to confirm that the tumor vasculature has been restricted following arterial clamping by assessing the change in parameters produced with SPY imaging analysis (quantitatively) and the visual fluorescence of the tissue [14]. When all the feeders to the tumor are properly cross-clamped, the tumor and surrounding parenchyma should hypofluoresce. Overall, fluorescent imaging of renal vasculature during partial nephrectomies allows for a more directed approach for tumor resection, leading to less overall damage to normal kidney parenchyma and better patient outcomes.

Urothelial Carcinoma and Urinary Diversion

Fluorescent imaging has two main potential uses in urothelial carcinoma of the bladder: the first is to map out regional lymph nodes associated with resected masses and the other is to ensure well-vascularized anastomoses, viable bowel, and identification of stricture should they occur at the anastomotic site.

Standard treatment for muscle-invasive bladder cancer remains radical cystectomy with pelvic lymph node dissection (PLND) [20]. SPY angiography may allow for quicker and more easy identification of SLN. ICG can be administered IV to visualize vasculature, but it can also be injected into the submucosa and smooth muscle to be taken up into the lymphatics [21]. This technique allows for easy identification of sentinel lymph nodes, which require resection in all cystectomies performed for malignancy [22].

Manny et al. describe the use of submucosal and detrusor ICG injected circumferentially with a cystoscope in 10 patients undergoing robotic radical cystectomy. Intraoperative identification of tumor was possible in 90% of patients using NIRF, only not achieved in a single patient noted to have circumferential bladder wall thickening, with bladder wall measuring >2 cm in thickness. Sentinel lymph node drainage was also identified in 90% of patients, all of whom had multiple areas of drainage, with bilateral sentinel drainage in eight of nine patients. Importantly, of the three patients with node positive disease on final pathology, nodal fluorescence was 100% sensitive, but only 47% specific for identification of node positivity [21]. While this technique does allow for a quick and simple understanding of tissue, its use for extended lymph node dissections may be less dependable [23]. The main constraint of ICG in identifying lymph nodes is its ability to flow easily through the lymphatic vessels. One potential problem with high tumor burden is that vessels may become obstructed by metastatic disease, leading to areas of hypo-fluorescence where metastases are present [23]. The sensitivity for ICG and fluorescent dye's use in SNL dissection ranges widely from 44% to 100% depending on the study and for that reason should not be used alone for identification and resection lymph nodes [23–25]. Overall, fluorescent imaging of tissue lymphatics is an emerging field, and as more advancements in technology and surgical technique arise, its practicality and utility will become more apparent.

As often used intraoperatively by general surgeons, IV ICG can be utilized to visualize mesenteric vasculature in both the laparoscopic and open setting when performing urinary diversion, be it in the form of a neobladder, ileal conduit, or otherwise. The above group who utilized submucosa ICG for sentinel node identification also describes use of IV ICG for identification of mesenteric arcades when performing robotic intracorporeal diversion. Real-time visualization of vasculature guides stapling of the bowel and mesentery, and in 100% of cases (eight total), no complications related to diversion ischemia were observed, including anastomotic stricture and stomal stenosis [21].

Another advancing use of SPY imaging is allowing for better visualization and quantitative assessment of vasculature in anastomoses. For instance, ureteroenteric strictures (UES) are a common consequence of radical cystectomies and any surgery involving ureteral diversions [1]. Various surgical techniques have been developed to reduce stricture, but few have led to any substantial risk reduction, maintaining a complication rate of approximately 9% [1, 26, 27]. Ischemia is thought to be a major contributing factor to the development of UES. Thus, it was theorized that by assessing distal perfusion at each on the anastomoses using SPY angiography, fewer strictures may occur [1]. Shen et al. compared UES rates before (47 patients) and after (47 patients) implementing SPY into their practice for radical cystectomies. The stricture rate for patients prior to SPY implementation was 7.5%, diagnosed with either hydronephrosis, lack of reflux on loopogram, or Lasix renal scan showing $t^{1/2} > 20$ min. After implementation of SPY and ICG, 0% of cases developed UES over a 12-month period. Through the use of SPY's vasculature analysis, their team identified poor distal perfusion in 34.4% of ureters requiring a more proximal anastomosis; however, use of SPY did not lead to a significantly more proximal anastomosis [1]. Doshi et al. conducted a similar study assessing rates of stricture in patients with or without the use of SPY imaging ($n = 31$ and 30, respectively). They found that only 3.2% of patients ($n = 1$) developed stricture when fluorescent imaging was used, compared to 13% ($n = 5$) with conventional methods [28]. Robotic-specific data is provided by Ahmadi et al., who analyzed 179 patients who underwent robotic-assisted laparoscopic radical cystectomy with intracorporeal diversion. When comparing the 132 patients in the non-ICG group to the 47 in the ICG group, those in the ICG group were likely to have more ureter excised based on concern for ischemia and were more likely to have long segment (>5 cm) ureteral excision. However, at 14 and 12 months average follow-up, respectively, no UESs were noted in the ICG group, compared to a per-patient stricture rate of 10.6% and per-ureter stricture rate of 6.6% in the non-ICG group [29]. This practice for assessing ureteral anastomoses can also be applied when creating a neobladder to prevent anastomotic leak.

Bowel anastomotic leak develops in 5–19% of urinary diversion cases and leads to significant increases in hospital stays, healthcare cost, and morbidity and mortality [2, 3, 30]. Like UES, they are thought to be caused by a variety of factors, one of which is tissue ischemia [2]. The use of fluorescent imaging may allow for better assessment of the vasculature to ensure healthy bowel prior to anastomosis, potentially leading to better outcomes. De Nardi et al. conducted a randomized controlled trial ($n = 240$) to assess leakage rates between patients who received intraoperative ICG fluorescent imaging, with those evaluated using conventional methods. While they did find 5% of the ICG patients (compared to 9% in the control) developed anastomotic leak, it did not reach statistical significance [2]. Interestingly, 11% of the ICG patients required additional resection due to poor perfusion, and none of these patients went on to develop anastomotic leak. Another case series assessed leakage rates using SPY angiography ($n = 139$) and found rates to be only 1.4%, again demonstrating that no patients who required additional resection (8% ($n = 11$)) went on to develop leaks [30]. While these surgeries focus on the gastrointestinal rather than genitourinary tract, their conclusions can still be extrapolated for neobladder formation and bowel anastomoses. Overall, the evidence regarding the clinical benefit of SPY angiography for anastomoses is still conflicting; however, its use has minimal side effects, low cost, and no increase in operative time and can still providing quality assessment of tissue perfusion, which can be beneficial to the surgeon and the patient.

Prostate Cancer

The utilization of SPY angiography in prostate surgery is still relatively new. As in urothelial cell carcinoma of the bladder, ICG dye can be injected directly into the prostatic tissue to visualize regional nodes requiring resection. One study found that fluorescent imaging allowed detection of lymph nodes outside of the standard region of excision in 18.5% of cases during prostatectomy [31]. Eleven patients were injected preoperatively with radiotracer-tagged ICG via transrectal ultrasound. In these cases, gamma camera images were fused with SPECT/CT to identify sentinel nodes, and a combination of imaging, laparoscopic gamma probe, and NIRF was used for node dissection. Fifty-five percent of patients had nodes identified on imaging 15 minutes following injection, which increased to 91% after 2 h. Of the 27 nodes identified preoperatively, only 1 was unidentifiable intraoperatively using the gamma probe and NIRF, while four (15%) could not be identified on NIRF alone. This was attributed to overlying fat, blood, and tissue, which obscured lymph nodes, as NIRF was reliable in the last millimeter to centimeter in areas where the radiotracer had weak signal on gamma probe [31]. Although technically complex, ICG and its combination with radiotracer provide promise in pelvic lymph node identification and dissection in adenocarcinoma of the prostate.

Another emerging use for prostatic surgery is to identify the landmark artery for the neurovascular bundle when conducting nerve-sparing prostatectomies for preservation of erectile function [32]. Visualization of the artery allows surgeons to better identify and avoid damage to reduce risk of damage and improve nerve function postoperatively. ICG utilization for landmark artery identification is still very new, with most publications only being case reports and proof of concept. However, Mangano et al. describe use of IV ICG in 26 consecutive patients with visualization of the neurovascular bundle in 100% of patients. No complications related to use of ICG occurred, and in the hands of a single surgeon, no increased operative time was noted with addition of ICG [33]. Although no functional outcomes are provided in the above study, it provides the groundwork for further studies evaluating long-term effects of increased visualization of the NVB using ICG. Uses of ICG in prostate cancer, and potentially benign prostate surgeries, abound.

Lymphatic-Sparing Varicocelectomy

When performing varicocelectomy, be it for pain, subfertility, or testicular undergrowth, the concept of structural identification and avoidance of the testicular artery and lymphatics are paramount.

Such sparing reduces the risk of postoperative hydrocele profoundly, which is known to be an all-too-common complication, particularly in pediatric patients. Esposito et al. describe use of intratesticularly injected ICG during laparoscopic Palomo varicocelectomy in 25 patients, with an average age of 13.7 years. They report reliable illumination under NIRF of the lymphatics of the spermatic cord 20–30 s after injection in 100% of patients. Two or three lymphatics were able to be identified in all patients, allowing for effective sparing. No adverse events related to ICG were reported, and no patient reported pain related to the testicular injection site. Importantly, at 18 months follow-up, no recurrence or persistence of varicocele occurred and no hydroceles were observed. This is in comparison to larger datasets showing a 20–30% postoperative hydrocele rate in allcomers, often requiring repeat surgical intervention [34].

Similarly, Fukui et al. describe a case of IV ICG use intraoperatively (in combination with intratesticular ICG as above) for identification of the gonadal artery and vein. Specifically, they note illumination of the artery 20–30 s following IV injection and illumination of the vein about 20 s following that, allowing efficient division of the artery from the surrounding veins, which were to be ligated with the addition of very little time to the case [35]. Obviously, both percutaneous and IV use of ICG present opportunity for use in urologic cases and the above highlight uses in both pediatric and adult patients.

Kidney Transplant

Healthy kidneys available for transplantation are a scarce resource. Sufficient organ perfusion is a main prognostic factors for proper allograft function and is vital to ensure proper vessel anastomosis intraoperatively [8]. Hypoperfusion may not be apparent intraoperatively with only visual inspection. While angiography, duplex sonography, and renal tissue oxygenation can be used to assess the quality of anastomosis, they have been found to be more expensive, time-consuming, and less practical when compared to using ICG and SPY [8]. Rother et al. quantitatively compared SPY fluorescent angiography to intrarenal resistance index from duplex sonography during kidney transplants and found that ICG serves as a good alternative with a more objective assessment of microperfusion [36]. They found that a lower intrarenal resistance index (RI) correlated with a significantly higher ingress (IN) and ingress rate (InR) (objective representations of inflow of blood to the organ) on SPY imaging analysis. Interestingly, these findings were only significant for the upper pole of the kidney and not the lower. However, while IN and InR are objective measurements from the imaging equipment (derived from the SPY's analysis of the tissue), RI depends on the skill of the operator and may vary based on the surgeon's experience. They went on to compare histological changes of the kidney, measured by the interstitial fibrosis and tubular atrophy score (IFTA), to SPY analyses and found a significant inverse correlation between IFTA scores and IN and InR, showing that with decreased blood flow into the kidney, there was increased histological fibrosis and atrophy [36]. This study demonstrates how a quantitative measure derived from SPY angiography and imaging correlates to microvascular changes and is a cheap and more accessible alternative to past methods. ICG dosing is estimated to cost only $8–80 per patient, depending on how many doses of ICG can be given per vial [16, 18], and only requires a few minutes during surgery to capture high-quality, informative images [4]. Furthermore, given the anatomy of kidney vasculature and the superficial distribution of renal arteries, the 10–20 mm visualization depth given by ICG and SPY is sufficient to view most microvascular hypoperfusion [4]. SPY imaging provides the surgeon with a real-time qualitative assessment of potential occlusion or problems with the graft while also providing computational analysis to further assess tissue quantitatively [37]. Overall, the utilization of SPY during kidney transplants allows for quick and easy subjective and objective measurement of kidney vasculature to assess intraoperative success of the transplantation.

Technical Considerations

Ureteral Identification

Efficient ureteral identification is crucial not only in urologic procedures involving its reimplantation or ligation but also in colorectal and gynecologic cases, in which identification can help prevent iatrogenic ureteral injury. Currently, placement of open-ended ureteral catheters, double-J ureteral stents, and lighted ureteral stents is common practice for ureteral identification. However, these methods often only facilitate identification, as opposed to prevention, of ureteral injuries, particularly in laparoscopic/robotic cases in which tactile sensation is limited. Current practices involve creating a solution of 10–25 mg ICG in sterile water and injecting 10 cc of this solution through a 6 Fr open-ended ureteral catheter advanced 3–5 cm into the ureteral orifice cystoscopically. Should significant resistance be met or immediate efflux of the injected ICG be appreciated, we recommend obtaining retrograde pyelogram through the same open-ended catheter. If no significant ureteral stricture is visualized on retrograde pyelogram, a sensor wire can be used to facilitate advancement of the open-ended catheter to the level of the renal pelvis. ICG injection can be performed as a slow infusion over 5 min, or as a bolus. Maximal fluorescence can be expected between 9 and 20 min following injection and is known to persist for up to 3 h post-injection. It is likely that fluorescence continues beyond this time, but our experience in this area is limited. Maintaining the open-ended ureteral catheter after injection is not necessary but can further facilitate ureteral identification by direct palpation. Should this be performed, we recommend placement of the ureteral catheter into an Edelman urethral catheter [9] (Fig. 15.1).

Ureteral Reconstruction

Ureteral reimplantation, although used for a large variety of pathologies within urology, has a common dreaded complication: anastomotic stricture. Distal ureteral ischemia, generally caused by compromising blood supply during skeletonization, is a contributing factor to anastomotic stricture. This is further complicated by a history of pelvic radiation in many instances as the etiology of distal stricture. Distal ureteral ischemia is also of concern in the creation of urinary diversions in any context (oncologic or otherwise) as distal ureteral dissection is essentially always performed to allow adequate ureteral length for diversion anastomosis. The use of laparoscopic/robotic technology in ureteral reimplantation is another complicating factor, as a "no touch technique" and meticulous tissue handling is more difficult without delicate tactile feedback. Thus, use of ICG in assessment of distal ureteral viability is becoming increasingly accepted and utilized in assessment of perfusion following skeletonization and ligation. To assess this, following distal ureteral dissection and ligation, 3 mL of ICG is injected intravenously followed by 10 cc saline with use of color-segmented fluorescence mode to provide a "heat map" view of the distal ureter. This can be repeated following anastomosis to ensure adequate perfusion. Should there be concern for distal ureteral ischemia on heat map, we recommend marking the distal most area of adequate ureteral perfusion with a stitch and performing proximal ligation of the ureter [1].

Intraluminal injection of ICG in the setting of benign ureteral strictures has also been reported for visualization of the extent of ureteral stricture when performing ureteroureterostomy. In this setting, 10 mL of 2.5 mg/mL ICG is injected via a 6 Fr open-ended ureteral catheter above and below the level of ureteral stenosis, unless the patient also has nephrostomy tube, in which case 5 mL is injected antegrade and 5 mL retrograde. The ureteral catheter is then clamped. This allows for visualization of the healthy ureteral segments under NIRF vision with a robotic or laparoscopic camera, as these segments will fluoresce under NIRF, prior to transection [12].

Partial Nephrectomy

The widely accepted gold standard for identification of tumor during robotic-assisted laparoscopic partial nephrectomy is intraoperative ultrasound. However, use of ICG for tumor identification has been described. One advantage in this context is that ICG also allows for assessment of renal artery anatomy and facilitates selective clamping should anatomy be conducive. In this context, we recommend injection of 5–7.5 mg of ICG following proximal-to-distal hilar dissection with use of topical papaverine if vasospasm is encountered and clamping the vessel likely supplying the tumor with a bulldog clamp. ICG injection allows for visualization of flow in both the main renal artery and vein as well as the tumor and adjacent parenchyma. After ensuring the area of planned resection (the tumor and surrounding normal parenchyma) is hypoperfused, it is safe to proceed with resection. Should persistent perfusion of the tumor and surrounding parenchyma be encountered, we recommend clamping of the main renal artery. In both cases, re-bolusing of the above dose of ICG is recommended following resection and removal of the bulldog clamp to ensure adequate reperfusion of the remaining parenchyma [38] (Fig. 15.4).

Similar dosing should be used in tumor differentiation using ICG. In this context, the kidney should be defatted and the tumor margin scored using electrocautery under ultrasound guidance. Two doses of ICG are often used in this context. One test dose should be given immediately when the tumor and a small amount of surrounding parenchyma are identified to anticipate the amount that should be given during tumor resection. This dose is typically 1.25 mg but can be as small as 0.625 mg in smaller patients. After administration of ICG, the tumor should not fluoresce, while normal parenchyma should have adequate ICG uptake and fluoresce

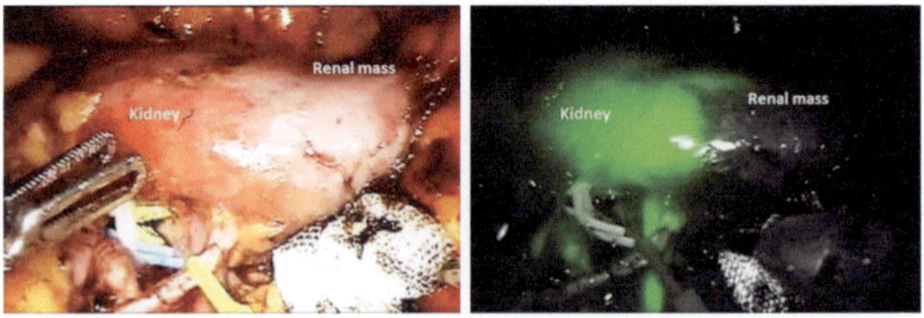

Fig. 15.4 ICG-guided selective clamping during robotic-assisted laparoscopic partial nephrectomy [13]

under NIRF. Following administration and prior to clamping, the scored area should be confirmed adequate or rescoring performed if the tumor margins (areas of hypofluorescence) protrude beyond the area marked under ultrasound guidance. Alternating between the NIRF camera and white light camera at the deep margin can be helpful in confirming resection of all gross tumor present. The entire resection bed should be "green" under near-infrared camera, and any area that appears to be hypoperfused should be resected [17] (Fig. 15.5).

Urothelial Carcinoma and Urinary Diversion

As highlighted previously, distal ureteral viability will determine the fate of a urinary diversion, regardless of whether or not it involves a bowel segment, and can be the difference between long-term indwelling diversions stents secondary to anastomotic stricture and a naturally patent anastomosis. It is also crucial in the avoidance of another more acute and often more complicated issue: anastomotic breakdown and urine leak. However, another potential cause of reoperation that is often overlooked by urologists is bowel viability, whether used for an ileal conduit, Indiana pouch, or neobladder. Bowel ischemia in these cases can also cause breakdown and lead to urine/bowel leak and stomal stenosis. Thus, it is crucial to prove viability following division of the mesentery prior to ureteral anastomosis. In urothelial cell carcinoma, ICG is not only valuable in avoidance of surgical complications but also tumor identification and sentinel node dissection.

Tumor identification is performed cystoscopically, with injection of 2 mL of 2.5 mg/mL ICG solution through an 18 Fr cystoscopic injection needle. This solution should target superficial detrusor and submucosa, to minimize risk of perforation and tumor spillage. Foley catheter placement is recommended following injection to facilitate decompressor and minimize possible bladder injury while gaining access endoscopically. The recommendation is then to perform examination of the surgical field every 5 min with a NIRF camera to document sentinel node drainage and to ensure adequate nodal dissection. The area occupied by

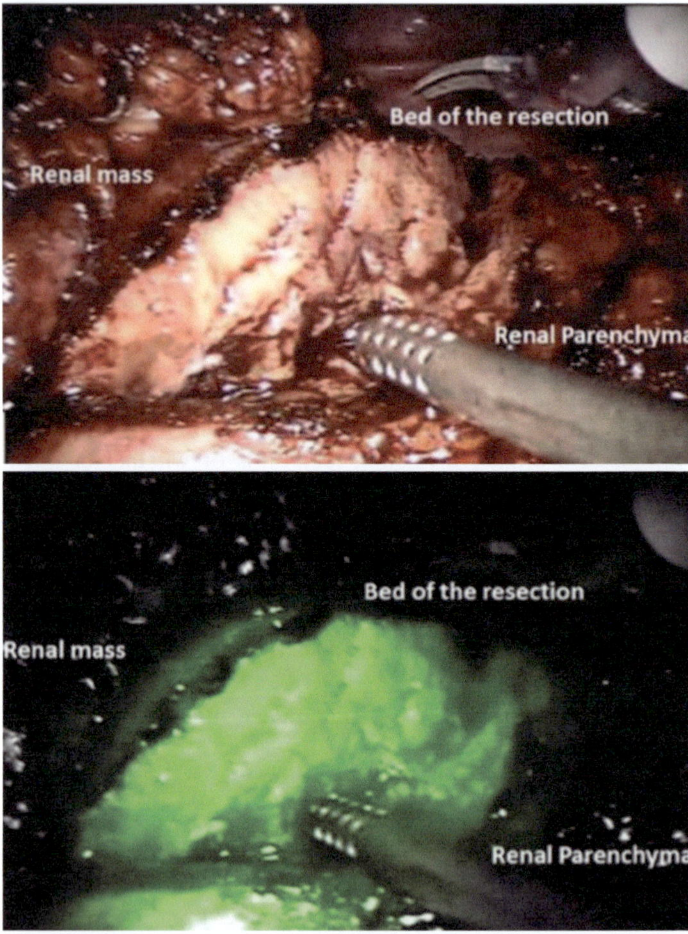

Fig. 15.5 ICG-guided renal mass resection during robotic-assisted laparoscopic partial nephrectomy with hypofluorescence of mass and normal perfusion of renal parenchyma [13]

bladder tumor is typically identifiable in 15 min (Fig. 15.6), while sentinel nodes generally take 30 min to illuminate under NIRF (Fig. 15.7). However, complete node dissection using a traditional template should not be omitted [21].

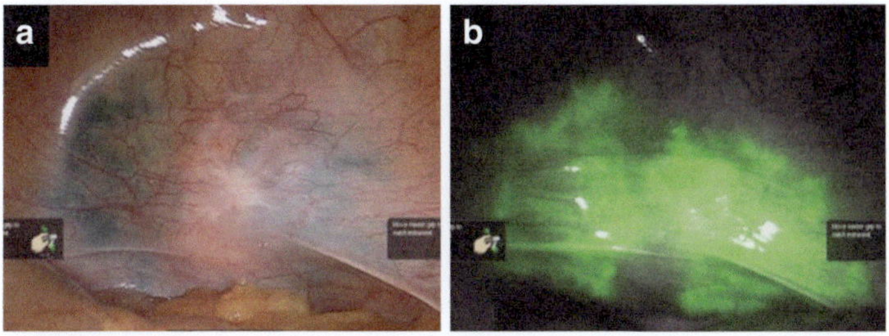

Fig. 15.6 Robotic view after immediate docking of robot following interstitial cystoscopic injection of tumor margins with ICG [21]

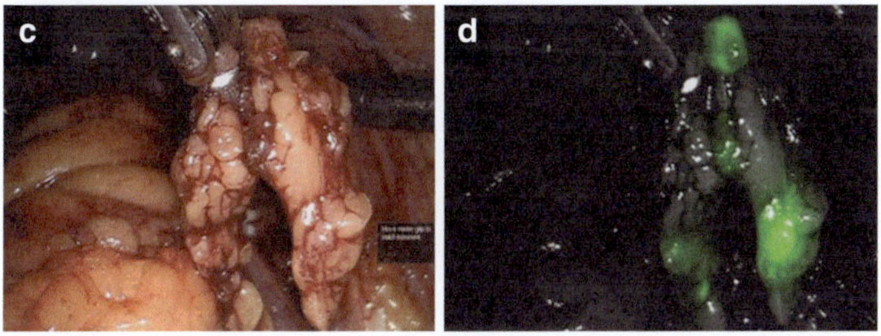

Fig. 15.7 Right common iliac lymph node packet in the setting of muscle-invasive bladder cancer following interstitial injection of tumor margins cystoscopically prior to robotic-assisted laparoscopic radical cystectomy with pelvic lymph node dissection [21]

Mesenteric angiography can be performed similarly by intravenous injection of 2 mL of 2.5 mg/mL ICG. Mesenteric arteries should transilluminate under NIRF within 30 s, assisting in harvest of a well-vascularized segment for conduit or other urinary diversions. Similar angiography can be repeated following stapling of the bowel to assess the viability of the proximal and distal ends of the conduit as well as the bowel anastomosis [21] (Figs. 15.8 and 15.9). Distal ureteral evaluation is also well defined and should be performed prior to spatulation and anastomosis, but after transfer of the left ureter to the right side through a retro-mesenteric window. A similar concentration to the above is recommended, but 10 mL given intravenously is the recom-

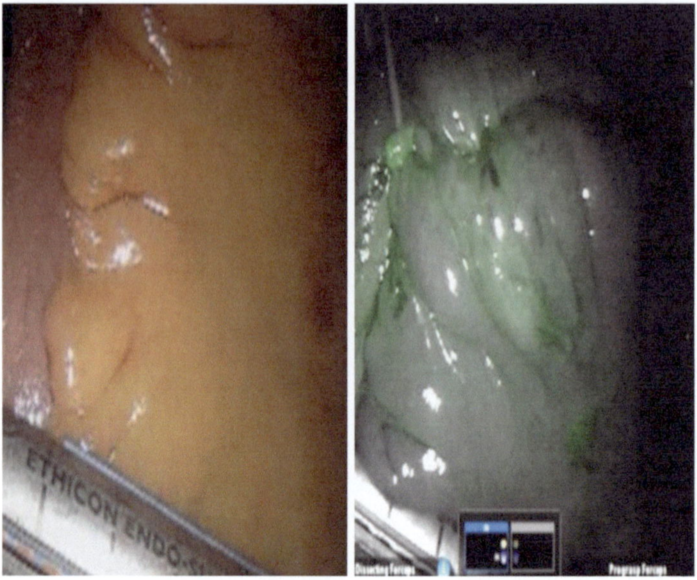

Fig. 15.8 Mesenteric angiography during creation of ileal conduit with ICG using NIRF to ensure preservation of mesenteric arcades (blood supply to conduit and anastomotic site) [21]

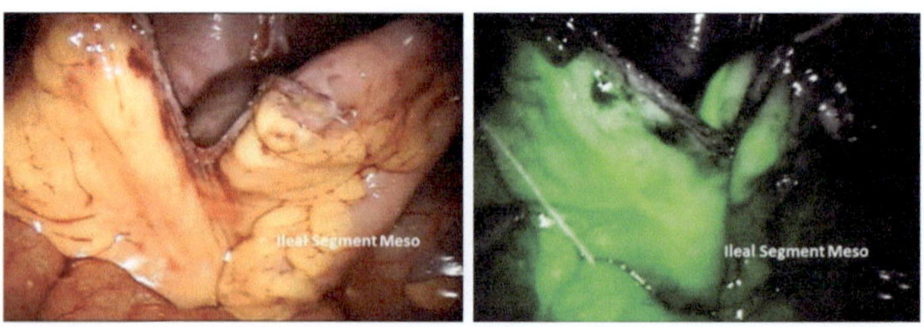

Fig. 15.9 NIRF-guided assessment of ileal segment used for conduit following ICG injection during robotic-assisted laparoscopic radical cystectomy with ileal conduit [13]

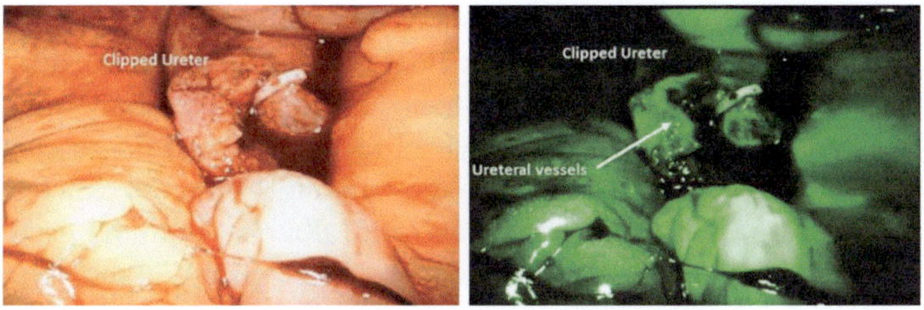

Fig. 15.10 Assessment of distal ureteral viability/vascularity during robotic-assisted laparoscopic radical cystectomy [13]

mended dose. To assess both the arterial and perfusion phases of the ICG, assessment of the distal ureters at 30 s and ~ 5 min is recommended using NIRF. In segments that do not demonstrate good arterial angiography, proximal transection is recommended prior to uretero-enteric anastomosis to minimize the risk of stricture [29] (Fig. 15.10).

Prostate Cancer

Although cancer control is of upmost importance when performing radical prostatectomy, conservation of erectile function generally remains a high priority. This cannot be overlooked by surgeons, and novel techniques for preservation of erectile function must be explored. Injection of 1.25 mL ICG following incision of the bladder neck and dissection of the seminal vesicles allows for optimal visualization and sparing of the "benchmark artery," which should theoretically lead to a more optimal nerve spare by improving hemostasis and visualization of the neurovascular bundle (NVB). Importantly, use of ICG for NVB identification has been not been shown to lengthen operative times and or lead to any identifiable complication in a series of 26 patients, eliminating possible drawbacks of its use [33].

Techniques for use of ICG in sentinel pelvic lymph node dissection abound. This is of particular importance for patients with unfavorable intermediate- or high-risk prostate cancer, in whom pelvic lymph node dissection is universally recommended at the time of RALP. Various protocols have been shown to increase the yield of positive nodes. Van der Poel et al. describe use of ICG noncovalently bound to ^{99m}Tc-nanocolloid, a commonly used radioactive tracer, to create a hybrid radioactive and fluorescent tracer. ^{99m}Tc-Nanocoll is generated by mixing 1 mL pertechnetate in saline to a vial containing Nanocoll (albumin colloidal particles) and allowing for 30 minutes of incubation. 1 mL of this solution is mixed with 0.050 mL (0.250 mg) ICG (solution of 25 mg solid ICG in 5 mL sterile water). 0.4 mL of this solution is injected to the peripheral zone of the prostate 3 h preoperatively under transrectal ultrasound guidance and flushed with 0.7 mL saline. A portable gamma camera is used to confirm adequate concentration within the prostate, and gamma camera images are further obtained at 15 min and 2 h post-injection. SPECT/CT is performed at 2 h and fusion of images is performed. This allows for dissection in accord with imaging using a laparoscopic gamma probe combined with high-definition laparoscopic fluorescence imaging [31]. Filters allowing for this imaging in the context of a white light background for anatomic delineation provide an effective measure to optimize and ensure adequate lymph node dissection. Effectively, use of ^{99m}Tc-nanocolloid offers the ability to both use lymphoscintigraphy and single-SPECT/CT imaging for preoperative nodal mapping (Fig. 15.11). In the absence of ^{99m}Tc-nanocolloid, ICG can be used alone, with 5 mg injected transperineally in the preoperative setting (Fig. 15.12).

Lymphatic-Sparing Varicocelectomy

Laparoscopic repair of varicocele, particularly in pediatric patients, is an important treatment modality used to address both testicular hypotrophy and symptomatic varicoceles. A commonly used and efficacious route for repair of varicoceles is the Palomo technique, which boasts a success rate of >95%. However, a common complication is postoperative hydrocele, which occurs in 20–30% of patients. Lymphatic-sparing surgery is known to reduce the rate of hydrocele and have better andrological outcomes, increasing its use among surgeons. Technically, this

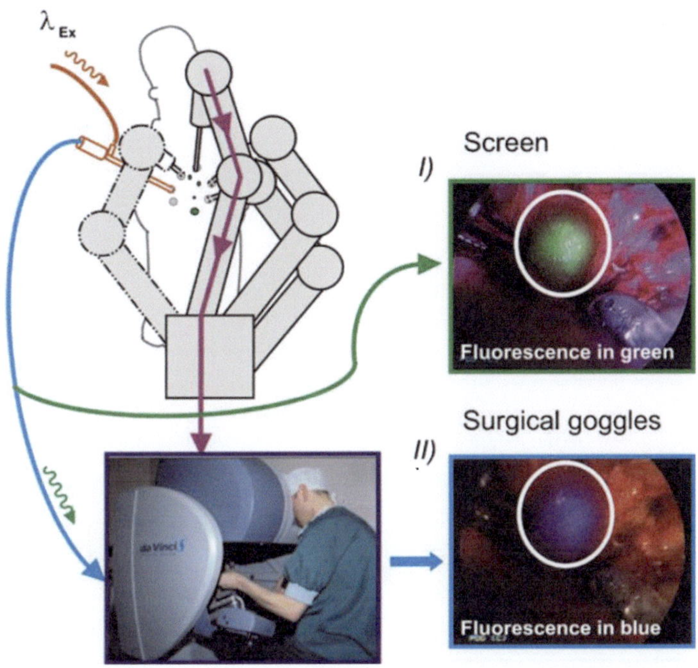

Fig. 15.11 Intraoperative sentinel lymph node detection during robotic-assisted laparoscopic prostatectomy following intraprostatic injection of ICG preoperatively using transrectal ultrasound guidance. (I) Using NIRF-laparoscopic D-light angiofluorescence system and (II) using da Vinci TilePro system [31]

involves diluting a vial of ICG (5 mg/dL) with 10 cc sterile water and injection of 2 cc of this solution into the body of the ipsilateral testicle with a 23G needle. This provides almost immediate visualization of lymphatic vessels in near-infrared mode on a laparoscopic camera and green appearance of lymphatics under standard white light mode, allowing for efficient identification and ligation of the spermatic bundle and sparing of lymphatics [34].

Similarly, a combination of both intravenous and subcutaneous injection of ICG for visualization of the spermatic vessels has been described to ensure laparoscopic ligation of only the sper-

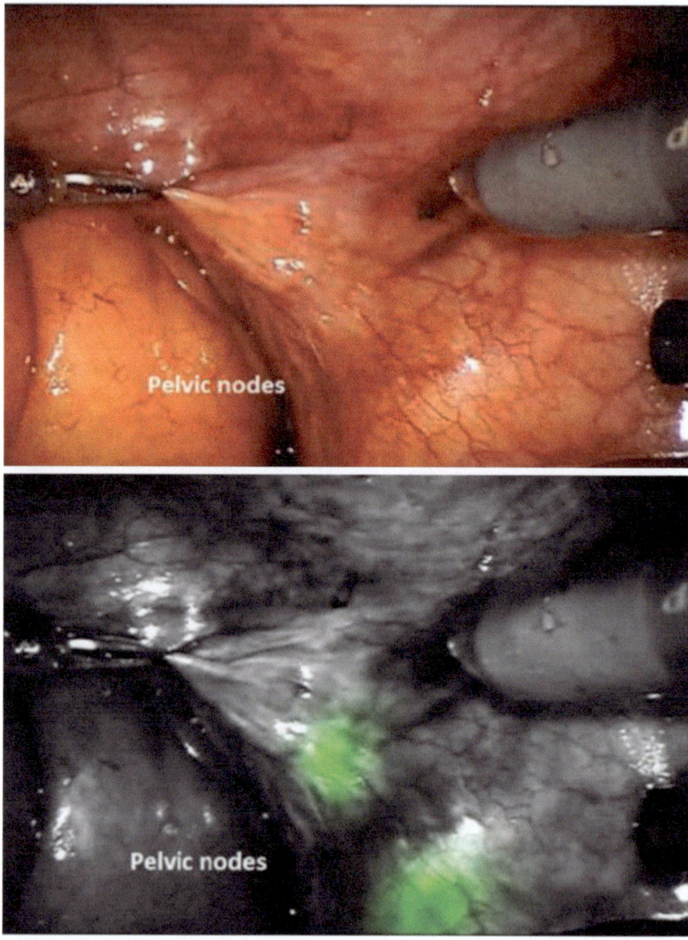

Fig. 15.12 NIRF-guided lymphadenectomy following intraprostatic of ICG during radical prostatectomy [13]

matic veins. To perform this, ICG is dissolved in sterile water at 2.5 mg/mL. 1 mL of this solution is injected intravenously for each desired angiography. The gonadal arterial flow can be visualized about 20–30 s following a shot, and 20 s following that, the gonadal vein is observed. At this concentration and volume, multiple angiographies can be performed during dissection with toggling between white light and near-infrared fluorescence to optimize dissection visualization. Lymphatic drainage can be effectively visualized by injection of 1 mL of solution subcutaneously in the desired hemiscrotum prior to cut and another 1 mL about 10 min prior to desired visualization to allow for reliable visualization [35].

Conclusion

Herein, we describe use of near-infrared technology in urologic surgery, oncologic and otherwise. Its use in both assessment of ureteral location and viability is crucial for pelvic surgeons and provides a method of limiting ureteral ischemia and minimizing risk of anastomotic strictures in urologic reconstruction. In partial nephrectomy, fluorescence guidance is helpful in identifying hilar vasculature and tumor margins and ensuring tumor and parenchymal ischemia following clamping prior to resection. Direct injection of ICG is imperative in lymph node dissections for nodal identification in urothelial carcinoma and prostatic adenocarcinoma. It is also being used for identification of the neurovascular bundle in nerve-sparing radical prostatectomy. Similarly, ICG can be used for lymphatic-sparing in varicocelectomy to limit the risk of hydrocele postoperatively. The uses of ICG in urologic surgery abound and will only continue to enhance surgical technique and further minimize risk of intra- and postoperative complications.

References

1. Shen JK, Jamnagerwalla J, Yuh BE, Bassett MR, Chenam A, Warner JN, et al. Real-time indocyanine green angiography with the SPY fluorescence imaging platform decreases benign ureteroenteric strictures in urinary diversions performed during radical cystectomy. Ther Adv Urol. 2019;11:175628721983963.
2. De Nardi P, Elmore U, Maggi G, Maggiore R, Boni L, Cassinotti E, et al. Intraoperative angiography with indocyanine green to assess anastomosis

perfusion in patients undergoing laparoscopic colorectal resection: results of a multicenter randomized controlled trial. Surg Endosc. 2020;34:53.
3. Kudszus S, Roesel C, Schachtrupp A, Höer JJ. Intraoperative laser fluorescence angiography in colorectal surgery: a noninvasive analysis to reduce the rate of anastomotic leakage. Langenbecks Arch Surg. 2010;395:1025.
4. Hoffmann C, Compton F, Schäfer JH, Steiner U, Fuller TF, Schostak M, et al. Intraoperative assessment of kidney allograft perfusion by laser-assisted Indocyanine green fluorescence videography. Transplant Proc. 2010;42:1526.
5. Karliczek A, Harlaar NJ, Zeebregts CJ, Wiggers T, Baas PC, van Dam GM. Surgeons lack predictive accuracy for anastomotic leakage in gastrointestinal surgery. Int J Color Dis. 2009;24:569.
6. Kaplan-Marans E, Fulla J, Tomer N, Bilal K, Palese M. Indocyanine green (ICG) in urologic surgery. Urology. 2019;132:10.
7. Olsen TW, Lim JI, Capone A, Myles RA, Gilman JP. Anaphylactic shock following indocyanine green angiography. Arch Ophthalmol. 1996;114:97.
8. Rother U, Gerken ALH, Karampinis I, Klumpp M, Regus S, Meyer A, et al. Dosing of indocyanine green for intraoperative laser fluorescence angiography in kidney transplantation. Microcirculation. 2017;24:1.
9. Keller D, Ishizawa T, Cohen R, Chand M. ICG fluorescence in colorectal surgery: reviewing the current literature, applications, and future direction. Lancet Gastroenterol Hepatol. 2017;2(10):757–66.
10. Bjurlin MA, Gan M, McClintock TR, Volpe A, Borofsky MS, Mottrie A, et al. Near-infrared fluorescence imaging: emerging applications in robotic upper urinary tract surgery. Eur Urol. 2014;65(4):793–801.
11. Siddighi S, Yune JJ, Hardesty J. Indocyanine green for intraoperative localization of ureter. Am J Obstet Gynecol. 2014;211(4):436.e1–2.
12. Lee Z, Simhan J, Parker DC, Reilly C, Llukani E, Lee DI, et al. Novel use of Indocyanine green for intraoperative, real-time localization of ureteral stenosis during robot-assisted Ureteroureterostomy. Urology. 2013;82(3):729–33.
13. Cacciamani GE, Shakir A, Tafuri A, Gill K, Han J, Ahmadi N, et al. Best practices in near-infrared fluorescence imaging with indocyanine green (NIRF/ICG)-guided robotic urologic surgery: a systematic review-based expert consensus. World J Urol. 2020;38(4):883–96.
14. Borofsky MS, Gill IS, Hemal AK, Marien TP, Jayaratna I, Krane LS, et al. Near-infrared fluorescence imaging to facilitate super-selective arterial clamping during zero-ischaemia robotic partial nephrectomy. BJU Int. 2013;111:604.
15. Hsu M, Gupta M, Su LM, Liao JC. Intraoperative optical imaging and tissue interrogation during urologic surgery. Curr Opin Urol. 2014;24:66.
16. Mitsui Y, Shiina H, Arichi N, Hiraoka T, Inoue S, Sumura M, et al. Indocyanine green (ICG)-based fluorescence navigation system for dis-

crimination of kidney cancer from normal parenchyma: application during partial nephrectomy. Int Urol Nephrol. 2012;44:753.

17. Angell JE, Khemees TA, Abaza R. Optimization of near infrared fluorescence tumor localization during robotic partial nephrectomy. J Urol. 2013;190(5):1668–73.
18. Manny TB, Krane LS, Hemal AK. Indocyanine green cannot predict malignancy in partial nephrectomy: histopathologic correlation with fluorescence pattern in 100 patients. J Endourol. 2013;27:918.
19. Shao P, Qin C, Yin C, Meng X, Ju X, Li J, et al. Laparoscopic partial nephrectomy with segmental renal artery clamping: technique and clinical outcomes. Eur Urol. 2011;59:849.
20. Alfred Witjes J, Lebret T, Compérat EM, Cowan NC, De Santis M, Bruins HM, et al. Updated 2016 EAU guidelines on muscle-invasive and metastatic bladder cancer. Eur Urol. 2017;71:462.
21. Manny TB, Hemal AK. Fluorescence-enhanced robotic radical cystectomy using unconjugated indocyanine green for pelvic lymphangiography, tumor marking, and mesenteric angiography: the initial clinical experience. Urology. 2014;83:824.
22. Cahill RA, Ris F, Mortensen NJ. Near-infrared laparoscopy for real-time intra-operative arterial and lymphatic perfusion imaging. Color Dis. 2011;13:12.
23. Harke NN, Godes M, Wagner C, Addali M, Fangmeyer B, Urbanova K, et al. Fluorescence-supported lymphography and extended pelvic lymph node dissection in robot-assisted radical prostatectomy: a prospective, randomized trial. World J Urol. 2018;36:1817.
24. KleinJan GH, van den Berg NS, de Jong J, Wit EM, Thygessen H, Vegt E, et al. Multimodal hybrid imaging agents for sentinel node mapping as a means to (re)connect nuclear medicine to advances made in robot-assisted surgery. Eur J Nucl Med Mol Imaging. 2016;43:1278.
25. Wit EMK, Acar C, Grivas N, Yuan C, Horenblas S, Liedberg F, et al. Sentinel node procedure in prostate cancer: a systematic review to assess diagnostic accuracy. Eur Urol. 2017;71:596.
26. Anderson CB, Morgan TM, Kappa S, Moore D, Clark PE, Davis R, et al. Ureteroenteric anastomotic strictures after radical cystectomy—does operative approach matter? J Urol. 2013;189:541–7.
27. Davis NF, Burke JP, McDermott T, Flynn R, Manecksha RP, Thornhill JA. Bricker versus Wallace anastomosis: a meta-analysis of ureteroenteric stricture rates after ileal conduit urinary diversion. Can Urol Assoc J. 2015;9:284.
28. Doshi CP, Wozniak A, Quek ML. Near-infrared fluorescence imaging of ureters with intravenous Indocyanine green during radical cystectomy to prevent ureteroenteric anastomotic strictures. Urology. 2020;144:220.
29. Ahmadi N, Ashrafi AN, Hartman N, Shakir A, Cacciamani GE, Freitas D, et al. Use of indocyanine green to minimise uretero-enteric strictures after robotic radical cystectomy. BJU Int. 2019;124(2):302–7.

30. Jafari MD, Wexner SD, Martz JE, McLemore EC, Margolin DA, Sherwinter DA, et al. Perfusion assessment in laparoscopic left-sided/anterior resection (PILLAR II): a multi-institutional study. J Am Coll Surg. 2015;220:82.
31. Van Der Poel HG, Buckle T, Brouwer OR, Valdés Olmos RA, Van Leeuwen FWB. Intraoperative laparoscopic fluorescence guidance to the sentinel lymph node in prostate cancer patients: clinical proof of concept of an integrated functional imaging approach using a multimodal tracer. Eur Urol. 2011;60:826.
32. Kumar A, Samavedi S, Bates A, Coelho R, Rocco B, Marquinez J, et al. Using Indocyanine green and near-infrared fluorescence technology to identify the "landmark artery" during robot-assisted radical prostatectomy. Videourology. 2015;29:1.
33. Mangano M, Gobbi A, Beniamin F, Lamon C, Ciacci M, Maccatrozzo L. Robot-assisted nerve-sparing radical prostatectomy using near-infrared fluorescence technology and indocyanine green: initial experience. Urolo J. 2018;85(1):29–31.
34. Esposito C, Turrà F, Del Conte F, Izzo S, Gargiulo F, Farina A, et al. Indocyanine green fluorescence lymphography: a new technique to perform lymphatic sparing laparoscopic palomo varicocelectomy in children. J Laparoendosc Adv Surg Tech. 2019;29(4):564–7.
35. Fukui K, Saito T, Fuchimoto Y. Pediatric laparoscopic varicocelectomy using indocyanine green (ICG) fluorescence imaging. J Pediatr Surg Case Rep. 2021;67:101818.
36. Rother U, Amann K, Adler W, Nawroth N, Karampinis I, Keese M, et al. Quantitative assessment of microperfusion by indocyanine green angiography in kidney transplantation resembles chronic morphological changes in kidney specimens. Microcirculation. 2019;26:e12529.
37. Sekijima M, Tojimbara T, Sato S, Nakamura M, Kawase T, Kai K, et al. An intraoperative fluorescent imaging system in organ transplantation. Transplant Proc. 2004;36:2188–90.
38. Borofsky MS, Gill IS, Hemal AK, Marien TP, Jayaratna I, Krane LS, et al. Near-infrared fluorescence imaging to facilitate super-selective arterial clamping during zero-ischaemia robotic partial nephrectomy: near-infrared fluorescence imaging in zero ischaemia RPN. BJU Int. 2013;111(4):604–10.

Use of Fluorescence Guidance in Gynecology

16

Lioudmila Lipetskaia, Barbara Diane Gillis, and Courtney Griffiths

Introduction

Gynecological surgery in the United States comprises about 25% of inpatient surgical procedures for women over the last 20 years, with 64% classified as solely obstetric, 29% as solely gynecologic, and 7% as both [1]. Up to one third of all women in the United States undergo hysterectomy by age 60 [2]. This massive surgical field is also growing with the increased incidence of gynecologic cancer, specifically endometrial cancer whose rates have steadily risen since the 1990s [3]. Endometrial cancer is closely linked with obesity, with approximately 57% of endome-

L. Lipetskaia (✉)
Division of Urogynecology, Department of Obstetrics and Gynecology, Cooper Medical School for Rowan University, Camden, NJ, USA
e-mail: lipetskaia-lioudmila@cooperhealth.edu

B. D. Gillis
West Virginia University School of Medicine, Morgantown, WV, USA
e-mail: bdg0001@mix.wvu.edu

C. Griffiths
Division of Gynecology Oncology, Cooper Medical School for Rowan University, Camden, NJ, USA
e-mail: griffiths-courtney@cooperhealth.edu

N. Szoka et al. (eds.), *The SAGES Manual of Fluorescence-Guided Surgery*, https://doi.org/10.1007/978-3-031-40685-0_16

trial cancers in the United States attributable to obesity [4]. Therefore, gynecological surgery for both benign and oncologic cases will likely continue to grow.

Fluorescence-guided surgery (FGS) is on the forefront of medicine with at least 85 clinical trials in the United States, and numerous applications already implemented across the world [5]. Fluorescence-guided surgery utilizes fluorescent dye or a near-infrared emitting light source to identify anatomic structures during surgical procedures. This chapter will describe uses of FGS in gynecologic oncology for lymphatic mapping, sentinel lymph node identification, and tumor margin detection, and in benign gynecology, for the management of endometriosis and during complex pelvic reconstruction, as well as for improving identification of anatomical structures and augmenting intraoperative navigation.

Disease-Specific Applications of Fluorescence Imaging

Gynecologic Oncology

Tumor Lymphatic Imaging in Gynecologic Cancers

Endometrial cancer (EC): Indocynanine Green (ICG) dye is clinically used to monitor the lymphatic vessels and sentinel lymph nodes (SLN) of uterine tumors [6]. It can reduce lymphedema and other associated morbidities to selectively remove SLNs which can prevent tumor metastasis. ICG improved the detection rate of pelvic SLN compared to conventional dyes and may be considered as the superior technique [7]. In clinical practice, the rate of systematic LND further decreased after incorporating SLN mapping with ICG. The National Comprehensive Cancer Network (NCCN) recommends fluorescent SLN mapping for endometrial cancer by cervical ICG injection directly [8]. The NCCN guidelines have approved sentinel node localization as a staging technique for EC, as grade 2B evidence. Prospective and retrospective clinical studies have shown that sentinel lymph node mapping (SLNM) combined with pathologic ultra-staging has satisfactory detection rate, sensitivity, and negative predictive value of SLN in patients with early low-risk endometrial carcinoma and does not affect progression-free and overall survival rates. However, the prognostic effect of SLN mapping in high-risk EC patients still needs to be further verified by larger studies. In the earlier version, NCCN guidelines suggested SLN mapping should be cautious for high-risk EC patients. In the latest version, it is believed that SLN mapping may also have a high detection rate and diagnostic accuracy in high-risk EC. Pelvic/para-aortic sentinel lymph nodes were three times more likely to be extracted than non-SLNs, providing accurate staging for optimized postoperative patient management [8]. To date, no published randomized study has investigated the survival benefit. Therefore, although the use of ICG and fluorescent detection cameras is considered the most appropriate for obtaining the best detection rates in lymphatic mapping in endometrial cancer, the SLN technique still is considered as experimental (Fig. 16.1).

Imaging techniques: 1.25 mg/mL concentration, 4 mL (1 mL deep and 1 mL superficial), was injected into the cervix (3 and 9 o'clock position) with 10 min waiting time before dissection. Alternatively, ICG can be injected into tumor directly (via hysteroscopy) or fundally/subserosally. The latter approach increases para-aortic LN detection rate but decreases pelvic LN detection rate and can lead to intraabdominal dispersion of the dye [9] (Fig. 16.2).

Cervical cancer: Cervical cancer is not as prevalent as endometrial cancer, and data on SLN mapping is limited and frequently derived from the studies analyzing SLN detection in cases of cer-

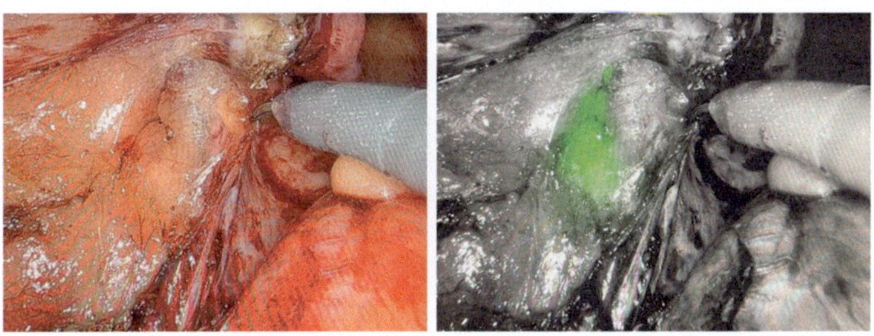

Fig. 16.1 Endometrial cancer: right obturator sentinel lymph node regular light (left) and infrared light (right)

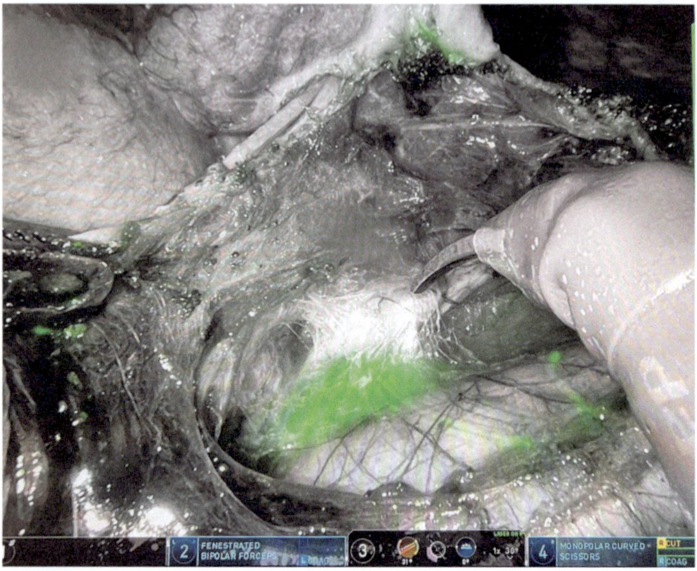

Fig. 16.2 High-resolution image of para-aortic sentinel lymph node mapping for endometrial cancer during robotic LND

vix and endometrial cancer. The assumption is made that migration to the pelvic nodes is similar in both cancers. With this caveat, the studies demonstrate the effectiveness of ICG during SLN biopsy using robotic, laparoscopic surgery and laparotomy, concluding that the method is feasible, safe, time-efficient, and seemingly reliable for lymphatic mapping in early-stage cervical cancer [10]. Two-meta-analyses concluded that in cervical and endometrial cancer, ICG SLN-mapping seems to be equivalent or superior to the conventional dyes [11, 12].

Imaging technique: No standardized technique was reported. Concentrations of ICG have ranged from 0.5 to 5.0 mg/mL, and injected volumes have varied from 0.2 to 4.0 mL. The study in healthy female pigs identified 250–500 μg ICG dose as optimal in identification of a SLN with more distinction from the surrounding tissues [13]. Cervix is injected in 2–4 quadrants (12, 3, 6, and

9 h or 3 and 9). Slow injection is recommended to prevent damage to lymphatic vessels. Optimal time for starting dissection is unclear. In the studies, the median time between injection and the start of dissection is approximately 30 min.

Vulvar cancer: In the vulva bilateral SLN sampling should be assured in central tumors only. If tumor is located at least 1 cm lateral to the clitoris, unilateral dissection is sufficient. A standard technique for dissection involves the use of double tracer (blue dye and Tc-99 m-labeled radiocolloid) and requires a lymphoscintigraphy. The use of ICG in vulvar cancer is limited as near-infrared (NIR) fluorescence can detect targets up to 5–8 mm deep [14]. A deeper target at 25 mm would be invisible by NIR fluorescence imaging alone; hence, majority studies combine NIR fluorescence imaging with radioscintigraphy which enables visualization of deeper inguinal SLNs, especially in patients with obesity. The robotic video endoscopy inguinal lymphadenectomy is emerging technique for diagnosis of vulvar cancer, but so far only one case report with SLN mapping with ICG followed by systematic inguinal lymphadenectomy is described [15]. So far, the best results in mapping are achieved using a combination of ICG and technetium-99 m nanocolloid. Once overlying tissue is removed, as guided by radioscintigraphy, NIR fluorescence is used for more precise image guidance to compensate for relatively poor spatial and temporal resolution of radioscintigraphy. Body mass index seems to be a limitation for using ICG alone as a tracer.

Imaging technique: Concentration of 0.5/2.5 mg/mL. A total of 4 mL (1 mL at 4 sites) was injected directly into the tumor (intracutaneously) with dissection starting in 10 min. Alternatively, ICG can be injected around the scar at prior excision site in case of cancer recurrence.

Ovarian cancer (OC): The incidence of lymph node metastases in early OC ranges between and 30%, and pelvic and paraaortic lymphadenectomy is recommended. In early ovarian cancer, lymph node metastases are found as isolated para-aortic nodes in 50% of patients, as isolated pelvic nodes in 20% of patients, and in both in the remaining 30% of patients [16]. The three major ovarian lymphatic drainage pathways (infundibulopelvic ligament, the ovarian ligament, and the round ligament) explain the wide geography of the metastatic disease and point out to the potential injection sites for tracers. So far, two ongoing prospective, multicenter studies attempt to determine efficacy and safety of ICG in SLN mapping. Both SELLY (SLN in early-stage ovarian cancer) and SENTOV ((sentinel lymph node technique in ovarian cancer) evaluate ICG in conjunction with Tc-99 m. The Tc-99 m remains trapped in the lymph nodes for a long period and is injected before the oophorectomy. The small ICG molecule migrates rapidly through lymphatic vessels and makes it difficult to accurately identify the first node; hence, ICG is injected after an ovary is removed. The preliminary data from SELLY and SENTOV concluded that SLN mapping in early-stage ovarian cancer is feasible without major intraoperative or safety concerns [17] [18]. The data on accuracy and detection rate of this technique is not available yet; hence, no recommendation can be given because this procedure still is experimental.

Imaging technique: Concentration of 1.25 mg/mL. A total of 0.5–1 mL was injected into infundibulopelvic and ovarian ligament with dissection starting almost immediately. Alternative injection sites are mesovarium, hilum of the ovary, and ovarian cortex.

Tumor Margin Detection

Free surgical margin is the main challenge in vulvar and vaginal cancer surgery. In solid tumors, incomplete surgery results in high risk of tumor recurrence. The real-time detection of tumor margins helps achieve complete resection and decrease risk of recurrence. Case reports present ICG use in vulvar and vaginal cancer for surgical resection guidance. In the first case after primary incomplete resection of vulvar cancer, an intravenous ICG injection determined the free margin after resection. In the second case, peritumoral ICG injection 1 cm around the upper vagina cancer showed a clear resection margin on the final pathological finding after robotic colpo-hysterectomy with LND [19].

Imaging technique: For vulvar cancer, 2 cc of diluted ICG IV immediately before surgery and for vaginal cancer, 2 mL peritumoral injection with 1 cm radius. No uterine manipulator is used, and a vaginal probe is inserted to develop the fornix. Techniques need to be validated on a large scale.

Management of Bowel and GU Anastomosis as a Part of Cytoreductive Surgery

Several patient and surgical factors influence the risk of anastomotic leak after bowel resection during pelvic exenteration. Surgeons typically rely on subjective methods to identify anastomotic leaks such as palpation of vessels and assessment of tissue vitality in white light. The addition of intraoperative ICG assessment of colorectal anastomoses demonstrated reduced risk of anastomotic leakage in treatment of GI malignancies in ten studies. In seven studies, resection of the colon or rectum was extended into more vital tissue if ICG detected an insufficient perfusion at the proposed anastomosis site. Three studies concluded that ICG perfusion assessment reduced the risk of anastomotic leakage significantly. One study found no difference in anastomotic leakage rate between the control group and the ICG group [20]. This concept was adopted in the management of anastomosis in gynecologic cancers requiring wide organ resection as a part of cytoreduction strategy. ICG was used to evaluate perfusion of ileum-ileum, right and left ureter with small bowel, and colorectal sides of anastomosis to assess vascularity of urinary diversion after pelvic exenteration for gynecologic cancers (Fig. 16.3). Out of 15 subjects, 3 patients had postoperative complications due to poor perfusion of anastomosis (ureteral and ileal anastomosis leaks and ureteric stricture); all these cases had a suboptimal intraoperative ICG perfusion [21] (Fig. 16.4).

Imaging technique: IV ICG bolus before and/or after anastomosis construction 0.2–0.5 mg/kg (total ranging from 0.2 to 0.5 mg/kg). In order to achieve a more objective perfusion assessment, scoring systems were developed and intraoperative pixel brightness analysis was performed. Unfortunately, the quantification did not lead to a cutoff value.

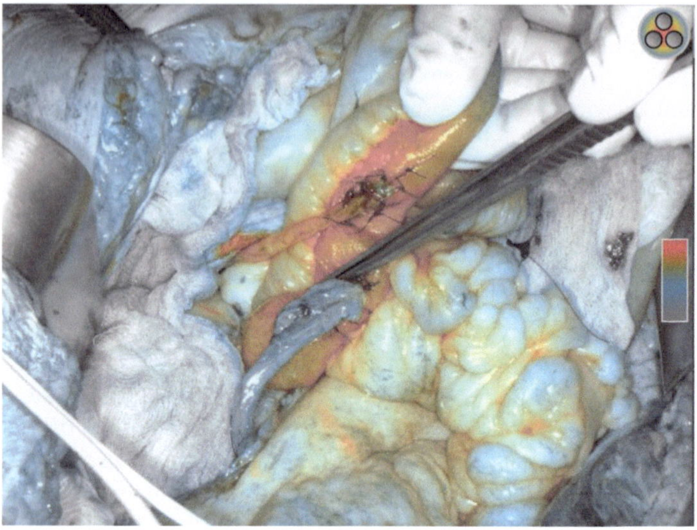

Fig. 16.3 Bricker ileal conduit uretero-enteric anastomoses demonstrating right ureter with optimal indocyanine green (ICG) perfusion (+++) vs. left ureter with poor ICG perfusion (– – -). (*Bizzai* et al. *Indocyanine Green to Assess Vascularity of Ileal Conduit Anastomosis During Pelvic Exenteration for Recuent/Persistent Gynecological Cancer: A Pilot Study. Front Oncol. 2021 Dec 7;11:727725. doi: 10.3389/fonc.2021.727725. PMID: 34950574; PMCID: PMC8691262*)

Surgical Management of Endometriosis

Detection of Endometriotic Lesions

Endometriosis has three clinical forms: peritoneal superficial endometriosis, ovarian endometriosis and deeply infiltrating endometriosis in the rectovaginal septum [22]. Identifying endometriosis lesions may be challenging due to variable appearances, small size, and concealed localization. ICG green highlights the location of endometriotic lesions as they are associated with increased areas of vascularization and inflammation. The endometriotic lesion patterns observed during surgery are described as diffuse or abundant fluorescence (hypervascular pattern) in 40% women and poor or absent (hypovascular pattern) in 60% women with endometriosis. Although some studies report excellent sensi-

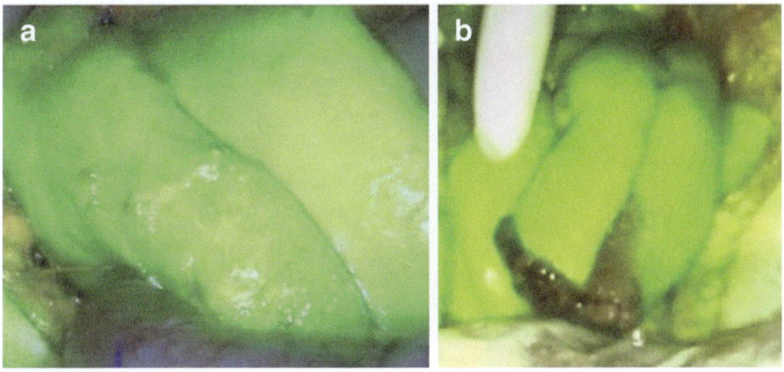

Fig. 16.4 Transabdominal anastomotic perfusion assessment using the SPY-PHI system (Stryker, USA). (**a**) Transabdominal perfusion assessment showing well-perfused bowel. (**b**) Transabdominal perfusion assessment showing perfusion defect (*Nguyen JMV* et al. *The use of indocyanine green fluorescence angiography to assess anastomotic perfusion following bowel resection in surgery for gynecologic malignancies – A report of 100 consecutive anastomoses. Gynecol Oncol. 2020 Aug;158* (2)*:402–406. Doi: 10.1016/j.ygyno.2020.05.008. Epub 2020 May 15. PMID: 32423604*)

tivity and specificity in identifying the lesions, others conclude that the single use of ICG shows no improvement in the detection of endometriosis [22]. It appears that ICG performs better in providing demarcation of deep endometriotic lesions assisting with more complete resection, but its diagnostic value is controversial.

Imaging technique: 0.25 mg/kg ICG i.v. with time intervals varying between a minimum of 5 and a maximum of about 30 min.

Management of Bowel Involvement During Surgery for Endometriosis

ICG green is used to evaluate the bowel vascularization after endometriosis rectal shaving surgery. Separating the healthy rectal tissue from the rectovaginal deep nodules aids in decision whether to enlarge the resection to the posterior vaginal fornix [23]. Deep lesion excision and rectal shaving techniques required for successful endometriosis treatment can jeopardize rectal wall integrity and lead to rectovaginal fistula formation. Visual assessment of the rectal shaving area is labeled as fluoresced with the visual Likert-type scale. Oversewing of rectal muscularis is performed if there is a concern for rectal tissue integrity (Fig. 16.5).

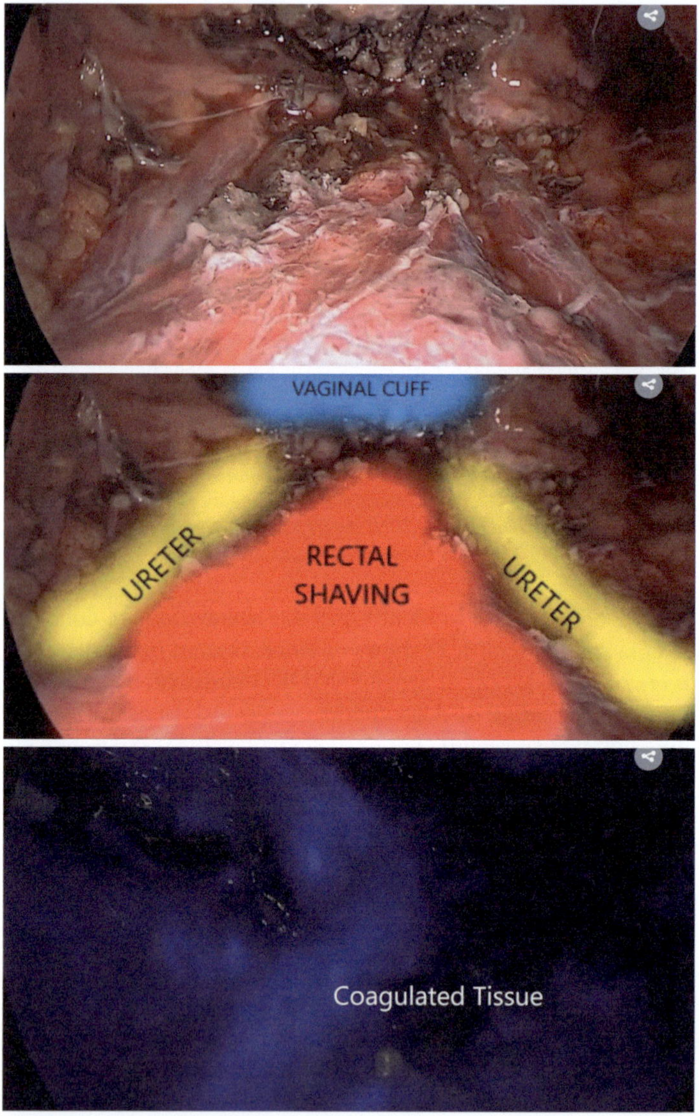

Fig. 16.5 Coagulated tissue appears dark and non-perfused in the area where rectal shaving was performed (*Bar-Shavit Y, et all Use of indocyanine green in endometriosis surgery. Fertil Steril. 2018 Jun;109* (6)*:1136–1137. doi: 10.1016/j.fertnstert.2018.02.113. Epub 2018 Jun 6. PMID: 29885885*)

The RCT study is underway to assess if this technique leads to decrease fistula formation [24]. Another study demonstrated that when full-thickness bowel resection is necessary for nodule excision, ICG perfusion mapping can be performed in the same manner as in colorectal surgery [25].

Imaging technique: A IV bolus of 0.2 mg/kg of indocyanine green after dilution (2.5 mg/mL) at the end of a rectal shaving.

Complex Pelvic Reconstructive Procedures

Demarcating Retropubic Space Anatomy in Burch Colposuspension

Retropubic colposuspension is a surgical treatment which involves lifting the tissues near the bladder neck and proximal urethra and attaching them to Cooper's ligament in attempt to treat stress urinary incontinence. Procedure is traditionally performed via open approach and tension of the sutures attaching vagina to Cooper's ligament adjusted by palpation. With advent of robotic surgery and lack of haptic feedback, new methods of tension adjustment are needed. Bladder neck can be identified by tagging on Foley balloon inserted into the bladder and inflated with 30 cc of ICG tinged medium. Foley balloon highlighted by ICG demarcates bladder wall from underlying vaginal tissue plain allowing for more precise dissection and adequate suspension suture.

Imaging technique: 100 cc of intralipid TPN solution mixed with 0.5 mL of ICG green (2.5 mg/mL in distilled water) and 30 cc instilled in 18F Foley balloon inserted into the bladder [26].

Neovagina Construction in Congenital Anomalies and Transgender Surgery

Patients with vaginal agenesis undergo vaginoplasty using a mold that had been wrapped with skin graft (McIndoe technique) or external traction device placed over the abdominal wall (Vecchietti procedure). Trans-female patients might require laparoscopic sigmoid vaginoplasty if standard penile-scrotal flap inversion technique is not feasible. In either case, creation of neovagina is a highly complex surgery requiring meticulous dissection of complex anatomical spaces. ICG can be used intraoperatively in laparoscopic sigmoid vaginoplasty to determine sigmoid segment perfusion and viability prior to committing to neovagina construction. In the study of five patients, ICG green demonstrated poor viability of sigmoid segment in one patient and procedure was aborted [27]. In another study, ICG green was helpful in identifying upper urinary tract anatomy, thus guiding safer and faster dissection during Vecchietti procedure [28].

Imaging technique: Cystoscopic intraureteral ICG injection lasted 3.4 min, improving the anatomic identification of the ureters, with the additional benefit of having the bladder highlighted in case of congenital anomaly.

Revisions of Prior Reconstructive Surgeries

Frequently pelvic reconstructive procedures use permanent grafts (polypropylene mesh or Gore-Tex sutures) to increase longevity of the repair and prevent prolapse or incontinence recurrence. Although the risks of complications associated with graft use are low, occasionally excision of permanent materials from pelvic structures is required to treat graft related complications. In case of erosion or infections due to foreign body, it is important to minimize the damage to adjacent organs while dissecting implant away from vagina. The tissue planes are frequently distorted due to inflammation and scarring, and highlighting adjacent structures with the ICG helps to delineate the tissue planes and prevent injury (Fig. 16.6).

Fig. 16.6 Revision of prior pelvic reconstructive surgery complicated by Gore-Tex suture erosion (Parts **a**–**c**) (**a**) Attempt to remove Gore-Tex stitch eroding in vagina. Stitch is located in the area of vagina adjacent to left ureterovesical junction. (**b**) Foley balloon filled with ICG mix enhances bladder visualization. (**c**) Foley balloon manipulated with robotic instruments into the area of left ureterovesical junction allows to safely continue dissection avoiding injury to bladder and ureter

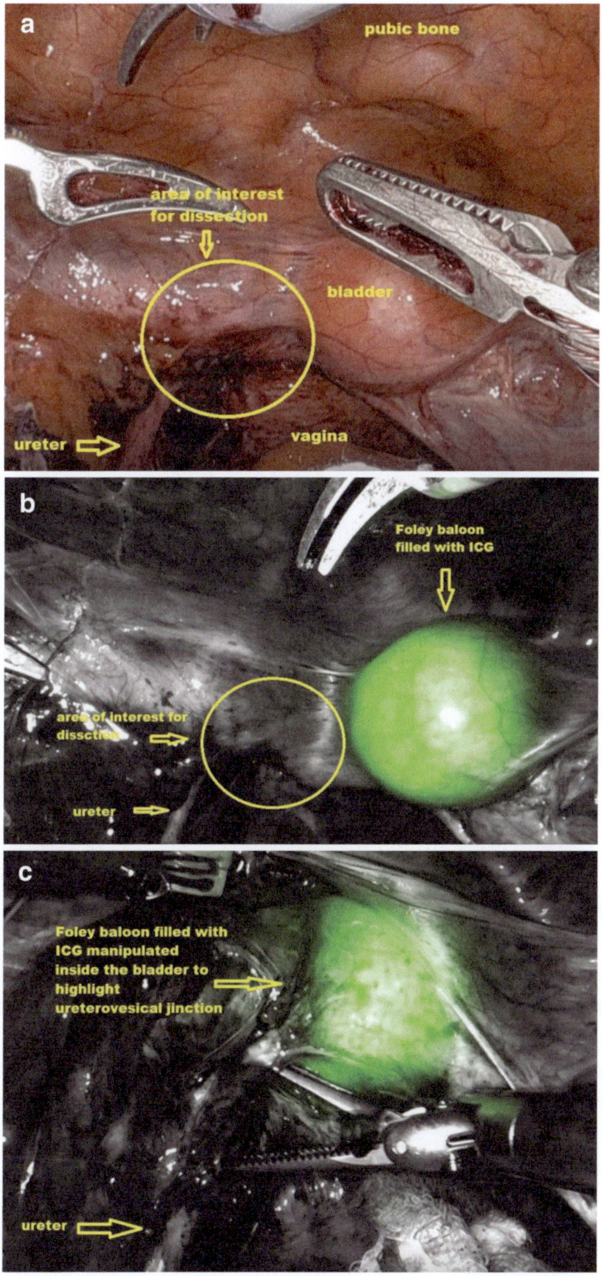
a
pubic bone
area of interest
for dissection
bladder
ureter
vagina
b
Foley baloon
filled with ICG
area of interest for
dissction
ureter
c
Foley baloon filled with
ICG manipulated
inside the bladder to
highlight
ureterovesical jinction
ureter

Imaging technique: 100 cc of intralipid TPN solution mixed with 0.5 mL of ICG green (2.5 mg/mL in distilled water) and 30 cc instilled in 18F Foly balloon inserted into bladder.

Fluorescent Angiography

Vaginal Cuff Angiography in an Attempt to Assess Devascularization Due to Thermal Injury After Total Robotic Hysterectomy

Minimally invasive hysterectomy compares favorably to laparotomy in overall complication rate but is notorious for increased vaginal cuff dehiscence. Both energy used during colpotomy and suturing techniques for cuff closure were implicated in higher dehiscence rate [29]. Vascular perfusion plays a role in cuff healing along with other factors. Developing techniques for quantification of thermal damage impact on perfusion can come in handy while we are attempting to find solutions for this problem. ICG angiography represents an emerging technology for real-time evaluation of the vaginal cuff during laparoscopic hysterectomy with potential to limit the incidence of vaginal cuff dehiscence through design of further research studies.

Imaging technique: 2.5–5 mg ICG IV bolus followed by 10 mL saline flash. ICG dye appeared in surgical field in 11 s. Repeated administration was required in 11 min. Most participants show fluorescence all the way to the cuff edge, but the width of thermal injury brim varies around the cuff. The calculation of cuff perimeter percentage with adequate perfusion is required to assess the extent of devascularized zone [30] (Fig. 16.7).

Ovarian Artery Perfusion to Assess Ovarian Torsion

Ovarian torsion is defined as partial or complete rotation of the ovarian vascular pedicle and causes obstruction to venous outflow and arterial inflow. It presents as acute abdominal pain and diagnosed during surgical exploration. The ultimate goal of sur-

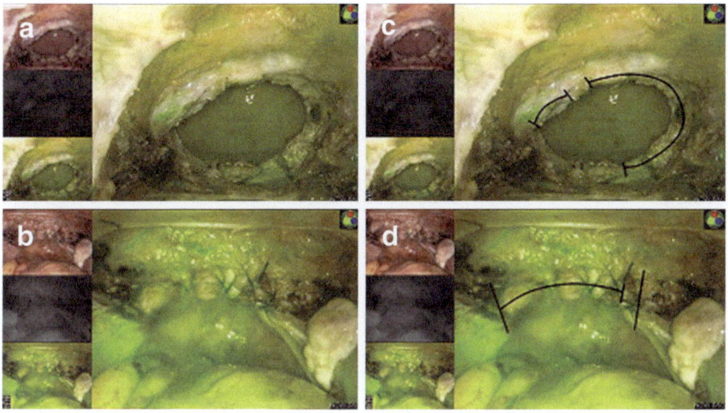

Fig. 16.7 Samples of images used for perfusion analysis (**a, b**) with representative markings demonstrating adequate perfusion (**c**, **d**) at the cuff. The short perpendicular bars delineate transition from perfused to nonperfused regions. The parallel curve demonstrates areas with adequate perfusion. The long perpendicular bars in D delineate the total length of the closed vaginal cuff (*Beran* et al *Laser Angiography with Indocyanine Green to Assess Vaginal Cuff Perfusion during Total Laparoscopic Hysterectomy: A Pilot Study. J Minim Invasive Gynecol. 2017 Mar-Apr;24* (3)*:432–437. doi: 10.1016/j.jmig.2016.12.021. Epub 2017 Jan 4. PMID: 28063908*)

gery is restoration of blood flow to the ovary and ovarian preservation whenever possible. Potential viability of torsed ovary is traditionally assessed visually by observing twisted and black-and-blue adnexa, and decision on surgical removal needs to be made in real time. One study assessed feasibility of ICG use in diagnosis of detorsed adnexa viability. Perfusion was achieved in ten patients (83%) in a median time of 1 min, resulting in ovarian conservation. Perfusion was absent in two cases, and post-oophorectomy histologic necrosis was confirmed in one case [31].

Imaging technique: A loading dose of 8 cc of ICG dye was injected IV and untwisted ovary was observed for 10 min after ICG dye administration. Perfusion was defined as visualization of ICG dye in the involved ovary and/or fallopian tube, causing the structures to turn green. If no perfusion was visualized 10 min after the initial bolus injection, an additional 4 cc bolus of ICG dye could be administered, and the ovary was observed for another 10 min. This process could be repeated an additional three times, if necessary, resulting in a maximum volume of 20 cc of ICG dye.

Fluorescence Imaging-Guided Surgical Navigation

Ureter Visualization

Iatrogenic bladder injuries are the most frequent urologic injuries, but they are usually recognized and repaired immediately, and potential complications are typically minor. In contrast, 50–70% of iatrogenic ureteral injuries are diagnosed postoperatively with gynecologic surgery accounting for 52% to 82% of those injuries [32]. The ureter is injured in roughly 0.5–2% of all hysterectomies and routine gynecologic pelvic operations [33, 34]. The lack of precise haptic feedback in robotic and laparoscopic surgery has previously been associated with increasing rates of inadvertent ureteral injuries across various surgical specialties [35]. Clear identification of the pelvic ureter can be difficult but remains essential to avoid inadvertent iatrogenic ureteral injury. The preventative ureteral stents placement is controversial in gynecological surgery due to the lack of clear evidence of efficacy. Illuminating catheters have been designed to improve visualization of ureters intraoperatively but did not gain popularity [36].

· Injection technique: Three techniques involving NIR entail IV use of NIR dye, direct instillation of NIR solution into ureteral orifice via cystoscopy, and use of ureteral catheter with NIR properties in construction material.

(a) 0.06 mg/kg of nerindocianine sodium administered IV. Ureter is imaged at 10 and 30 min post-infusion. Lower (0.042 mg/kg) and higher (0.12 mg/kg) doses perform poorer by diminishing visualization time or decreasing the efficacy [37] (Fig. 16.8).
(b) Cystoscopy is performed at the beginning of the surgery to insert the tip of a 6-Fr ureteral catheter and instill 8 mL of

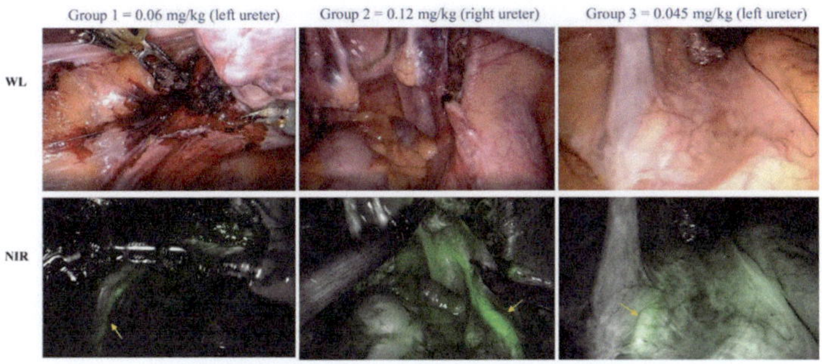

Fig. 16.8 A. Intraoperative ureteral identification by nerindocianine sodium use via IV administration (*Huh* et al. *Fluorescence Imaging of the Ureter in Minimally Invasive Pelvic Surgery. J Minim Invasive Gynecol. 2021 Feb;28*(2)*:332–341.e14. doi: 10.1016/j.jmig.2020.06.022. Epub 2020 Jun 29. PMID: 32615331*)

ICG (1.25 mg/mL solution). Finally, the catheters are removed because the fluorescence remains in the ureters up to 6 h. This method can be applied retroactively if injury is suspected at the end of surgery. Ureteral injury is identified by observing extravasation of the dye after instillation (Fig. 16.9).

(c) The ureteral catheter constructed with near-infrared dye similar to ICG embedded in its wall does not require intraoperative dye administration. This technique is user- friendly and can be utilized by the novice surgeons with little experience in laparoscopic surgery [38] (Fig. 16.10).

Fluorescent Medical Devices

By creating medical and surgical devices that fluoresce under NIR imaging, the number of patients benefiting from fluorescence assisted surgery will increase. There are a few medical device companies (EndoGlow, Rochester, NY.) that have been innovative in developing surgical devices that fluoresce under NIR imaging (Fig. 16.11). For instance, fluorescent imbedded rectal and vaginal manipulators take the place of traditional bougies or end-to-end anastomosis sizers in pelvic surgeries. Pilot studies have

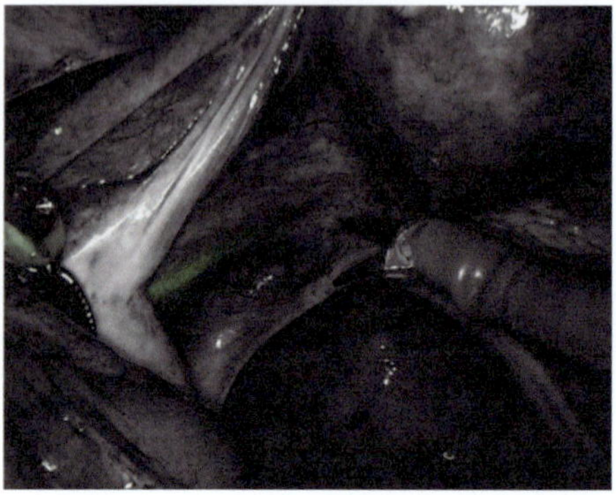

Fig. 16.9 Intraoperative ureteral identification by indocyanine green use via catheter infusion (*Shibata R* et al. *Intraoperative dyes, fluorescence and enhanced imaging in benign gynaecologic surgery. Cu Opin Obstet Gynecol. 2022 Aug 1;34* (4)*:237–243. doi: 10.1097/GCO.0000000000000793. PMID: 35895966*)

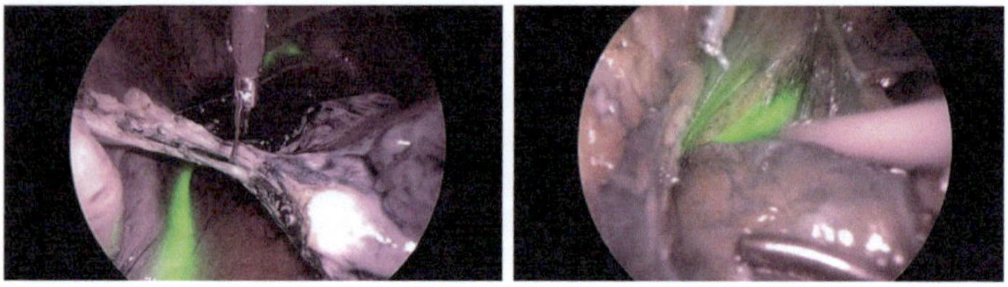

Fig. 16.10 Intraoperative ureteral identification by indocyanine green use via NIR-embedded novel ureteral catheter infusion (*Fujita H,* et al. *Use of a Novel Fluorescent Catheter to Locate the Ureters during Total Laparoscopic Hysterectomy. J Minim Invasive Gynecol. 2021 Jul;28* (7)*:1420–1424. doi: 10.1016/j.jmig.2021.04.004. Epub 2021 Apr 19. PMID: 33887490*)

demonstrated several benefits to the transillumination effect of using a fluorescent manipulator [39]. Surgeons were able to identify deep infiltrating rectal endometriosis, better recognize surgical planes in complex anatomy, and visualize relative tissue depth. The ability to transilluminate vaginal tissue aided in post-hysterectomy bladder dissections during sacrocolpopexies and rectopexies. An unexpected benefit was the increased communication between the attending surgeon and surgical learners (fellows/residents) or surgical assists. The enhanced visualization allowed the surgical learner or first-assist to see and understand the intricacies of the dissection more easily.

The manipulator can be placed in the vagina (Fig. 16.11) or rectum (Fig. 16.12) to manipulate tissue and highlight tissue plains, therefore guiding dissection.

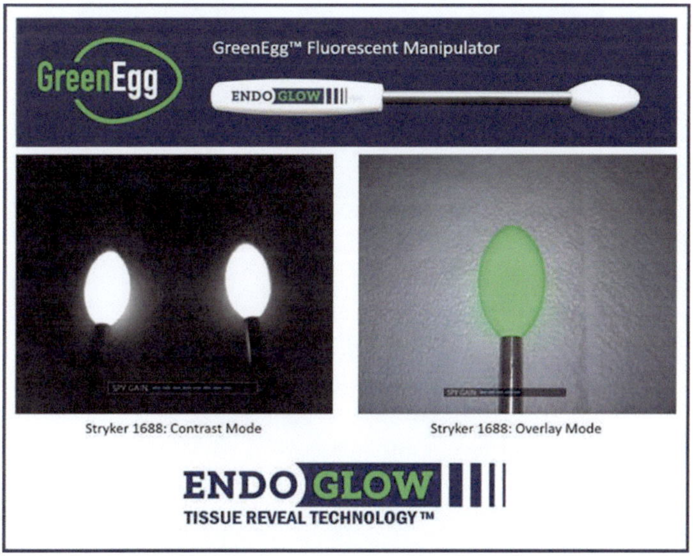

Fig. 16.11 EndoGlow device placed into vagina to guide dissection between vagina and bladder (regular light view on left and infrared view on the right)

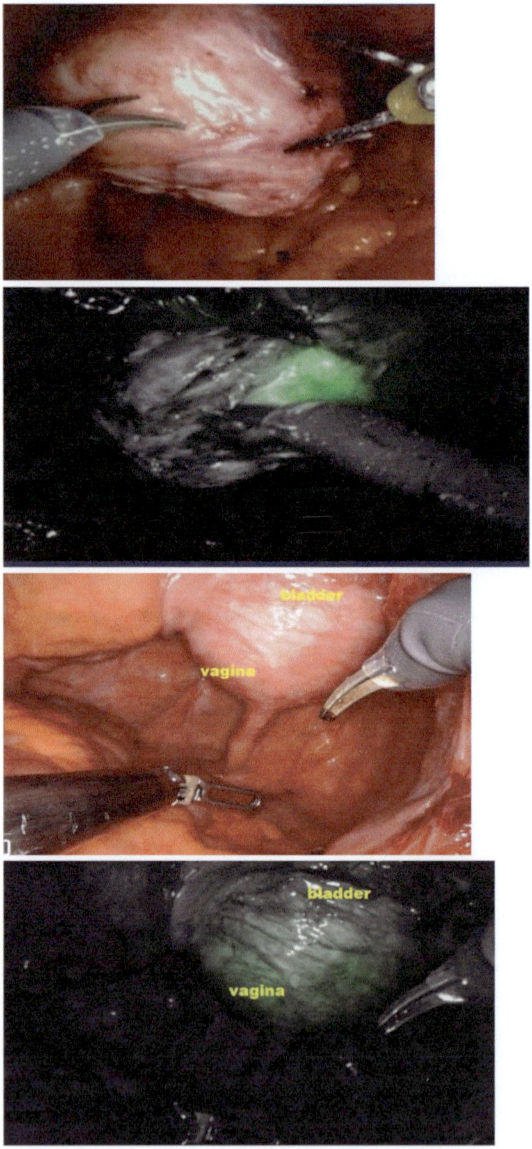

Fig. 16.11 (continued)

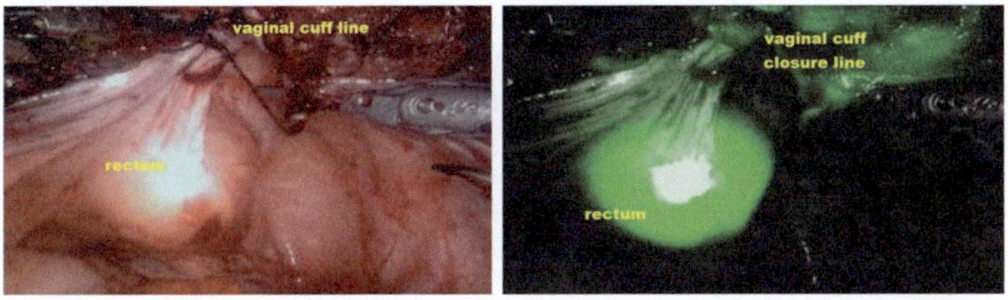

Fig. 16.12 EndoGlow device placed into rectum to guide dissection between rectum and closed vaginal cuff after hysterectomy (regular light view on left and infrared view on the right)

Conclusion

FGS has numerous clinical applications in gynecological surgery from SLN mapping, anatomic visualization of ureters or tissue planes, and perfusion assessment of anastomoses or specific arteries. These tools aid surgeons intraoperatively in real time and provide essential visual feedback that has previously been inaccessible. FGS continues to rapidly evolve and improve surgical care; however, further well-powered studies are needed to establish the value of fluorescence guidance in gynecologic surgery.

References

1. Oliphant SS, Jones KA, Wang L, Bunker CH, Lowder JL. Trends over time with commonly performed obstetric and gynecologic inpatient procedures. Obstet Gynecol. 2010;116(4):926–31. https://doi.org/10.1097/AOG.0b013e3181f38599.
2. Gupta S, Maghsoudlou P, Ajao M, Einarsson JI, King LP. Very low rates of ureteral injury in laparoscopic hysterectomy performed by fellowship-trained minimally invasive gynecologic surgeons. J Minim Invasive Gynecol. 2022;29(9):1099–103.
3. Towner M, Kim JJ, Simon MA, Matei D, Roque D. Disparities in gynecologic cancer incidence, treatment, and survival: a naative review of outcomes among black and white women in the United States. Int J Gynecol Cancer. 2022;32(7):931–8. Published 2022 Jul 4.
4. Onstad MA, Schmandt RE, Lu KH. Addressing the role of obesity in endometrial cancer risk, prevention, and treatment. J Clin Oncol. 2016;34(35):4225–30.
5. Stewart HL, Birch DJS. Fluorescence guided surgery methods. Appl Fluoresc. 2021;9:4. https://doi.org/10.1088/2050-6120/ac1dbb.

6. Pölcher M, Matz S, Braun M, Brambs C, Beer M, Hamann M. Sentinel lymph node mapping with indocyanine green compared to blue dye tracer in gynecologic malignancies-a single center experience of 218 patients. J Surg Oncol. 2021;123(4):1092–8. https://doi.org/10.1002/jso.26338.
7. Bodurtha Smith AJ, Fader AN, Tanner EJ. Sentinel lymph node assessment in endometrial cancer: a systematic review and meta-analysis. Am J Obstet Gynecol. 2017;216(5):459–476.e410. https://doi.org/10.1016/j.ajog.2016.11.1033.
8. Abu-Rustum NR, Yashar CM, Bradley K, Campos SM, Chino J, Chon HS, Chu C, Cohn D, Crispens MA, Damast S, et al. NCCN guidelines® insights: uterine neoplasms, version 3.2021. J Natl Compr Cancer Netw. 2021;19(8):888–95. https://doi.org/10.6004/jnccn.2021.0038. From NLM.
9. Peone AM, Casadio P, Formelli G, Levorato M, Ghi T, Costa S, Meriggiola MC, Pelusi G. Cervical and hysteroscopic injection for identification of sentinel lymph node in endometrial cancer. Gynecol Oncol. 2008;111(1):62–7. https://doi.org/10.1016/j.ygyno.2008.05.032.
10. Rocha A, Domínguez AM, Lécuru F, Bourdel N. Indocyanine green and infrared fluorescence in detection of sentinel lymph nodes in endometrial and cervical cancer staging—a systematic review. Eur J Obstet Gynecol Reprod Biol. 2016;206:213–9. https://doi.org/10.1016/j.ejogrb.2016.09.027.
11. Ruscito I, Gaspai ML, Braicu EI, Bellati F, Raio L, Sehouli J, Mueller MD, Panici PB, Papadia A. Sentinel node mapping in cervical and endometrial cancer: Indocyanine green versus other conventional dyes-a meta-analysis. Ann Surg Oncol. 2016;23(11):3749–56. https://doi.org/10.1245/s10434-016-5236-x.
12. Ulain Q, Han L, Wu Q, Zhao L, Wang Q, Tuo X, Wang Y, Wang Q, Ma S, Sun C, et al. Indocyanine green can stand alone in detecting sentinel lymph nodes in cervical cancer. J Int Med Res. 2018;46(12):4885–97. https://doi.org/10.1177/0300060518803041.
13. Levinson KL, Mahdi H, Escobar PF. Feasibility and optimal dosage of indocyanine green fluorescence for sentinel lymph node detection using robotic single-site instrumentation: preclinical study. J Minim Invasive Gynecol. 2013;20(5):691–6. https://doi.org/10.1016/j.jmig.2013.03.013.
14. Vahrmeijer AL, Hutteman M, van der Vorst JR, van de Velde CJ, Frangioni JV. Image-guided cancer surgery using near-infrared fluorescence. Nat Rev Clin Oncol. 2013;10(9):507–18. https://doi.org/10.1038/nrclinonc.2013.123.
15. Naldini A, Vizzielli G, Peone E, Gallotta V, Scambia G. Robotic video endoscopic inguinal lymphadenectomy (R-VEIL) for vulvar cancer with sentinel node mapping using indocyanine green and near-infrared fluorescence imaging technology. Gynecol Oncol. 2018;150(1):203–4. https://doi.org/10.1016/j.ygyno.2018.04.568.
16. Kleppe M, Wang T, Van Gorp T, Slangen BF, Kruse AJ, Kruitwagen RF. Lymph node metastasis in stages I and II ovarian cancer: a review.

Gynecol Oncol. 2011;123(3):610–4. https://doi.org/10.1016/j.ygyno.2011.09.013.
17. Lago V, Bello P, Montero B, Matute L, Padilla-Iserte P, Lopez S, Marina T, Agudelo M, Domingo S. Sentinel lymph node technique in early-stage ovarian cancer (SENTOV): a phase II clinical trial. Int J Gynecol Cancer. 2020;30(9):1390–6. https://doi.org/10.1136/ijgc-2020-001289.
18. Uccella S, Nero C, Vizza E, Vargiu V, Coado G, Bizzai N, Ghezzi F, Cosentino F, Turco LC, Fagotti A, et al. Sentinel-node biopsy in early-stage ovarian cancer: preliminary results of a prospective multicentre study (SELLY). Am J Obstet Gynecol. 2019;221(4):324.e321–10. https://doi.org/10.1016/j.ajog.2019.05.005.
19. Nguyen-Xuan HT, Montero Macias R, Bonsang-Kitzis H, Deloménie M, Ngô C, Koual M, Bats AS, Hivelin M, Lécuru F, Balaya V. Use of fluorescence to guide surgical resection in vulvo-vaginal neoplasia: two case reports. J Gynecol Obstet Hum Reprod. 2021;50(6):101768. https://doi.org/10.1016/j.jogoh.2020.101768.
20. Degett TH, Andersen HS, Gögenur I. Indocyanine green fluorescence angiography for intraoperative assessment of gastrointestinal anastomotic perfusion: a systematic review of clinical trials. Langenbeck's Arch Surg. 2016;401(6):767–75. https://doi.org/10.1007/s00423-016-1400-9.
21. Bizzai N, Foschi N, Loveo M, Tortorella L, Santullo F, Rosati A, Gueli Alletti S, Costantini B, Gallotta V, Feandina G, et al. Indocyanine green to assess vascularity of ileal conduit anastomosis during pelvic exenteration for recuent/persistent gynecological cancer: a pilot study. Front Oncologia. 2021;11:727725. https://doi.org/10.3389/fonc.2021.727725.
22. Nisolle M, Donnez J. Peritoneal endometriosis, ovarian endometriosis, and adenomyotic nodules of the rectovaginal septum are three different entities. Fertil Steril. 1997;68(4):585–96. https://doi.org/10.1016/s0015-0282(97)00191-x.
23. De Neef A, Cadière GB, Bourgeois P, Barbieux R, Dapri G, Fastrez M. Fluorescence of deep infiltrating endometriosis during laparoscopic surgery: a preliminary report on 6 cases. Surg Innov. 2018;25(5):450–4. https://doi.org/10.1177/1553350618785486.
24. Bar-Shavit Y, Jaillet L, Chauvet P, Canis M, Bourdel N. Use of indocyanine green in endometriosis surgery. Fertil Steril. 2018;109(6):1136–7. https://doi.org/10.1016/j.fertnstert.2018.02.113.
25. Raimondo D, Mastronardi M, Mabrouk M, Cafagna G, Salucci P, Arena A, Iodice R, Borghese G, Casadio P, Del Forno S, et al. Rectosigmoid endometriosis vascular patterns at intraoperative Indocyanine green angiography and their coelation with clinicopathological data. Surg Innov. 2020;27(5):474–80. https://doi.org/10.1177/1553350620930147.
26. Lipetskaia LV. Near infrared imaging in robotically assisted urogynecologic surgery. AJOG. 2017;216:S619.
27. van der Sluis WB, Bouman MB, Al-Tamimi M, Meijerink WJ, Tuynman JB. Real-time indocyanine green fluorescent angiography in laparoscopic sigmoid vaginoplasty to assess perfusion of the pedicled sigmoid seg-

ment. Fertil Steril. 2019;112(5):967–9. https://doi.org/10.1016/j.fertnstert.2019.08.063. From NLM.
28. Fontoura Oliveira A, Feeira H. Neovagina creation in congenital vaginal agenesis: new mini-laparoscopic approach applying intraoperative indocyanine green fluorescence. Surg Innov. 2021;28(1):24–32. https://doi.org/10.1177/1553350620968990.
29. Fuchs Weizman N, Einarsson JI, Wang KC, Vitonis AF, Cohen SL. Vaginal cuff dehiscence: risk factors and associated morbidities. JSLS. 2015;19(2):1. https://doi.org/10.4293/jsls.2013.00351. From NLM.
30. Beran BD, Shockley M, Arnolds K, Escobar P, Zimberg S, Sprague ML. Laser angiography with Indocyanine green to assess vaginal cuff perfusion during total laparoscopic hysterectomy: a pilot study. J Minim Invasive Gynecol. 2017;24(3):432–7. https://doi.org/10.1016/j.jmig.2016.12.021. From NLM.
31. Nicholson K, Urh A, Demertzis K, Holubyeva A, LaPier Z, Cisneros-Camacho A, Goldberg GL, Schwartz B. Intraoperative Indocyanine green dye use in ovarian torsion: a feasibility study. J Minim Invasive Gynecol. 2022;29(6):738–42. https://doi.org/10.1016/j.jmig.2022.01.008. From NLM.
32. Ostrzenski A, Radolinski B, Ostrzenska KM. A review of laparoscopic ureteral injury in pelvic surgery. Obstet Gynecol Surv. 2003;58(12):794–9. https://doi.org/10.1097/01.Ogx.0000097781.79401.0b. From NLM.
33. McGeady JB, Breyer BN. Cuent epidemiology of genitourinary trauma. Urol Clin North Am. 2013;40(3):323–34. https://doi.org/10.1016/j.ucl.2013.04.001. From NLM.
34. Dallas KB, Rogo-Gupta L, Elliott CS. Urologic injury and fistula after hysterectomy for benign indications. Obstet Gynecol. 2019;134(2):241–9. https://doi.org/10.1097/aog.0000000000003353. From NLM.
35. Saidi MH, Sadler RK, Vancaillie TG, Akright BD, Farhart SA, White AJ. Diagnosis and management of serious urinary complications after major operative laparoscopy. Obstet Gynecol. 1996;87(2):272–6. https://doi.org/10.1016/0029-7844(95)00411-4. From NLM.
36. Redan JA, McCarus SD. Protect the ureters. JSLS. 2009;13(2):139–41. From NLM.
37. Huh WK, Johnson JL, Elliott E, Boone JD, Leath CA 3rd, Kovar JL, Kim KH. Fluorescence imaging of the ureter in minimally invasive pelvic surgery. J Minim Invasive Gynecol. 2021;28(2):332–341.e314. https://doi.org/10.1016/j.jmig.2020.06.022.
38. Fujita H, Kikuchi I, Nakagawa R, Katano M, Nakano E, Kitayama R, Tanaka Y. Use of a novel fluorescent catheter to locate the ureters during Total laparoscopic hysterectomy. J Minim Invasive Gynecol. 2021;28(7):1420–4. https://doi.org/10.1016/j.jmig.2021.04.004.
39. Ris F, Liot E, Buchs NC, Kraus R, Ismael G, Belfontali V, Douissard J, Cunningham C, Lindsey I, Guy R, et al. Multicentre phase II trial of near-infrared imaging in elective colorectal surgery. Br J Surg. 2018;105(10):1359–67. https://doi.org/10.1002/bjs.10844.

Future Directions in Fluorescence-and Image-Guided Surgery

17

Gene Yang

Introduction

Fluorescence- and image-guided surgery are rapidly growing fields of research with a wide range of potential applications to bridge the gap between preoperative imaging and the operative environment. Fluorescence guidance systems have been utilized in many clinical applications across several disciplines to improve surgical outcomes, including tumor localization, anatomy identification, perfusion assessment, and lymphatic mapping [1]. Since the development of near-infrared fluorescent agents indocyanine green (ICG) and methylene blue, several additional fluorophores with varying fluorescence properties have been developed and validated for use in fluorescence guided surgery [2]. More recently, molecular and activatable fluorophores have emerged as alternatives to traditional fluorophores to expand the translation of this technology to additional surgical indications [3, 4].

Novel applications of several imaging technologies have provided additional methods for surgeons to make intraoperative image-based decision-making. A promising example is laser

G. Yang (✉)
Department of Surgery, Jacobs School of Medicine and Biomedical Sciences, University at Buffalo, Buffalo, NY, USA
e-mail: geneyang@buffalo.edu

N. Szoka et al. (eds.), *The SAGES Manual of Fluorescence-Guided Surgery*, https://doi.org/10.1007/978-3-031-40685-0_17

speckle contrast imaging. Laser speckle contrast imaging (LSCI) is a noninvasive, real-time imaging technique that allows for perfusion assessment. This technology has been applied in the fields of cardiology, neurology, and dermatology. Validation studies have demonstrated LSCI as a potential valuable tool for perfusion assessment in laparoscopic surgery [5].

Augmented reality (AR) is another technology that is demonstrating increasing utility in image-guided surgery. AR can aid surgeons in the rapid identification of subsurface targets and structures, reduce surgeon's cognitive load from mentally matching preoperative imaging to the operative environment, and guide resections with overlay of a virtual model onto the patient [6]. The purpose of this review is to provide an overview of the technology and recent developments in targeted fluorophores, LSCI, and AR.

Fluorescence-Guided Surgery

Fluorescence-guided surgery (FGS) has developed into a validated method to augment surgeon's ability to identify anatomic landmarks, localize tumors, and assess perfusion. Since the initial use of fluorescein in 1948 to localize intracranial neoplasms during neurosurgery, several additional fluorescent agents have been used for a variety of surgical applications. ICG initially used for quantitative measurement of hepatic and cardiac function has demonstrated clinical applications for perfusion assessment, cholangiography, lymphography, and tumor imaging. Methylene blue has been evaluated for ureter, thyroid, and neuroendocrine tumor assessment [7]. Five-Aminolevulinic acid and its derivative are clinically approved for imaging of malignant gliomas and bladder cancer with randomized controlled phase 3 trials demonstrating improved resection margin and increased progression-free survival for patients in these applications [8].

Recent focus has shifted from structural and functional fluorescence to molecular fluorescence, with subsequent developments resulting in fluorophores with increased specificity. In this method, tumor-specific ligands are conjugated to fluorescent dye, taking advantage of proven molecular probes and well-developed molecular pathology to aid in lesion detection and margin assessment during surgery and enable molecular targeted therapy with drug and photo-absorber conjugates [9].

Several therapeutic monoclonal antibodies have been repurposed for FGS by fluorescence conjugation. Bevacizumab conjugated with the fluorophore IRDye800CW has been applied in clinical feasibility studies to target tumors that overexpress vascular endothelial growth factor. The use of bevacizumab-IRDye800CW during cytoreductive surgery for peritoneal carcinomatosis of colorectal origin demonstrated additional detection of malignant lesions [10]. Application in breast surgery has demonstrated the ability of bevacizumab-IRDye800CW to assess tumor-positive margin during back-table assessment after breast conserving surgery [11]. Similar applications in head and neck surgery have demonstrated the ability of cetuximab-IRDye800CW to assess positive tumor margins on ex vivo back-table imaging, and panitumumab-IRDye800CW demonstrated feasibility in performing both in situ tumor imaging and ex vivo tumor margin assessment [12, 13].

An alternative approach is the use of activatable fluorescent probes. Activatable fluorescent probes seek to limit background signal by activating fluorescence after engaging the target. Compared to traditional fluorescent probes, activatable probes typically yield higher fluorescent signal and higher tumor-to-background fluorescence ratio. A promising example of an activatable fluorescent probe is LUM015. LUM015, a PEGylated cathepsin-activated fluorescent imaging probe, is currently being investigated for detection of breast, gastrointestinal, brain, and prostate cancers. Initial studies demonstrated feasibility in tumor-specific fluorescence of sarcoma and breast cancer during ex vivo imaging and intraoperative detection of residual breast cancer [14]. Subsequent phase 2 study demonstrated improvement in final margin status sensitivity over standard pathology assessment of lumpectomy specimen. This was associated with reduced need for second surgery in patients who underwent intraoperative excision of fluorescence guided shaves [15].

Limitations to Clinical Translation

Molecular fluorescence imaging can provide additional information that augments the ability of a surgeon to see and treat pathology, but this technology remains in the early stages of development. Clinical studies consist mostly of early-phase trials conducted to evaluate the safety and optimal dosing of fluorescent agents and feasibility of intraoperative lesion detection. Further large, multicenter, randomized controlled trials are required to evaluate the diagnostic accuracy of fluorescence molecular imaging and impact on surgical outcomes. As the field of intraoperative molecular imaging matures, concurrent development of universal protocol for calibration and benchmarking of imaging devices to standardize the development and comparison of novel fluorescent agents will be essential [16, 17].

Laser Speckle Contrast Imaging

LSCI has developed into a promising technology for image-guided surgery with current emphasis on intraoperative perfusion assessment. LSCI is based on the concept that tissue illuminated with coherent laser light backscatters in a random interference pattern, known as speckle pattern, onto a detector. When the speckle pattern is captured over an exposure time, movement of particles inside the tissue causes speckle pattern fluctuations resulting in changes in the speckle image. Fluctuations in tissue images due to movement of red blood cells allow for the assessment of tissue perfusion. The first in vivo application of LSCI on visceral organ perfusion in open surgery was reported by Eriksson et al., demonstrating the feasibility of LSCI to measure hepatic microcirculation [18]. Subsequent studies with applications in porcine gastrointestinal tract and microvascular perfusion measurements of gastric conduit during esophagectomy further demonstrate the feasibility of using LSCI during gastrointestinal surgery [19, 20].

More recent studies apply LSCI to the laparoscopic setting. Heeman et al. demonstrated feasibility of a laparoscopic laser speckle contrast imaging setup to measure tissue perfusion during colon resection [21]. Comparison study of LSCI to ICG fluorescence imaging in intraoperative perfusion assessment during laparoscopic vascular occlusion of porcine intestine, stomach, and kidney demonstrated precise and accurate identification of demarcation between perfused and non-perfused tissue with both LSCI and ICG imaging. LSCI demonstrated an advantage over ICG with time-dependent perfusion assessment. Discordance in demarcation identification was noted in the ICG imaging group when images were assessed after 5 min from ICG administration [22].

Other novel developments in FGS include Activ Surgical, a company pioneering digital surgery imaging who has developed ActivSight, a modular imaging device which integrates with standard laparoscopic visualization systems to provide multimodal advanced visual intelligence. ActivSight enables visualization of ICG via its ActivICG module, as well as LCSI visualization via is ActivPerfusion module [23, 24].

Limitations to Clinic Translation

Several limitations remain obstacles to the clinical use of LSCI. Initially introduced, LSCI was a qualitative method of perfusion assessment. Technical advancements such as introduction of multi-exposure speckle imaging now allow for quantitative assessments [25, 26]. LSCI is sensitive to motion as unwanted motion can be incorporated into the measured signal. In particular applications, such as intra-abdominal organ perfusion assessment, creating the required highly controlled environment is not always easily amenable. Recent studies have been published on motion artifact correction, but the need for a universal, real-time motion correction algorithm remains [5].

Augmented Reality

AR is a technology that superimposes computer-generated objects onto real images and video in real time, often described on a virtuality continuum between real environment (direct view of real environment) and virtual reality (immersion in a fully digital environment). Recent definitions of AR platforms require the combination of real and virtual environments to be interactive in real time and registered in 3D [27]. The application of AR to medical imaging data offers several advantages. Compared to the traditional method of viewing imaging data on a separate monitor, AR visualization eliminates the need for physicians to mentally transform imaging data onto a patient. This has broad applications within medicine but further profound implications for image-guided interventions. By using AR-guided surgery, the proceduralist's attention is not divided between navigation method and the patient resulting in improved hand-eye coordination, accuracy, and time efficiency [28]. In addition, AR platforms enable stereoscopic/3D visualization of volumetric data to improve physician perception of imaging data to support the clinical decision-making process. Following is a review of current implementation of AR technology in surgery, as well as a brief description of the key technologies involved in developing AR platforms: medical imaging segmentation and modeling, tracking, registration, and visualization.

AR systems are currently best implemented during surgery when there is little to no movement of the real environment and when tissue deformation is minimal, as these use cases require less tracking and processing power as compared to applications on mobile organs where tracking and display are significantly more complicated. Thus, clinical application of AR systems has been successfully implemented in the fields of neurosurgery, orthopedics, and otolaryngology, including for bone dissection, clipping of cerebral aneurysms, microvascular decompression, and placement of pedicle screws [29, 30]. AR systems have demonstrated accurate registration (0.2–3 mm), but increased operative time and potential associated financial costs have been reported with the use of AR systems for intraoperative guidance [31].

AR has been difficult to apply to abdominal surgery due to the amount of organ movement. Successful use cases have been reported for liver and pancreatic surgery, where AR has been used to compare the reconstructed virtual model with intraoperative ultrasound to identify lesions for resection [32]. Successful superimposed 3D representation of the patient's hepatobiliary structures over the surgeon's field of view has been studied during open liver surgery [33]. Intraoperative AR has been used to accurately detect sentinel lymph node using preoperative SPECT/CT scan [34]. Recently, RSIP Vision, a company specializing in image analysis and artificial intelligence for medical imaging, has developed RSIP Neph, an intraoperative AR tool that assists surgeons during partial nephrectomy to accurately locate and resect intracapsular renal lesions [35].

Image Segmentation

The datasets presented from medical imaging are large, making them challenging to manipulate in real time. Image segmentation is the processing of medical imaging to isolate regions of interest and generate a model to interactively visualize the area. Identifying the relevant anatomy has traditionally been achieved by marking structures either manually or semi-autonomously within each individual image. Although several open-source packages are available to facilitate this process, image segmentation remains a limiting factor to clinical application of AR surgical guidance. Significant research efforts are underway to develop generalizable autonomous image segmentation; however, a proven and clinically accepted method is yet to be established because of similar contrast intensity between neighboring tissue, unclear lesion/target boundary, and variation in lesion/target shape [36].

Registration

The exact alignment of the virtual image to the real environment is crucial to the clinical application of AR platforms. Image registration is the process to determine the spatial correspondence of two or more image sets. In image-guided surgery, the two image sets are defined as a static and a moving set, and an algorithm is applied to determine the optimal translation that would minimize the difference seen between the virtual and real environment. The accurate alignment of both images can be achieved with a coordinate of trackers, used to determine the exact position and orientation of the camera and the patient's body. Marker-based registration relies on rigid calibration of markers to real objects to allow for precise estimation of the real object as detected by either an external or internal sensor. Marker-free registration exploits the natural features observed by the tracking device within the real environment. An example of this is the simultaneous localization and mapping (SLAM) technique. More recent registration techniques integrate 3D surface information constructed directly by observing the real environment with stereoscopic cameras and time-of-flight depth sensors. The acquired surface can then be registered with a 3D model of the target [37].

Registration is complicated when the organ of interest does not behave as expected. This issue is particularly highlighted in general surgery where target anatomy is not rigid and deforms in a dynamic manner (ex. deformations with heartbeat and respiration). In addition, preoperative imaging is difficult to register to the real environment when attempting image-guided surgery during minimally invasive procedures as organs shift with laparoscopic insufflation and physical manipulation [38].

Limitations to Clinical Translation

Although AR application in surgery has shown great promise through individual specialty applications and preclinical research, several issues limit the clinical translation of AR systems. Medical imaging continues to advance to provide more detail for preoperative planning, but the amount of data to be processed to segment image datasets are large, and current segmentation methods are time intensive. Further research is needed to identify generalizable segmentation methods [39].

Additional research is required to understand the challenges surgeons may encounter in utilizing augmented information in the operating room. Head-mounted displays may unintentionally obscure vision of the surgical field by decreasing the field of view or create visual clutter from the virtual model overlay. In addition, overlay displays may distract surgeons from the procedure. Surgeons may also encounter visual clutter or information overload where overlay outputs contain more information than the surgeon can meaningfully comprehend [40, 41]. Poor ergonomics with head-mounted displays may lead to fatigue, and virtual overlays may cause simulator sickness exhibited by nausea, headache, and vertigo [42, 43].

Conclusion

Fluorescence- and image-guided surgery are evolving fields of study that have the potential to transform surgical care and improve patient outcomes. Development of novel targeted molecular fluorophores offer the possibility of accurate and precise in vivo tumor localization and margin assessment to guide complete resection. LSCI provides a noninvasive, real-time method to intraoperatively assess perfusion without the need for fluorophore administration. Advancements in image processing and registration are bringing surgeons closer to realizing reliable and accurate use of AR in the operating room. Significant barriers exist to the clinical translation of these technologies to the operative environment; however, these technologies remain areas of robust research, and the next decade will likely bring solutions which address said limitations and allow a larger audience to access these disruptive innovations.

References

1. Alander JT, et al. A review of indocyanine green fluorescent imaging in surgery. J Biomed Imaging. 2012;2012:7–7.
2. Stewart HL, Birch DJS. Fluorescence guided surgery. Methods Appl Fluoresc. 2021;9(4):042002.
3. Haque A, et al. Next generation NIR fluorophores for tumor imaging and fluorescence-guided surgery: a review. Bioorg Med Chem. 2017;25:7.
4. Zhang Y, et al. Activatable molecular probes for fluorescence-guided surgery, endoscopy and tissue biopsy. Chem Soc Rev. 2022;51(2):566–93.
5. Heeman W, et al. Clinical applications of laser speckle contrast imaging: a review. J Biomed Opt. 2019;24(8):080901–1.
6. Barcali E, et al. Augmented reality in surgery: a scoping review. Appl Sci. 2022;12(14):6890.
7. Hillary SL, Guillermet S, Brown NJ, Balasubramanian SP. Use of methylene blue and near-infrared fluorescence in thyroid and parathyroid surgery. Langenbecks Arch Surg. 2018;403(1):111–8. https://doi.org/10.1007/s00423-017-1641-2. Epub 2017 Dec 11. PMID: 29230539; PMCID: PMC5805804.
8. Stummer W, Pichlmeier U, Meinel T, Wiestler OD, Zanella F, Reulen HJ, ALA-Glioma Study Group. Fluorescence-guided surgery with 5-aminolevulinic acid for resection of malignant glioma: a randomised controlled multicentre phase III trial. Lancet Oncol. 2006;7(5):392–401. https://doi.org/10.1016/S1470-2045(06)70665-9. PMID: 16648043.
9. Nagaya T, et al. Fluorescence-guided surgery. Front Oncol. 2017;7:314.
10. Harlaar NJ, et al. Molecular fluorescence-guided surgery of peritoneal carcinomatosis of colorectal origin: a single-centre feasibility study. Lancet Gastroenterol Hepatol. 2016;1(4):283–90.
11. Lamberts LE, et al. Tumor-specific uptake of fluorescent bevacizumab–IRDye800CW microdosing in patients with primary breast cancer: a phase I feasibility study targeted near-infrared fluorescence imaging in breast cancer. Clin Cancer Res. 2017;23(11):2730–41.
12. Rosenthal EL, et al. Sensitivity and specificity of cetuximab-IRDye800CW to identify regional metastatic disease in head and neck cancer. Clin Cancer Res. 2017;23(16):4744–52.
13. van Keulen S, et al. Rapid, non-invasive fluorescence margin assessment: Optical specimen mapping in oral squamous cell carcinoma. Oral Oncol. 2019;88:58–65.
14. Smith BL, et al. Real-time, intraoperative detection of residual breast cancer in lumpectomy cavity walls using a novel cathepsin-activated fluorescent imaging system. Breast Cancer Res Treat. 2018;171:413–20.

15. Hwang ES, et al. Clinical impact of intraoperative margin assessment in breast-conserving surgery with a novel pegulicianine fluorescence–guided system: a nonrandomized controlled trial. JAMA Surg. 2022;157(7):573–80.
16. Souza D, Alisha V, et al. Review of fluorescence guided surgery systems: identification of key performance capabilities beyond indocyanine green imaging. J Biomed Opt. 2016;21(8):080901–1.
17. Pogue BW, et al. Perspective review of what is needed for molecular-specific fluorescence-guided surgery. J Biomed Opt. 2018;23(10):100601–1.
18. Eriksson S, et al. Laser speckle contrast imaging for intraoperative assessment of liver microcirculation: a clinical pilot study. Med Devices. 2014;7:257–61.
19. Ambrus R, et al. Evaluation of gastric microcirculation by laser speckle contrast imaging during esophagectomy. J Am Coll Surg. 2017;225(3):395–402.
20. Milstein DMJ, et al. Laser speckle contrast imaging identifies ischemic areas on gastric tube reconstructions following esophagectomy. Medicine. 2016;95:25.
21. Heeman W, et al. Application of laser speckle contrast imaging in laparoscopic surgery. Biomed Opt Express. 2019;10(4):2010–9.
22. Nwaiwu CA, et al. Feasibility and comparison of laparoscopic laser speckle contrast imaging to near-infrared display of indocyanine green in intraoperative tissue blood flow/tissue perfusion in preclinical porcine models. Surg Endosc. 2022;37:1–10.
23. Sanders CM, Nwaiwu CA, Liu YZ, Panchal AN, Butsch JL, Hoffman AB, Posner AR, Falvo MA, Visco J, Ortolani JB, Barone SM, Burstein MD, DeJesus C, Bouvy ND, Boni L, Shah SK, Wilson EB, Dechert AF, Buharin VE, Schwaitzberg SD, Kim PCW. ActivSightTM dye-less visualization of tissue perfusion in MIS surgery: interim analysis of first clinical (n=66) and preclinical (n=20) Studies with ICG comparison. World Congress of Endoscopic Surgery/European Association of Endoscopic Surgery 2021. Presentation date: November 24, 2021.
24. Shah SK, Nwaiwu CA, Agarwal AK, Bajwa KS, Felinksi MM, Walker PA, Wilson TD, Dechert AF, Kim PCW, Wilson EB. First-In-Human (FIH) Safety, feasibility, & usability trial (NCT# 04633512) of a laparoscopic imaging device using laser speckle contrast imaging (LSCI). In: Visualizing real-time tissue perfusion and blood flow without fluorophore in colorectal and bariatric patients, vol. 233. Boston: American College of Surgeons Clinical Congress; 2021. p. S45. Presentation date: October 24, 2021.

25. Parthasarathy AB, et al. Robust flow measurement with multi-exposure speckle imaging. Opt Express. 2008;16(3):1975–89.
26. Richards LM, et al. Intraoperative multi-exposure speckle imaging of cerebral blood flow. J Cereb Blood Flow Metab. 2017;37(9):3097–109. https://doi.org/10.1177/0271678X16686987.
27. Gupta A, Ruijters D, Flexman ML. Augmented reality for interventional procedures. In: Digital surgery. Cham: Springer; 2021. p. 233–46.
28. Shuhaiber JH. Augmented reality in surgery. Arch Surg. 2004;139(2):170–4.
29. Gmeiner M, Dirnberger J, Fenz W. Virtual cerebral aneurysm clipping with real-time haptic force feedback in neurosurgical education. World Neurosurg. 2018;112:e313–23.
30. Xin B, Chen G, Wang Y. The efficacy of immersive virtual reality surgical simulator training for pedicle screw placement: a randomized double-blind controlled trial. World Neurosurg. 2018;124:e324–30.
31. Kang X, et al. Stereoscopic augmented reality for laparoscopic surgery. Surg Endosc. 2014;28(7):2227–35.
32. Tanagho YS, Andriole GL, Paradis AG, Madison KM, Sandhu GS, Varela JE, Benway BM. 2D versus 3D visualization: impact on laparoscopic proficiency using the fundamentals of laparoscopic surgery skill set. J Laparoendosc Adv Surg Tech A. 2012;22(9):865–70. https://doi.org/10.1089/lap.2012.0220. Epub 2012 Oct 16.
33. Gavaghan KA, et al. A portable image overlay projection device for computer-aided open liver surgery. IEEE Trans Biomed Eng. 2011;58(6):1855–64.
34. Wendler T, et al. First demonstration of 3-D lymphatic mapping in breast cancer using freehand SPECT. Eur J Nucl Med Mol Imaging. 2010;37(8):1452–61.
35. https://www.rsipvision.com/rsip-neph/.
36. Herline AJ, Stefansic JD, Debelak JP, et al. Image-guided surgery: preliminary feasibility studies of frameless stereotactic liver surgery. Arch Surg. 1999;134:644.
37. Mountney P, Yang G-Z. Motion compensated SLAM for image guided surgery. Medical image computing and computer-assisted intervention–MICCAI. In: 13th international conference, Beijing, China, September 20–24, 2010, proceedings, part II 13. Berlin: Springer; 2010. p. 2010.
38. Bernhardt S, Nicolau SA, Soler L, Doignon C. The status of augmented reality in laparoscopic surgery as of 2016. Med Image Anal. 2017;37:66–90.
39. Vávra P, et al. Recent development of augmented reality in surgery: a review. J Healthc Eng. 2017;2017:1.
40. Guanà R, Ferrero L, Garofalo S, Cerrina A, Cussa D, Arezzo A, Schleef J. Skills comparison in pediatric residents using a 2-dimensional versus a 3-dimensional high-definition camera in a pediatric laparoscopic simulator. J Surg Educ. 2017;74(4):644–9. https://doi.org/10.1016/j.jsurg.2016.12.002. Epub 2016 Dec 27.

41. Pratt P, Stoyanov D, Visentini-Scarzanella M, Yang GZ. Dynamic guidance for robotic surgery using image-constrained biomechanical models. In: In international conference on medical image computing and computer-assisted intervention. Springer; 2010. p. 77–85.
42. Condino S, Carbone M, Piazza R, Ferrari M, Ferrari V. Perceptual limits of optical see-through visors for augmented reality guidance of manual tasks. IEEE Trans Biomed Eng. 2020;67(2):411–9.
43. Edwards PJ, et al. The challenge of augmented reality in surgery. In: Digital surgery. Cham: Springer; 2021. p. 121–35.

Index

N. Szoka et al. (eds.), *The SAGES Manual of Fluorescence-Guided Surgery*, https://doi.org/10.1007/978-3-031-40685-0

B

Q

R

MIX
Papier aus verantwortungsvollen Quellen
Paper from responsible sources
FSC® C105338

If you have any concerns about our products,
you can contact us on
ProductSafety@springernature.com

In case Publisher is established outside the EU,
the EU authorized representative is:
Springer Nature Customer Service Center GmbH
Europaplatz 3, 69115 Heidelberg, Germany

Printed by Libri Plureos GmbH
in Hamburg, Germany